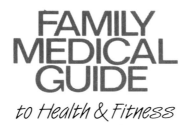

FAMILY
MEDICAL
GUIDE
to Health & Fitness

Volume 3

The Systems of the Body and Their Disorders

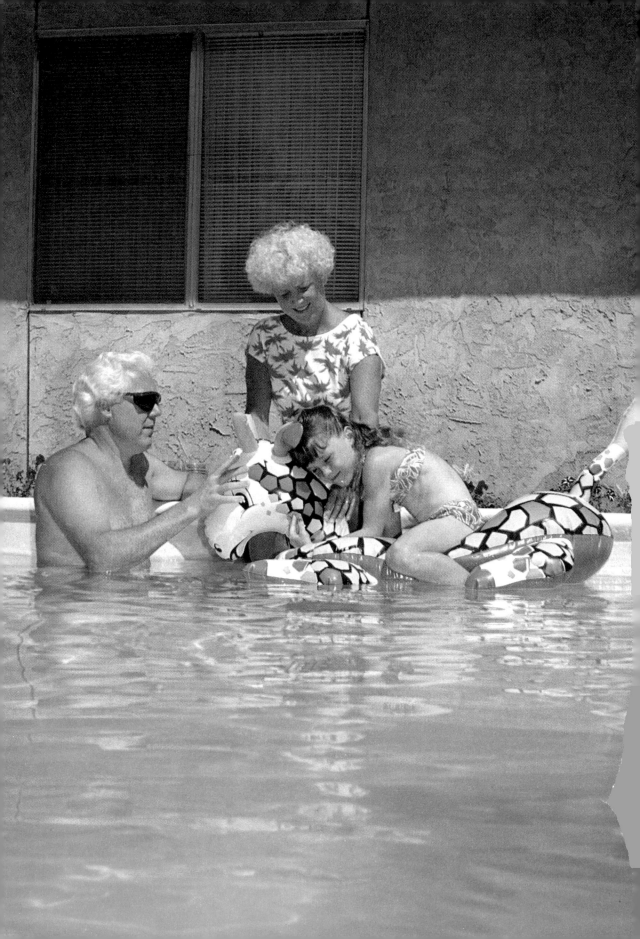

Volume **3**

The Systems of the Body and Their Disorders

FAMILY MEDICAL GUIDE

to Health & Fitness

in three volumes, illustrated

Mervyn G. Hardinge, M.D., Dr.P.H., Ph.D.
Harold Shryock, M.A., M.D.

In collaboration with 28 leading medical specialists

Published jointly by

Pacific Press Publishing Association
Boise, ID 83707
Oshawa, Ontario, Canada

Review and Herald Publishing Association
Washington, D.C. 20039-0555
Hagerstown, MD 21740

PHOTOS AND ILLUSTRATIONS

Credits for illustrations used in Volume 3 of Family Medical Guide:

Pages x, 766, 834, 836, 934, 1056, 1060, 1062, 1122, 1124 by Betty Blue.
Pages 822, 824, 973, 980, 1009, 1010 by Public Health Service Audiovisual Facility.
Pages 827, 829, 885, 983, 999, 1130, 1131, 1132, 1134, 1135, 1136 by Lucille Innes.
Pages 847, 1116 by Chas. Pfizer and Company, Inc.
Pages 850, 851, 857, 863 by © CIBA.
Page 871 by Veterans Administration.
Page 874 by Loma Linda University School of Medicine.
Page 893 by Dental Society.
Pages 898, 924 by The Upjohn Company.
Pages 900, 909 by Review & Herald Publishing Association.
Pages ii, 936, 998, 1064 by Duane Tank/Betty Blue.
Page 984 by Eli Lilly and Company.
Pages 1029, 1143 by Lederle Laboratories.

Please Note: Although the information contained in *The Family Medical Guide* is based on accurate, reliable medical knowledge, it is designed to be of a general nature and for informational purposes only. *The Family Medical Guide* is not intended to be used for self-diagnosis of medical problems nor to determine treatment apart from your physician. Always consult your physician when medical attention is indicated.

Edited by Marvin Moore and Bonnie Widicker
Designed by Ira Lee
Cover photo by Duane Tank and Betty Blue
Inside art by Kim Justinen
Typeset in 11/13 Century Old Style

Copyright © 1991 by
Pacific Press Publishing Association
Printed in United States of America
All Rights Reserved
Revised Edition 1994

Library of Congress Catalog Number: 90-60852

ISBN 0-8163-0880-2: Volume 3
ISBN 0-8163-0926-4: Volumes 1-3

94 95 96 97 98 ● 6 5 4 3 2

Contents

Volume 1—Lifestyle

Section 1—A healthy lifestyle

Section 2—Mental and spiritual health

Section 3—Nutrition: Charts and recipes, disorders

Volume 3—The systems of the body and their disorders

Section 1—The cardiovascular and lymphatic systems and their disorders

Section 2—The digestive and respiratory systems and their disorders

Section 3—The skeletal and cutaneous systems and their disorders

Section 4—The endocrine and nervous systems and their disorders

Section 5—The reproductive and urinary systems and their disorders

Section 6—The sense organs and their disorders

Introduction to volume 3

People who have a basic knowledge of how a car engine works have a distinct advantage over those who have no idea what makes an engine run. They are able to maintain their car more intelligently, and thus extend its life. And even though they would not attempt to repair their own car, they have a good idea what the mechanic is talking about when he explains a problem, and are better able to judge whether the repair he suggests is what they really want. A good mechanic always appreciates a customer who understands what the mechanic is talking about.

It's the same with your body. You are at a distinct advantage if you have a basic idea how it works. You can preserve your health more effectively, and thus extend your life. And even though you would not try to treat a major illness without medical advice, you have a good idea what the doctor is talking about when he explains a problem, and you are better able to judge whether the treatment he recommends is what you really want. A good doctor always appreciates a patient who understands what his doctor is talking about.

The purpose of this volume of the *Family Medical Guide* is to explain the organs and systems of the body, how they work, and how they can malfunction. Ten systems have been grouped by twos in five sections, and the sense organs are in a section by themselves. Each system is described first—how it works, and what it is like in good health. Following this is a discussion of the various ways in which that system and its organs can malfunction—the diseases and disorders that can afflict it.

Where a system of the body is quite complex, you will find an entire chapter describing how it works and another chapter that discusses its diseases and disorders. In the case of systems that require less explanation, the description of how the system works is in the same chapter with the discussion of its diseases and disorders.

The authors and publishers of the *Family Medical Guide* recommend that you take the time right away to study this volume carefully, learning how your body works and what can go wrong with it. This will give you many practical ideas on how to preserve your health. It will also help you to know when to consult your doctor about symptoms that you might otherwise overlook, and it may help you to avoid a life-threatening disease.

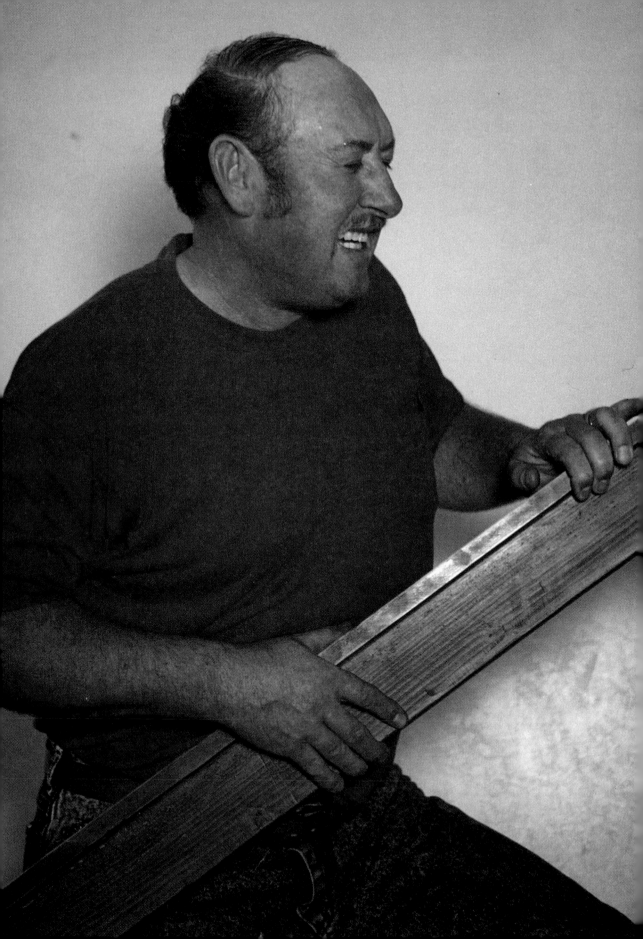

VOL. 3

SECTION 1

THE CARDIO-VASCULAR AND LYMPHATIC SYSTEMS

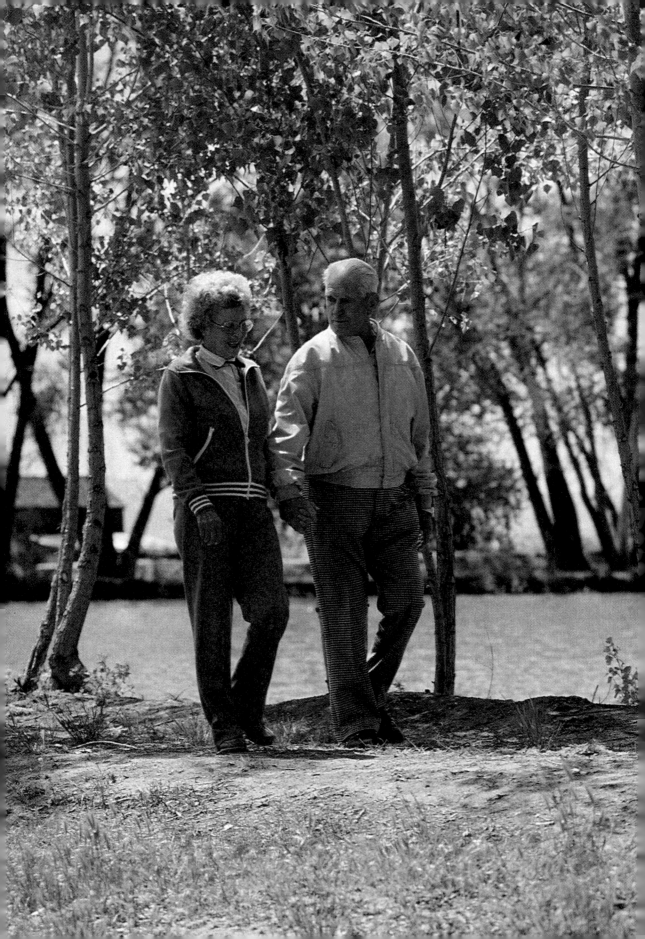

CHAPTER 1

The heart, blood vessels, and blood

The circulatory system is the main transportation system of the body. It consists of the **heart,** or pumping station, the **arteries, arterioles, and capillaries,** hollow tubes which gradually become smaller and smaller as they carry the blood away from the heart to the tissues of the body, and the **veinules and veins,** also hollow tubes which gradually get larger and larger as they convey the blood back to the heart.

The heart

The heart, doubtless nature's most efficient pump, is actually two pumps side by side, each made up of two chambers. Its walls consist almost entirely of heart muscle. The two upper chambers—right and left atria—are thin walled and act as catchment basins for the blood returning to the heart, from the body to the right and from the lungs to the left. From here the blood enters the thick-walled lower chambers of the right and left ventricles and is pumped from the right side to the lungs, and from the left side to the rest of the body.

Your heart is somewhat larger than the size of your clenched fist. In the average man it weighs about 10 ounces (350 grams), while in the average woman approximately 8.5 ounces (300 grams). A normal heart beats rhythmically sixty to eighty times each minute. While at rest, the blood cycles through the body's 60,000 miles of blood vessels once each minute, and each beat of each ventricle pumps about 4 ounces (120 milliliters) of blood or 2,100 gallons each day. Both the rate of beating and the amount of blood ejected with each beat may double when you are doing vigorous physical activity.

This is an enormous amount of work. If you were to lift a 10-pound weight 3 feet off the floor every thirty seconds (about the same as

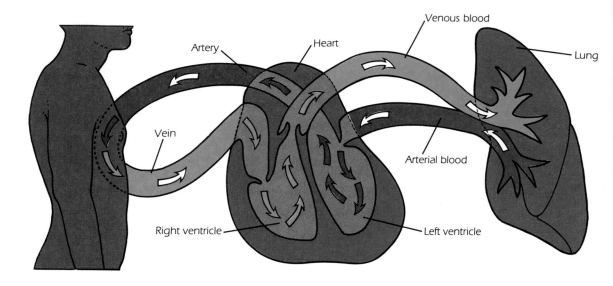

Artery   Heart   Venous blood   Lung

Vein   Arterial blood

Right ventricle   Left ventricle

Venous blood returning from the body enters the right side of the heart and is pumped to the lungs.

Arterial blood is returned to the left side of the heart and is pumped throughout the body.

lifting a 4.5 kilogram weight to a height of one meter), you would be doing as much work as your heart does regularly. It would be difficult enough to lift this weight twice a minute for an eight-hour day, but the heart keeps this up twenty-four hours a day, day after day, for an entire lifetime.

How can the heart accomplish this feat? One reason is that it rests between each beat. Scientific studies show that these rest periods add up to almost twice its work periods, or almost sixteen hours each day. Also, the heart's own tissues receive, weight for weight, about five times as much blood as the average of other tissues. The right and the left coronary arteries, so called because they encircle the heart as a crown does the head, provide blood directly to the heart muscle. And again, the organ

has a remarkably great reserve power. For a short time, in an emergency, it can do six times as much work as it has to do while the body is at rest.

The heart's rhythm is maintained by a unique control system. The pacemaker, located in the wall of the right atrium, sends an impulse to a group of specialized cells located between the auricles and ventricles (A-V node). From here the impulse travels onward a short distance (bundle of His) before spreading out over a network of conducting fibers lying on the inner surface of the ventricles, activating them to contract.

Your heart has four one-way valves to direct the flow of blood: one placed between each of the atria and ventricles, the inlet valves, and one located at the beginning of the two arteries that leave the heart, the outlet valves.

With a stethoscope you can listen to the **heart sounds**—the rhythmic contracting or beating of your heart. The heartbeat gives a double sound which is classically described as lubb-dup. After this double sound, there is an interval of quiet and then the lubb-dup occurs again and again: lubb-dup, lubb-dup, lubb-dup. The "lubb" sound is produced by the closing of the valves between the atria and the ventricles, which occurs as the ventricles begin to contract and the pressure within

them rises. As the ventricles continue to contract, the blood in them is forced out into the large arteries—the pulmonary artery going to the lungs, and the aorta to the rest of the body. Then as the ventricles relax in preparation for their next contraction, the pressure within them drops. The blood which has just been forced out into the arteries backs up against the outlet valves, closing them. The closing of the outlet valves accounts for the "dup." It is during the interval between one lubb-dup and the next that the heart rests.

The blood vessels, arteries, capillaries, and veins

Arteries are thick-walled vessels, composed largely of smooth muscle and elastic connective tissue. This allows for considerable change in their caliber. They can dilate or enlarge and narrow or constrict. Thus the flow of blood through the smaller arterioles can be regulated according to the needs of the tissues or organs which they supply.

The left ventricle pumps its blood into the aorta, which is the body's largest artery. The aorta branches so as to carry blood to all parts of the body. As the arteries continue to branch, the vessels become smaller and smaller. The smallest arteries, which regulate where the blood goes, are called arterioles, and their terminal branches are the smallest of all, the capillaries. The blood cells have to pass through these tiny vessels

single file. If the billions of capillaries in your body were placed end to end to make a single tube, the tube would extend more than twice around the earth!

Capillaries are composed mostly of a single layer of endothelial cells. Their walls are so thin that gases, such as oxygen and carbon dioxide, food nutrients, and other body chemicals can freely pass through them. Capillaries can be taken out of, or returned to service, as the needs of the tissue require. The more active the tissue, the greater number of capillaries in service. When a tissue is relatively inactive, capillaries take turns, working in relays, as they care for the tissue's needs.

Veins, unlike arteries, are thin walled—although also composed of smooth muscle and elastic tissue.

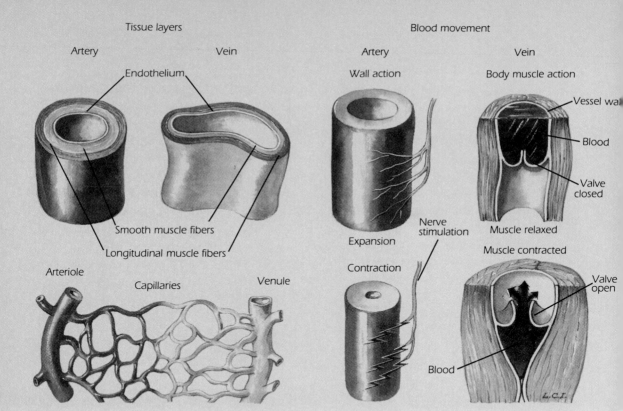

Tissue layers

Artery

Endothelium

Vein

Smooth muscle fibers

Longitudinal muscle fibers

Arteriole

Capillaries

Venule

Blood movement

Artery

Wall action

Expansion

Contraction

Nerve stimulation

Blood

Vein

Body muscle action

Vessel wall

Blood

Valve closed

Muscle relaxed

Muscle contracted

Valve open

Blood

Arteries have thick muscular walls. Veins have thin, less muscular walls and one-way valves. Capillaries are minute vessels connecting the smallest arteries (arterioles) to the smallest veins (venules).

Veins carry blood back to the heart. In a healthy body all the veins carry blood all the time, but sometimes they may be almost collapsed while at other times fully distended. Their walls can stretch or dilate sufficiently to carry to the heart all the blood carried to them by the arteries.

The pressure pushing the blood through the capillaries is almost zero as the blood leaves the capillaries. How, then, does the blood return to the heart, say from the soles of your feet? This is accomplished in an interesting way. The contraction of the body's muscles puts pressure on the vein walls, squeezing blood toward the heart. Most veins, unlike arteries, have small valves built into their walls that prevent blood from flowing backward. When your muscles relax, new blood flows in to fill the veins. So as you exercise, the contracting and relaxing of your muscles literally "pumps" the blood back to your heart.

Blood pressure

Moment by moment, the amount of blood leaving the heart is replaced by virtually the same amount entering the heart. So you can see that the heart and blood vessels are filled with blood all of the time. When the left ventricle of your heart contracts, it ejects or pushes out into the aorta, already full of blood, about 4 ounces of blood. This half cup of blood causes the arterial wall to stretch or bulge. Then, as the elastic tissue recoils and the smooth muscle contracts, the ball of blood passes down the arterial tree. The pressure required by the heart and arteries to accomplish this is called the **blood pressure.**

When a doctor examines you, he is interested, among other things, in finding what your blood pressure is. This he does by placing an inflatable cuff around your arm (just above your elbow), connecting a gauge to the cuff, and listening through a stethoscope placed just below the crease in front of your elbow. He then inflates the cuff. As the cuff becomes tighter and tighter, it acts like a tourniquet, squeezing the arm so tightly that the blood can no longer flow through the artery to reach your forearm. The sound of the blood flow ceases.

The physician now slowly releases the pressure in the cuff until the first sounds of blood flow are noted. By watching the pressure gauge, he can read the pressure at this moment. When the pressure within the cuff no longer restricts the flow of blood through the artery, the sounds of your heartbeats can no longer be heard. The pressure at this point is again recorded.

These two readings, the high and the low, are called the **systolic** and **diastolic** pressures. The systolic pressure is the highest pressure that the heart produces as it pumps blood into the arteries at the time of a heartbeat. The lowest reading represents the pressure that remains in the arteries just before the next heartbeat takes place.

In a normal, healthy young adult whose heart is working properly and whose blood vessels are not diseased, the systolic pressure is usually about 120 and the diastolic pressure about 80. This is commonly written as 120/80. These figures indicate the height, in millimeters, of a column of mercury if the other end of the tube were connected to the artery.

By the time the blood reaches the capillaries it is flowing slowly. This slow movement of blood through the capillaries allows time for the oxygen and food nutrients to enter the tissues and for the carbon dioxide and waste materials to enter the blood. The blood in the large arteries may move at a speed of about 100 feet (30 meters) per minute, which is more than a thousand times as fast as it moves through the capillaries. A drop of blood takes about two seconds to pass through a capillary which is about .025 inch (6 millimeters) long, and will be back in the heart, from a distant part of the body, within half a minute!

The level of blood pressure throughout your body and the volume of blood flow in any local region of the body are precisely influenced by the autonomic (or automatic) nervous system. This is accomplished by stimulating the smooth muscle in the arterioles. Contraction of these muscles narrows the caliber of the arteries, resulting in an increase in blood pressure.

The blood pressure in your body varies from time to time, and even from place to place. When you stand, your blood pressure is higher in your

771

legs than in your arms. It rises slightly when you sit up from lying down, or stand up from sitting. When you exert yourself, such as lifting a heavy suitcase or exercising vigorously, your blood pressure rises to met the demand for blood in the muscles involved in these tasks. During digestion, the digestive organs need more blood. This increase is provided by a reduction of the flow of blood to other parts of the body so that a correspondingly greater volume of blood flows through the digestive organs. When you are engaged in active thinking, the flow of blood through the brain accelerates slightly.

Blood pressure and the heart rate rise during emergencies, as the muscles attaching to the bones (skeletal muscles) are alerted to possible action. When you are frightened, your blood pressure rises, putting a greater workload on your heart and artery walls. But emergencies should be but for short periods. People who are nervous, anxious, and fearful tend to maintain a higher than desirable blood pressure. This may lead to serious problems (see under "high blood pressure" or "hypertension" on page 785). Generally a consistent pressure of 140/80 is considered borderline hypertension.

Blood

The **blood**, carried within the blood vessels, is the main transport system of the body. On the outward journey, blood brings the cells oxygen, nutrients, and chemical substances essential for their proper functioning. On its return trip, blood removes cellular wastes.

Your blood, some 10 to 11 pints in volume, consists of blood cells, or corpuscles, floating in a yellowish liquid called plasma. Plasma also contains a variety of salts, fats, proteins, hormones, blood sugar, blood-clotting agents, and antibodies. The major wastes are carbon dioxide and urea.

Six types of cells normally seen in the blood.

There are two kinds of blood cells: red and white. The **red cells** or erythrocytes number some 25 to 30 trillion in an adult, and outnumber the white cells about 600 to one. Smaller than white cells, they live about 120 days. To replace those that wear out, the bone marrow must produce about 200 billion new red cells daily, or from 2 to 3 million every second, twenty-four hours a day—and more if you have lost blood or given a

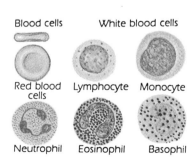

Blood cells   White blood cells

Red blood cells   Lymphocyte   Monocyte

Neutrophil   Eosinophil   Basophil

transfusion! Your body is an incredible structure and should never be taken for granted.

The major function of red cells is to carry oxygen from the lungs to the body cells, and carbon dioxide from the cells back to the lungs. The remarkable substance making this transfer—a red iron-containing pigment called hemoglobin—gives blood its red color.

The five different types of **white cells** constitute part of the body's police force, defending it against disease and any foreign invader. The bone marrow produces three different granulocytes that travel to all parts of the body hunting for trouble. They live a very short time because they often die fighting the enemy. In cases of infection or injury to the tissues, the white cells gather in large numbers to help prevent the spread of infection and to aid in the process of healing.

The bone marrow also produces a fourth type of white cell—a macrophage or monocyte. This large cell is a front-line defender and acts like a vacuum sweeper, engulfing debris entering the bloodstream. Encountering any foreign organisms, such as bacteria or viruses, it alerts the defense forces.

A fifth type of white blood cell is the lymphocyte, produced and stored in the lymph glands or lymph nodes, which is part of the lymphatic system. Lymphocytes also provide a defense against bacteria and foreign substances. Some of these are extremely long-lived, and once exposed to certain disease agents or foreign substances, they store this "biologi-

cal information" for years or a lifetime.

The body's marvelous defense mechanisms against an aggressor are still but partially understood. Here are some of the more obvious defense steps. A virus enters a cell. Immediately a macrophage moves over and engulfs the stricken cell. By some mysterious method of communication it immediately summons a helper T cell to the scene. This cell identifies the enemy and takes command of the defense forces. In the spleen and other lymph nodes it orders the production of killer T cells to fight the enemy. These killer T cells attack the cells that have been invaded.

The helper T cells also mobilize other lymphocytes, called B cells, to increase in numbers and to produce potent chemical substances called antibodies. These Y-shaped protein molecules rush to the site of infection. Here the antibodies either neutralize the enemy or mark it for attack by other defense cells or chemicals.

As an infection is overcome, another type of T cell slows down or stops the production and activity of B cells and T cells, bringing the defense forces to an on-duty peacetime footing. Formed sometime during the battle with the enemy, a so-called "memory cell" develops, which may travel in the blood or lymph for years. It is capable of immediately identifying the enemy and quickly mobilizing the body's defenses.

Platelets, small fragments of larger cells called megakaryocytes, are formed in the bone marrow. When a blood vessel wall is injured or

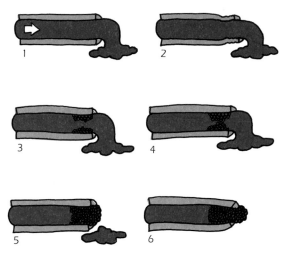

broken, permitting the loss of blood, platelets accumulate at the site of the damage. They stick to the injured surfaces and break apart, releasing a special chemical that stimulates the formation of tiny threads of fibrin, a protein present in the blood. The tangled mass of fibrin threads entraps blood cells in its meshes, and together with them forms a clot. This prevents further loss of blood from the cut or injured vessel. Circulating platelets live an average of ten days.

Steps in clot formation: (1) vessel when first cut, (2) cut end constricts and retracts, (3) platelets stick to injured surfaces, (4) fibrin appears, (5) clot forms in four to five minutes, (6) clot retracts within an hour.

Blood types or groups

Even though the blood from one person looks just like that from another person, it may differ significantly. Persons of the same race or even of the same family may have different "types" of blood. The genes you inherited from your parents determine your **blood type.**

On the surface of each person's red blood cells are specific protein molecules called **antigens,** and equally specific **antibodies** in the

Blood types and their frequencies				
Type	Antigen	Antibodies	Percent	Class
A	A	B	40	
B	B	A	10	
AB	A, B	none	5	Universal recipients
O	none	A, B	45	Universal donors

plasma. The chart on page 774 summarizes the four common blood types: A, B, AB, and O with their major characteristics.

Another system of blood classification has to do with whether an Rh antigen is present. About 85 percent of the people in the United States have this factor in their blood and are said to be "Rh positive." The remaining 15 percent are Rh negative.

A person who is Rh negative cannot tolerate Rh positive blood given as a transfusion. Such a mistake causes serious damage to the kidneys, with possible death. The reason is that the Rh negative person builds up antibodies that destroy the cells of the Rh positive blood. A further complication occurs when a woman with Rh negative blood becomes pregnant with a child who happens to have Rh positive blood.

Blood transfusions

In cases of severe hemorrhage, injury, certain types of surgery, and other situations in which it becomes necessary to restore or replace a person's blood, the transfusion of blood from another person (or from the same person given by himself in advance) may prove to be lifesaving.

If you need a transfusion, it is imperative that you be given blood that is compatible with your blood type. The donor's blood must be matched with yours in the laboratory to be sure that it is correct. If you receive the wrong type, your antibodies will attack the antigens in the donor's (incoming) blood, causing the donor's red blood cells to stick together (agglutinate), and the result could be kidney failure, shock, or even death. For example, if you are a type A, you cannot receive type B blood because your antibodies will attack the antigens in the incoming red blood cells. However, if you are type AB, you do not have antibodies to be triggered by the antigens of the blood you receive, and you will have no reaction. You are called a universal recipient. That means you can receive blood from any donor. People with type O blood are universal donors. That is, they can donate their blood to anyone, because they have no antigens to trigger the antibodies in the people to whom they donate. However, type O can only receive blood from another person with type O blood.

If you do not know your blood type, your physician can order a blood test that will tell you. The percent column tells approximately what percent of the population has that particular blood type (the type in the left-hand column).

Human blood cannot be manufactured outside the human body. Therefore healthy people interested in helping to save lives donate blood to be stored in blood banks for emergencies. The average adult can give one pint (450 ml) of blood at a time without endangering his health, provided he does not do it too often. It takes the donor's body about six weeks to regenerate this amount of blood.

CHAPTER 2

Disorders of the heart and blood vessels

Cardiovascular disease accounts for more than one third of all deaths in the developed nations of the world. The two most common forms of this disease are coronary heart disease and high blood pressure (hypertension). Another, stroke, is close behind. In the United States, for example, one out of every eight Americans has one or more of these diseases, with coronary heart disease being the number one killer. In Japan stroke is the leading cause of death.

In the Western world more people suffer and die from heart disease than from any other ailment. The most common vascular ailments—coronary heart disease, hypertension or high blood pressure, and stroke—account for close to a million deaths annually.

The underlying cause of these and other fairly common heart and blood vessel diseases is largely a disease process of the arteries called atherosclerosis. Since athero-sclerosis is a form of arterio-sclerosis, it will be discussed first. Until some forty years ago, people generally believed that heart disease was a natural result of aging, of some infectious disease such as rheumatic fever, or of heredity.

However, from the careful observation of the lifestyle of large groups of people, researchers have identified certain circumstances and conditions, called "risk factors," that cause people to be more susceptible to atherosclerosis and, as a result, to heart attacks. These risk factors, some major and others minor, some controllable and others not, are listed below and briefly discussed.

While the presence or absence of risk factors does not absolutely predict one's susceptibility to a heart attack, experience has shown that the more risk factors a person has, the more likely the occurrence of a coronary. Obviously, then, a person is wise to analyze his lifestyle and make

Risk factors	
Controllable	**Uncontrollable**
Major	
High blood cholesterol	Age
High blood pressure	Sex
Cigarette smoking	Heredity
Minor	
Emotional stress	
Lack of exercise	
Obesity	
Type A personality	
Diabetes	

a determined effort to eliminate as many of the risk factors as possible. Since lifestyles and risk factors will be discussed in more detail elsewhere, only a brief summary will be given here.

Controllable risk factors

Cholesterol, which is manufactured by the body, is a normal constituent of the cells and blood, and is actually essential to life itself. The problem arises when the amount in the body, as noted by the level in the blood, becomes excessive. Interestingly, foods of plant origin—fruits, vegetables, grains, and nuts—contain no cholesterol. But it is found in generous amounts in foods of animal origin—meat, fish, fowl, milk, and especially eggs, seafoods, and organ meats. Thus excessive levels of cholesterol in the blood result from the overmanufacture of cholesterol by the body or by unwise dietary practices, among other things.

Cholesterol, a fatlike substance, is attached to a protein, called lipoprotein, that is carried in the blood. The various lipoproteins are classified according to their densities. Very low density lipoproteins (VLDL), low density (LDL), and high density (HDL). HDL or "good" cholesterol is believed to carry fats out of the cells of the body and to protect the artery walls from atherosclerosis. LDL or "bad" cholesterol is thought to be the prime culprit in developing atherosclerosis. The higher the ratio of HDL to LDL, the better off the person is. For practical purposes, however, the total amount of cholesterol in the blood forms a good index of the person's susceptibility to atherosclerosis.

The level of cholesterol in the blood varies from time to time and from day to day in the same person, so for a precise determination a cholesterol test should be done more than once. However, a single test provides a valuable target range. Generally a level of 170 milligrams per 100 milliliters of blood (170 mg per 100 ml) or below is considered a good or "safe" level. But actually no absolutely safe or normal value exists, for with any value above 125 milligrams per 100 milliliters the risk increases. The average American has a blood cholesterol level of about 225 milligrams per 100 milliliters. With a value of 250 milligrams compared to 175 milligrams, the risk rises fourfold. With levels greater than 300, the risk of a coronary increases eight or more times.

High blood pressure (hypertension) occurs when the pressure within the arteries is consistently maintained above 140/85 while a person is at rest. Such pressures, over a period of years, will damage the walls of the arteries and contribute to their hardening (arteriosclerosis). Hardening of the coronary arteries of the heart results in diminished flow and places the person at a higher risk of a coronary.

Cigarette smoking, another major risk factor, greatly increases the risk of a heart attack. A number of constituents of tobacco smoke enter the blood, affecting the heart and blood vessels. Nicotine directly affects the heart, causing it to beat faster. At the same time it constricts or narrows the smaller arteries, thus raising the blood pressure, reducing available blood to the heart, and increasing the heart's workload. Carbon monoxide, a gas present in cigarette smoke, enters the blood, combining more strongly with hemoglobin than does oxygen. This displaces some of the oxygen which the blood normally carries, so the heart gets less oxygen for its needs while at the same time nicotine is making it work harder.

Beyond this, nicotine causes the body to react as it would to stress. Adrenaline (epinephrine) is secreted into the blood, increasing the heart rate, raising both the blood pressure and the level of cholesterol. The junction points of the cells lining the arteries buckle, allowing cholesterol and other lipoproteins to enter the walls, initiating, as some think, the process of atherosclerosis. While filter-tip cigarettes may slightly reduce the amount of nicotine entering the body, they may actually increase the concentration of carbon monoxide!

Emotional stress is part of everyday living, but when the level is high and its occurrence frequent, serious problems may arise. Stress is the body's response to some event or situation perceived to be undesirable or harmful. The responses parallel those of fear and anger—the "fight or flight" response—in which the body gears for action to stand up and meet the problem or to try to escape it. The heart speeds up; blood pressure rises; muscles tense; in the blood the levels of blood sugar, blood fats, and cholesterol rise; and adrenalin pours into the blood, which now clots more readily. The person feels fearful or anxious, tense, and nervous. Persons with type A personalities and others who respond adversely to everyday stresses are at a higher risk for a heart attack.

As with nicotine, so with stress. Cholesterol enters the artery walls where the junction points of cells lining the arteries buckle.

Lack of exercise is another major risk factor. Exercise strengthens the heart and blood vessels as the active muscles make demands for more oxygen and fuel. Inactivity, on the other hand, weakens the cardiovascular system and at the same time increases the occurrence of other risk factors such as obesity, hypertension, elevated cholesterol, and nervous tension.

Obesity, like sedentary living, is also considered a major risk factor. The workload of the heart increases, since blood has to be pumped through hundreds of miles of extra blood vessels to keep alive the pounds of extra body mass. Obesity is closely associated with hypertension, diabetes, elevated blood fats, and cholesterol.

Diabetes or "sugar diabetes" results from the body's inability to utilize insulin efficiently or from the production of insufficient amounts. Blood sugar rises to undesirable levels, and some spills over into the urine. High blood levels of fats (triglycerides) and cholesterol, along with atherosclerosis and arteriosclerosis, are common. Precise control by appropriate medication (insulin or insulin substitutes) and by diet and exercise is essential to avoid greatly increasing the risk of heart attack.

Uncontrollable risk factors

Age does not of itself cause heart disease. Instead, the slow destruction of the arterial wall with gradual narrowing that occurs over a period of twenty to thirty years may eventually result in a heart attack. So it is not surprising to find that heart disease is more common in older people. Many older people have strong, healthy hearts because their lifestyle avoided or minimized the controllable risk factors. Occasionally one hears of an individual who lives to a ripe old age and has done everything he shouldn't! However, nature's endowment of a robust cardiovascular system should get the credit, not his way of life.

Sex. Men are generally more prone to heart attacks than are women, especially males thirty-five to fifty years of age. Several factors appear to favor women. Female hormones or estrogens seem to be protective, for within a few years after menopause the susceptibility of women equals that of men. Women tend to carry a higher HDL level than men. And, until recently, women did not smoke to the same extent as did men. Unfortunately, this situation is changing.

Heredity. Some evidence exists that heart disease runs in families. A family record in which blood relatives have had coronary heart disease, especially between forty to fifty years of age, increases your risk of a heart attack. In some families very high cholesterol levels and/or high blood pressure appear to be inherited. These conditions add to the risk. Although you cannot choose your parents and close relatives, recognizing your inherited weaknesses and modifying your lifestyle may help you considerably.

Atherosclerosis

As already mentioned, arteries are musculo-elastic tubes that carry oxygen-laden blood to the tissues of the body. Their smooth inner lining minimizes friction. Sometimes fatty streaks appear on this inner lining, especially where the artery divides or is damaged. These streaks may enlarge, and muscle cells beneath them may multiply, causing the wall to bulge inward. This, in turn, sets up turbulence, which further damages the lining. The growing mass, which contains muscle cells, cholesterol, and calcium salts, along with fibrous tissue and collagen, is called an **atheroma** or **plaque.** The passageway is narrowed, blood flow is restricted, and if the process continues, the artery may become blocked. This hardening process, called **atherosclerosis,** contributes to a general form of hardening of the arteries called **arteriosclerosis,** and is the prime cause of coronary heart disease.

Although the causes of atherosclerosis are not fully understood, the disease is associated with elevated levels of blood cholesterol and blood fats. Certain lifestyle habits seem to be contributory: a diet rich in animal fats and cholesterol (fatty meats, butter, eggs, certain seafoods,

and organ meats), along with kidney failure and the other risk factors discussed above.

Symptoms. Since atherosclerosis occurs within an artery wall, the primary symptoms are disorders of the organ to which the artery provides blood. These symptoms appear as the blood supply to the affected organ is reduced, either gradually or abruptly.

If the arteries of your heart are affected, you may suffer from angina or a heart attack; if those of the brain, a stroke; if those of your legs, muscle cramps on walking, or if severe occlusion has developed, gangrene of your toes or foot. If your renal arteries are blocked, kidney failure will result.

An exception to this is the development of an aneurysm (see page 799) in the artery itself. Here

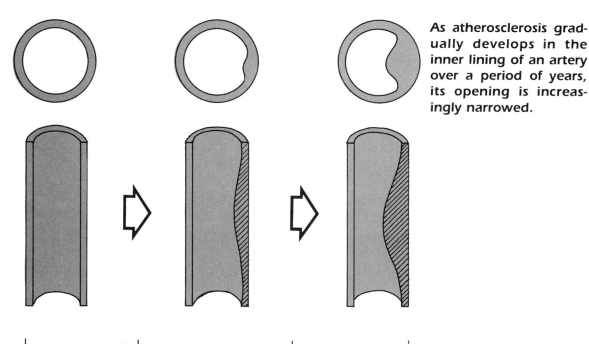

As atherosclerosis gradually develops in the inner lining of an artery over a period of years, its opening is increasingly narrowed.

Vessel narrowed over years

atherosclerosis has so weakened the artery wall that blood begins to seep between its layers, or the wall bursts.

What you can do. Since atherosclerosis develops over a period of years without any symptoms, when symptoms do appear, the process is well advanced. You should carefully evaluate your lifestyle and take the necessary steps to alter those factors that may lead to atherosclerosis (see under "risk factors," pages 777-779).

What your physician can do. Your physician can determine your blood pressure, the level of your cholesterol and blood fats (triglycerides), or whether your blood sugar is too high (diabetes). He can aid you with your diet and other lifestyle changes. He may recommend certain medications for conditions that do not respond to lifestyle changes.

Coronary heart disease (Ischemic heart disease, angina, heart attack)

An average healthy man living in the United States has about one chance in five of developing coronary heart disease before he reaches sixty-five. Notice that we mentioned the average *man*. Coronary heart disease is more common among men than among women.

Coronary heart disease accounts for practically all the instances of "heart attack" that strike suddenly.

Obstruction by a blood clot (thrombus) in a major branch of a coronary artery deprives a certain area of the heart wall of its blood supply, bringing on a heart attack (myocardial infarction).

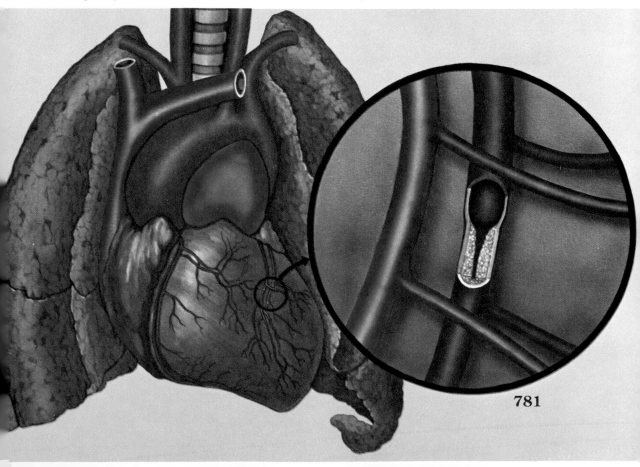

781

Of those suffering such an attack, 25 percent die within three hours. Another 10 percent die within the next four weeks. The survivors live with the knowledge that they remain vulnerable to another heart attack unless they drastically change their way of life.

Atherosclerosis is the basic cause of coronary heart disease. The coronary arteries are just as susceptible as any other arteries to the development of atherosclerosis. The right and left coronary arteries, as their name implies, encircle the heart like a crown, and supply the heart muscle with blood. As these arteries or their branches become blocked, the heart muscle they supply becomes deprived of oxygen. A state of myocardial ischemia occurs, with shortness of breath or chest pain (angina), especially on exertion or when a person is emotionally stressed. It is possible, however, to have ischemia of the heart muscle without pain.

Angina is a pain deep to the breastbone (angina pectoris) caused by a reduced flow of blood to some area of the heart muscle. It usually results from atherosclerosis in the wall of a coronary artery, though sometimes it is due to a spasm of the vessel. The pain, discomfort, or feeling of pressure or squeezing may be severe, and the intensity of the distress may vary. The pain may radiate to the shoulder and down the arm (usually on the left side), but may involve both arms, the neck, and even the lower face. These symptoms mimic those of a heart attack, but usually last only a few minutes and are relieved by rest or a drug such as nitroglycerine.

What you can do. If it is your first attack, assume that the situation is the more serious of the two possibilities, a heart attack rather than angina, and see your physician immediately. If he is not available, call the fire department or an ambulance. Remain calm, cease all physical activity, and remain quietly at rest, lying on your back.

If you have had previous episodes you doubtless have nitroglycerine tablets; place one or two under your tongue. This should relieve your anginal pain. If the pain and discomfort persist for more than five

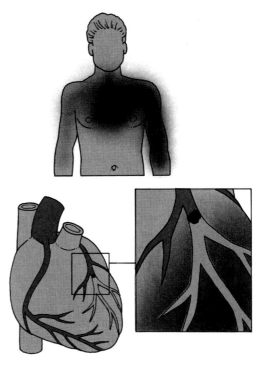

Restricted blood flow through a coronary artery may cause severe pain over the heart radiating to the shoulder, arm or arms, neck, and even the face.

minutes or become increasingly severe, you probably are having a heart attack, and the condition is very serious. Call for help. For the long term you need to examine your lifestyle and make the necessary changes suggested under "controllable risk factors" (see pages 777).

What your physician can do. Your physician can thoroughly evaluate your condition, both by a physical examination and by making a number of laboratory tests. These may include blood pressure, an electrocardiogram, blood tests to determine the level of your fats (triglycerides) and cholesterol, a chest X-ray to show the size of your heart, and an angiogram (by the injection of a dye) to estimate the blood flow through your coronary arteries.

Heart attack

A heart attack occurs when blood flow through one of the coronary arteries or its major branches is blocked by a thrombus or blood clot, due usually to advanced atherosclerosis. The area of heart muscle damaged by lack of blood is called an **infarct.** If the infarct is small and the conducting system of the heart is not affected, the chance of recovery is good. The attack may occur suddenly and without warning, or it may come on gradually.

The pain from a heart attack may parallel that experienced with severe angina (see page 782), but generally it is not relieved by rest or the elimination of the emotional stress that triggered it, and frequently will last for thirty or more minutes. The pain may vary

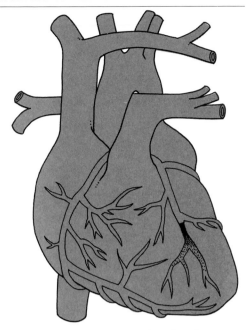

Note that a blood clot in the anterior branch of the left coronary artery has deprived the muscle of the heart wall of blood (mottled area). This is what happens in a heart attack.

widely, from agonizing to mild, with various combinations of symptoms. Usually the intense pain originates in the chest, with a crushing, squeezing feeling. The victim may experience sweating, cold, clammy skin, nausea, vomiting, weakness, shortness of breath, dizziness and fainting, and a feeling of impending death.

In the Western world heart attacks are the most common cause of death, one in three being fatal. The care given in the first few minutes may make the difference between life and death, so don't delay in getting medical help. The American Medical Association gives some good advice: "Don't you wait. If you think someone is having a

783

heart attack, call the fire department rescue squad immediately. Seconds count. Don't wait for severe pain, dizziness, fainting or sweating, or shortness of breath. . . . Don't let the fear of embarrassment delay your call. If you're wrong about the existence of a heart attack, it doesn't matter. If you're right, nothing could matter more." So any unexplained chest pain which persists for more than a few minutes should be examined by a physician.

What you can do. A heart attack is an emergency. If you are with someone who experiences severe chest pains, call for professional help: a physician, fire department rescue squad, or ambulance. Place the victim in a half-reclining position with head and shoulders slightly elevated. You may save a life if you or someone at hand can administer cardiopulmonary resuscitation (CPR)—mouth-to-mouth breathing with external heart massage—so oxygen can reach the brain and vital areas. Allow the victim to breathe fresh air. If oxygen is available, play a gentle stream over the face and nose. A nitroglycerine tablet, if available, can be placed under the tongue. The sooner the victim reaches a hospital or coronary-care unit, the better.

What your physician can do. While bed rest initially is mandatory, your physician will assess the severity of the attack and allow as much activity as he deems wise, since bed rest may increase the risk of abnormal clotting. He may order a platelet (thrombocyte) count and prescribe an anticoagulant to further reduce the risk of a blood clot forming, and

he will relieve pain when necessary. Oxygen may make breathing easier. He will order a number of tests, such as electrocardiograms (EKG), to monitor the type and extent of the injury and blood tests to measure the damage done to the heart muscle. If

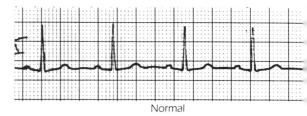
Normal

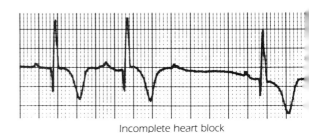
Incomplete heart block

Typical electrocardiogram (EKG) tracings, showing normal and irregular heart action.

the heart begins to fail or the heart rhythms are disturbed, he may prescribe other medications.

The long-term prospects depend on the extent of the damage and on the steps taken to actively modify all risk factors present in the lifestyle. In case of mild heart attack, without complications, full recovery can be expected. If severe, some loss of functional activity may result. Lifestyle modifications, which include stopping smoking, exercise, weight loss, dietary changes, and restyling of behavior, together with long-term medical follow-up, will largely determine the outcome.

Because many heart problems result from atherosclerosis, and the procedures of rehabilitation, coronary bypass surgery, and angioplasty apply to more than one problem, the details are presented at the end of this section (see page 790).

Hypertension

Because it affects the heart so frequently, hypertension or high blood pressure is discussed here rather than under vascular diseases. High blood pressure is the most common and dangerous underlying cause of heart and blood vessel disease, and it is the leading cause of death in industrialized nations. Hypertension, called the "silent killer," produces no symptoms during the first fifteen or so years and goes undetected without blood pressure measurements. Only in advanced stages, and not always then, will symptoms appear—headache, nosebleed, dizziness, fainting, and ringing of the ears. But despite the fact that no symptoms appear, high blood pressure silently, slowly, but surely, injures the heart, damages the arteries (especially those of the heart, brain, eyes, and kidneys), and cuts short the lifespan by ten to twenty years.

What is blood pressure? Blood pressure is the force required by the heart to pump blood against the resistance offered by the arteries. The arteries are always full of blood. Their walls consist of layers of muscle and elastic tissue, so they can expand and contract. When the heart contracts, it pushes 4 to 8 ounces of blood into already full vessels. The arteries must bulge outward to accept the heart's output, and then their musculo-elastic walls recoil, maintaining pressure to continue the flow. When the heart contracts, systolic pressure is highest; when the heart relaxes, diastolic pressure is the lowest. The normal range for blood pressure in healthy young adults is 90 to 140 for the systolic and 60 to 90 for the diastolic.

What is high blood pressure? Persistent readings above 160 systolic or above 95 diastolic fall into the range of high blood pressure. Notice the words *persistent readings* above these figures. A single reading may not indicate your average blood pressure. Blood pressure may abruptly rise under stress, excitement, or an emergency, but should drop back to normal when the cause is removed.

The cause of hypertension in the overwhelming majority of cases is idiopathic or of unknown cause. Secondary hypertension may result from chronic kidney disease, certain hormonal disorders, and, in certain women, becoming pregnant or taking oral contraceptives.

A certain form of hypertension (essential hypertension) has no known cause, though research suggests one possibility—that a gradual increase in the volume of blood accompanies a slow rise in blood pressure. Some inherited inability of the kidneys to excrete excess salt in the diet causes this increase in blood volume. This would explain why hypertension seems to run in families. The child of a parent with high blood pressure has twice the chance of developing hypertension as a child whose parents have normal blood pressure. Another observation is that overweight children seem more likely to have hypertension when they reach middle age than normal-weight children.

Undiscovered or uncontrolled hypertension can be a deadly disease. The increased pressure within the arteries accelerates the process of atherosclerosis in the coronary arteries, and in the arteries of the brain, kidneys, and other organs. The result is more than a twofold increase in heart attacks and sudden death, a sixfold increase in conges-

What you can do. As already mentioned, hypertension can be considered a symptomless disease. Should you discover you have the problem, you can reduce your salt intake, if it is high; you can lose weight, if you are obese. If you smoke, give it up because smoking contributes to atherosclerosis and heart disease. If you are a type A person on a tight schedule, reduce your emotional stress; include regular exercise in your program because exercise is relaxing; and seek help from your physician.

What your physician can do. Even mild high blood pressure is harmful over time. If your own efforts fail to reduce your blood pressure, a number of medications are

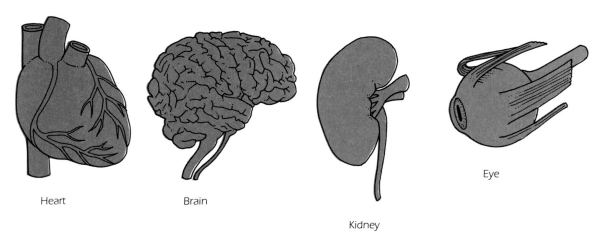

Heart   Brain

Eye

Kidney

Untreated high blood pressure accelerates the process of atherosclerosis in the arteries of the heart, **brain, kidneys, and eye, resulting in heart attacks, stroke, kidney failure, and retinal (eye) problems.**

tive heart failure, a fourfold increase in strokes, and a two-fold increase from fatal kidney disease in hypertensives as compared with those having normal blood pressure.

available. These must be taken under the guidance of your physician, who will determine which are most effective. Diuretics or "water pills" reduce the amount of salt and water in your

786

body. Others decrease the action of your sympathetic nerves, which cause your arteries to constrict or narrow. Other agents relax the blood vessels, allowing pressure to fall. Still others decrease the formation of naturally occurring substances that constrict blood vessels. Do not discontinue treatment without your physician's advice.

Heart failure

Heart failure or congestive heart failure occurs when the heart can no longer pump blood efficiently. This may result from a number of causes: a heart weakened by a heart attack or by a local disease, such as rheumatic fever or infectious endocarditis; prolonged high blood pressure, which increases the workload of the heart; faulty heart valves that fail to control the flow of blood within the heart's chambers, making its pumping action inefficient; and anemia, a condition in which the heart must pump extra blood to compensate for the smaller amounts of oxygen the blood can carry.

Congestive heart failure usually affects the entire heart, but at times may single out either the left or right side. The symptoms vary, depending on which side is affected. In **left-side failure** the pumping action of the left ventricle does not clear the blood coming from the lungs. As a result, blood backs up in the lungs. Mild exercise, climbing stairs, as well as lying flat in bed, will make the individual breathless. As the problem worsens, wheezing accompanies difficult breathing. Other symptoms include congested lungs, chest pain,

and coughing up blood-tinged phlegm or sputum. Susceptibility to infections, such as pneumonia and bronchitis, increases.

In **right-side failure** the blood returning from the body and limbs is not efficiently pumped to the lungs and, as a result, backs up. This causes swelling of the ankles and feet, especially by the end of the day. Poor general circulation causes lips, membranes, and nail beds to appear bluish (cyanotic) and causes the individual to feel tired and weak. If the person is bedridden, fluid may collect in his low back, and his liver may become swollen and tender.

Congestive heart failure generally affects both sides of the heart. This serious condition may be fatal; however, under wise management most sufferers can live relatively normal lives.

What you can do. You should place yourself under the care of a physician. Under his direction you should stay as physically active as possible, while avoiding strenuous exercise. When sitting or lying down, move your feet and arms frequently. This will promote circulation and minimize clot formation, especially in the legs and pelvis. Reduce your intake of salt, because salt tends to hold water in the tissues.

Remember, should you suddenly become acutely short of breath, this is an emergency. Call for a physician or paramedics, or go to a hospital. Do not delay.

What your physician can do. He can help you in a number of ways: eliminate excess fluid from your tissues by prescribing diuretics, which

787

will require you to pass more urine; strengthen the contraction of your heart muscle by using some form of digitalis, which improves the heart's work capacity; reduce the ability of your blood to clot by using an anti-coagulant; and eliminate or treat the factors that contributed to your heart failure—overweight, high blood pressure, defective heart valves, etc.

Heart disease: rehabilitation and prevention

What to do after a heart attack. A heart attack is a shocking experience. Even to be diagnosed as having a serious heart disease is frightening. You can deny there's a problem; you can give up and become an invalid; or you can go from where you are, recognizing that with appropriate adjustments in outlook and lifestyle, with realism and common sense, you, like most heart disease survivors, can live a relatively normal and productive life.

If you have had a heart attack, the first step is to make as satisfactory a recovery as possible. Cooperate with your physician. Enroll in a cardiovascular rehabilitation program as soon as feasible. Hospitals, YMCAs, and a number of private organizations offer well-supervised instruction. If you are having difficulty adjusting psychologically, seek professional help. And make the necessary lifestyle changes, for heart and blood vessel disease in the Western world results largely from the way life is lived. Changing your lifestyle may not be easy, but the future length and quality of your life are at stake.

The details of what constitutes a healthful lifestyle and how it will both prevent and rehabilitate cardiovascular disease are presented in another section (see page 117). However, the main points are summarized here.

1. Get appropriate and regular exercise (approved by physician)
2. Get adequate rest and sleep
3. Eat a nutritious diet
   a. No excess calories, only sufficient to maintain ideal weight
   b. Low in fat, especially saturated animal fats
   c. Low in refined carbohydrate foods, such as refined sugar and cereals
   d. High in dietary fiber—fruits, vegetables, legumes, and whole-grain cereals
   e. Low in salt
4. Avoid smoking, beverage alcohol, and caffeine-containing beverages
5. Avoid stressful situations
6. Work within your capacity on a reasonable schedule
7. Include relaxing, enjoyable, non-competitive recreation

Should you have some problem like diabetes, keep it well controlled. If you are obese, lose excess weight. A lifestyle change as suggested will help to lower blood cholesterol, if high; lower blood pressure, if elevated; and give you a zest for living.

Coronary artery bypass

Prior to bypass surgery, a careful study of blood flow through the coronaries is accomplished by an X-ray study (angiography), taking motion pictures while injecting a dye into the arteries. The dye is observed as it moves through the vessels, and the sites of narrowing noted. Some 200,000 bypass operations are performed in the United States each year. About one in fifty do not survive the procedure.

After anesthesia, the surgeon opens the chest, and the patient is put on a heart-lung machine (which both oxygenates and circulates the blood). The surgeon interposes a vein, usually taken from the leg, between the aorta and a point distant to the obstruction in the severely narrowed or blocked coronary artery. In this way blood flows in the usual channel to the restricted point, and through the bypass beyond this point, making the restricted artery

fully functional. One or more blockages may be bypassed.

Most recipients of bypass surgery obtain immediate relief from severe angina and are able to be much more physically active. However, not all patients with coronary artery disease are suitable candidates. More conservative medical management can help some; in others the narrowing of the arteries is too diffuse. Nor is the operation always successful in accomplishing its purpose.

One must remember that bypass surgery does not cure the underlying problem, that is, atherosclerosis. If changes in lifestyle are not made, the problem will recur. In fact, the vein used for the bypass is likely to become atherosclerotic more rapidly than did the coronary arteries themselves.

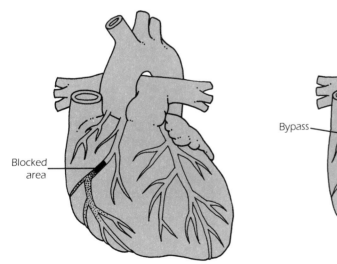 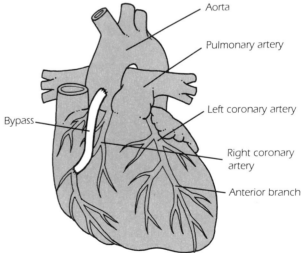

Note the venous graft extending from the aorta to the right coronary artery, bypassing the occlusion in the vessel.

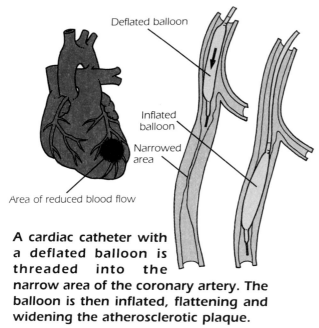

Deflated balloon

Inflated balloon

Narrowed area

Area of reduced blood flow

A cardiac catheter with a deflated balloon is threaded into the narrow area of the coronary artery. The balloon is then inflated, flattening and widening the atherosclerotic plaque.

Angioplasty

In this relatively new and promising treatment of coronary artery disease, a catheter with an inflatable balloonlike tip is passed into the artery until it is stopped by the obstruction. The balloon is then inflated, breaking the plaque and widening the restricted area. On occasion, because of unsatisfactory results, the procedure must be repeated. Although simpler, safer, and cheaper than bypass surgery, angioplasty is not suitable for all forms of coronary heart disease.

Disturbed heart rhythms

The rate at which your heart normally beats depends upon what you are doing and on your state of mind. During physical activity it will beat faster, as it will if you are nervous or excited. If you rest or sleep, it will slow down. Occasionally you may be aware of a skipped beat or palpitation. This is not unusual.

Your heart beats with a regular rhythm sixty to eighty times each minute when at rest, accelerating to a rate of 175 or more during vigorous exercise. However, a number of causes exist for unnecessary or undesirable irregularities, which include beating too fast (tachycardia), beating too slowly (bradycardia), and beating irregularly (arrhythmia). The more common causes include anxiety, high intakes of caffeine (from tea, coffee, and soft drinks), beverage alcohol, cigarette smoking, and problems and diseases related to the heart and its valves.

Most heart irregularities, like "skipping a beat" or having an "extra beat" are harmless though sometimes annoying. If, however, the irregularities are persistent and troubling, see your physician.

Palpitation. Normally you are unaware of your heartbeat, but when the heart begins to palpitate, you become conscious of it. Emotional stress, fear, anger, grief, anxiety, together with caffeine, alcohol, and tobacco produce palpitation, the most common disturbance of the heart. This type of forceful heartbeat is benign unless prolonged over long periods.

Tachycardia. During tachycardia the heart suddenly speeds up to rates of 160 or more per minute. The paroxysm, as it is sometimes called, may last from a few minutes up to several days. You become aware of your heart beating, which may be associated with chest pain, fainting spells, and difficulty in breathing. Sometimes some simple procedure

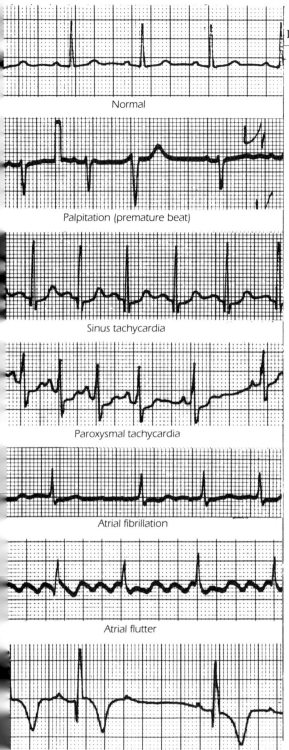

Normal

Palpitation (premature beat)

Sinus tachycardia

Paroxysmal tachycardia

Atrial fibrillation

Atrial flutter

Incomplete heart block

The electrocardiographic tracings show normal, rapid, and irregular heart rhythms.

may avert the spell, such as holding your breath, drinking a glass of cold water, or blowing up a balloon. Preventive measures would be to discontinue the use of caffeine-containing beverages, alcohol, and tobacco. Generally the condition is not serious, but should it persist, you should see your physician. He may put pressure on an artery in your neck, which may arrest the condition, or may advise the use of certain medications.

Atrial fibrillation. Here the beating of the atria or upper chambers of the heart are very rapid and irregular. In fact, the rate may be so fast that the muscle fibers only twitch and blood is not pushed into the ventricles, resulting in inadequate filling. This, along with the fact that the action of the atria and ventricles are uncoordinated, reduces the efficiency of the pumping action of the heart. In **atrial flutter** the rate of beating is slower and more regular.

Commonly, atrial fibrillation and flutter result from heart damage that is caused by coronary heart disease or rheumatic heart disease, although sometimes no cause can be found. Symptoms include dizziness, fainting spells, anginal attacks, and heart failure. Occasionally a clot may form on the wall of an atrium. If it is dislodged, the clot becomes an embolus and will travel in the blood to a point where the artery becomes too small for its further passage, preventing blood from flowing beyond this point. If the embolus arises in the right atrium, it will end up in the lungs; if from the left atrium, it may travel to any part of the body, including the brain, kidneys, intestines, etc.

791

Serious difficulties or even death may result.

Should you have either atrial fibrillation or flutter, place yourself under the care of your physician so that he can prescribe appropriate medications or other treatment.

Heart block. In heart block the contraction impulses are delayed or fail to get through from their source in the wall of the right atrium to the ventricles. While the ventricles continue to beat because of their natural rhythm, the rate, while regular, is very slow, perhaps forty or fewer beats per minute **(bradycardia).** Different degrees of heart block range from mild to severe. You may be unaware of mild forms of heart block. However, complete heart block is a serious condition. Consult your physician. You may experience extreme weakness, breathlessness, spells of unconsciousness, or heart failure. Prior to the use of artificial pacemakers, mortality was as high as 50 percent in a single year.

Pacemakers. These electronic devices have a small power source and pulse generator implanted beneath the skin below the collarbone, with tiny electrodes leading to the heart. Their relatively strong impulse replaces or overrides the irregular or weak natural impulse and provides a practical stimulation of the heart. With long-lived batteries, they operate without intervention for seven or more years. People wearing pacemakers must stay away from strong radio or radar transmitters and from locations where electromagnetic impulses are generated. Periodic checkups are a wise precaution.

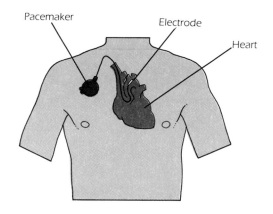

A pacemaker, implanted under the skin, is connected to an electrode in contact with the heart. The strong, regular impulses of the pacemaker now control the rhythm of the heart.

Cardiac arrest occurs when the heart stops beating. It may result from a severe heart attack or from one of the most serious of the arrhythmias—**ventricular tachycardia.** The rate of the rapidly beating ventricle may accelerate to the point where the muscle fibers no longer contract but merely twitch or fibrillate **(ventricular fibrillation),** and the heart no longer pumps blood. If within two or three minutes the beat is not reinstituted, brain damage or other serious injury may occur, or the outcome may be fatal. Immediate skilled help must be sought from an ambulance, fire department, or hospital emergency room. For ventricular fibrillation a defibrillator will often help. A trained person may apply cardiopulmonary resuscitation (CPR) till additional help arrives.

792

Sudden death. Some 400,000 sudden deaths occur in the United States each year. Of these, more than two-thirds result from heart attack caused by coronary heart disease. Other causes include heart failure resulting from one of several causes: pulmonary embolism in which a sizable clot originating in a vein finds its way into one of the large branches of the pulmonary artery; certain cases of stroke in which the blood supply to part of the brain is disrupted; rupture of an aneurysm; and the development of a dissecting aneurysm. All of these causes of sudden death are related either to the heart or to the blood vessels.

Heart valve disease

Four valves, composed of thin leaflets of tissue, direct the flow of blood through the chambers of the heart and outward through the arteries. Blood arriving at the heart from throughout the body enters the right atrium. From there it passes through the **tricuspid valve** to the right ventricle. At the same time blood returning from the lungs enters the left atrium and passes through the **mitral valve** to the left ventricle. As the ventricles contract and the pressure rises in their chambers, the tricuspid and mitral valves snap shut, preventing blood from flowing back into the atria. The right ventricle pumps its blood through the **pulmonary valve** via the pulmonary artery to the lungs. The left ventricle pushes its blood through the **aortic valve** via the aorta to all parts of the body. As the ventricles relax, blood tries to rush back into these chambers. Now

the pulmonary and aortic valves snap shut, confining the blood in their respective arteries.

When the valves are defective from birth, from an infection (rheumatic fever), or from some other heart disorder, the flow of blood through them is affected. If the leaflets are distorted and irregular, they fail to close properly and allow blood to back-flow, a condition known as **incompetence.** If they are thickened and fused together, the narrowed opening restricts the blood flow, a condition called **stenosis.**

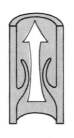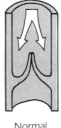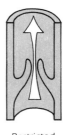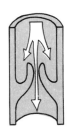

| Normal opening | Normal closing | Restricted opening | Backflow |

A normal valve opens and then closes completely. A damaged valve neither opens nor closes adequately, thus restricting outflow and permitting backflow.

Mitral stenosis. When the flow of blood coming from the lungs to the left atrium cannot freely pass through the narrowed mitral valve into the left ventricle, the atrium hypertrophies or enlarges. Pressure rises in the pulmonary veins, and the lungs become congested. The right ventricle now pumps harder, attempting to keep the blood passing through the lungs, and in time it enlarges.

The main symptoms—shortness of breath and congestion of the lungs—are aggravated by exercise or lying down. Blood-tinged sputum and cough, bronchitis, along with discomfort and pain in the chest, may be present. As the right side of the heart (bringing blood from throughout the body) begins to fail, the ankles swell, and fluid collects in the abdomen. Weakness and fatigue become constant; heart failure may occur. A more serious problem is atrial fibrillation, with a blood clot forming on the inside wall of the atrium and subsequently breaking loose as an embolus (see page 808).

What you can do. Frequently people are unaware they have diseased heart valves and remain symptom-free for many years while living normal lives. When a problem does develop, one can do little about it. Seek the advice of a physician.

What your physician can do. He can do a number of tests to specifically determine your problem. An echocardiogram is very helpful. If your ankles swell and you accumulate fluid, he may prescribe a diuretic to reduce salt and water. If you have heart failure, digitalis or some similar medication may prove helpful. For atrial fibrillation an antiarrhythmic agent and an anticoagulant may be used to correct the rhythm and prevent a clot from forming.

Diseased heart valves are highly susceptible to infections, such as endocarditis. When surgical or dental procedures are undertaken which may allow bacteria to enter the bloodstream, antibiotics can protect against infection. During open-heart surgery the defective heart valve may be surgically repaired (the opening enlarged) or replaced with an artificial valve. These have been perfected over the past few years and are made from a variety of materials: your own tendon tissue, animal parts, plastic materials, and metal.

Mitral incompetence. Because the leaflets of the valve do not fit perfectly together, blood from the left ventricle back-flows through the mitral valve into the left atrium. This requires the left ventricle to work harder, and in time it enlarges. One may be symptom-free for years, but eventually heart failure may develop. The resulting problems are very similar to those seen in mitral stenosis: shortness of breath, fatigue, and those associated with heart failure. Incompetent valves are more susceptible to bacterial infections.

Once symptoms develop, the care and treatment is similar to those discussed under mitral stenosis.

Aortic stenosis. Here the valve between the left ventricle and the aorta is narrowed, making the left ventricle work harder. Symptoms may be absent for years, until breathlessness occurs, especially after exercise. Later, when circulation to the brain, muscles, and heart itself are affected, dizziness, fainting, weakness, and angina may develop. Eventually the left heart will fail.

What you can do. In early stages you can live a normal life. As long as you can exercise, do so moderately, avoiding strenuous exercise. Work closely with your physician.

What your physician can do. Should you require dental or surgical

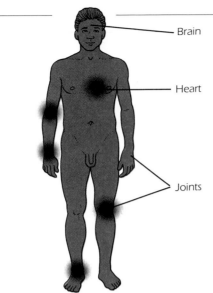

Rheumatic fever may affect the heart (rheumatic heart disease), the joints (migrating polyarthritis), and the brain (Sydenham's chorea).

work, your physician can cover you with an antibiotic. When the situation warrants it, a valve replacement is the only treatment (see "mitral stenosis").

Aortic incompetence. When the aortic valve cannot close efficiently, blood that has been pumped into the aorta leaks or flows back into the ventricle. This greatly increases the workload of the ventricle, which will gradually enlarge. Eventually left heart failure will occur. The symptoms and treatment parallel those seen in aortic stenosis.

Pulmonary and tricuspid valves, stenosis, and incompetence. Only a small percentage of people suffer from these disorders, which generally result either from a congenital abnormality or from rheumatic fever. The symptoms as well as treatment are similar to those that are discussed elsewhere under other heart valve

disorders. Should you have such a problem, see your physician.

Rheumatic heart disease

Rheumatic heart disease, a serious complication of rheumatic fever (see page 473), often follows a sore throat or some other infection caused by streptococcus bacteria. The heart becomes inflamed and may take the form of (1) **endocarditis** (inflammation of the lining of the heart or of the valves), (2) **pericarditis** (inflammation of the covering of the heart), or (3) **myocarditis** (inflammation of the heart muscle). But 60 percent of time the heart valves are involved. The inflammation of the lining of the heart (endocarditis) typically causes ulceration of the valves. This may lead to narrowing of the valve opening due to scar formation **(stenosis)**, or distortion of the valve leaflets so they no longer fit perfectly together and allow blood to flow through when closed **(incompetence)**.

Inasmuch as rheumatic heart disease is a complication of rheumatic fever and caused by an infection from the streptococcus germ, the treatment consists of combating the infection. This requires aggressive and continuing use of antibiotics, as the fever may recur. With each recurrence further damage to the heart valves occurs. The symptoms and treatment associated with each valve affected are discussed under the specific heart valve.

Infective endocarditis (bacterial endocarditis)

The membrane that covers the inner surface of the heart and heart

795

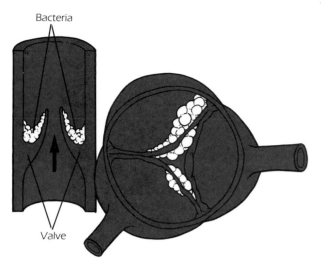

Bacteria

Valve

Bacterial endocarditis. Here colonies of bacteria are attached to the heart valves. If untreated, the valves are permanently damaged.

valves is called the endocardium. The inflammation of this lining by an infective organism is called endocarditis. The germs causing endocarditis are most commonly bacteria (streptococcus and staphylococcus), but fungi may be involved. The organisms (entering via the bloodstream) attach themselves to the endocardium, especially in previously blemished areas, such as congenital defects, heart valves previously damaged (as with rheumatic fever), or scars from previous surgery.

The heart valves, the main target of the bacteria, may eventually be destroyed. Blood cells and clotted blood attach to the colonies of bacteria, forming highly fragile growths. These growths may break apart, sending infected fragments as emboli throughout the circulation. These may lodge anywhere—the brain, the kidneys, the lungs, and even in the heart itself (arriving through the coronary arteries).

Two types of infective endocarditis exist, acute and subacute. The acute type, with more virulent germs, comes on suddenly, with rapid destruction of the heart valve, and, if untreated, will cause death within a few weeks. In the subacute type, the disease progresses gradually, sometimes undetected, with milder symptoms, until serious damage to the heart valves has occurred, with the outcome just as deadly.

The symptoms vary widely but usually include weakness, fatigue, loss of appetite, chills, low fever, headaches, and aching joints. If emboli are being scattered through the bloodstream, symptoms will depend on their size and where they lodge: if in the lungs or kidneys, an abscess; if in the brain, weakness or paralysis of one side; if in a coronary artery, a heart attack.

Those at highest risk are people who have already had some heart problem. Their physician can do the appropriate tests and prescribe an antibiotic effective against the particular organism. Those with damaged heart valves, congenital heart defects, or who have had open-heart surgery should guard against possible infection (by antibiotic therapy), when undergoing dental or surgical procedures. Should you be among any of the above and have symptoms of endocarditis, report to your physician promptly.

Myocarditis

Myocarditis, an inflammation of the heart muscle, usually occurs as a complication of some other disease, such as diphtheria, rheumatic fever, measles, mumps, and influenza, or from a direct injury. In mild cases the symptoms may be changes in heart rhythm, shortness of breath, and chest pain. These will clear up with recovery. In more serious cases, as with diphtheria or rheumatic fever, the result can be heart failure and death. Treatment is directed toward the underlying infection, together with rest and the avoidance of alcohol.

Pericarditis

Pericarditis is an inflammation of the pericardium, a membrane which covers the outside of the heart and lines the pericardial sac in which the heart beats. Pericarditis may result from a viral, bacterial, fungal, or parasitic infection, or from an injury, or it may arise subsequent to a heart attack. The inflamed membrane becomes thick and rough, and fluid collects in the sac.

Symptoms include sudden, severe pain over the heart that radiates to the left shoulder, and a friction rub that may be heard with a stethoscope. Deep breathing aggravates the pain, while leaning forward provides relief. Early treatment is important to prevent complications. The heart may be constricted by the pericardial sac becoming smaller as it becomes thickened and scarred, or by large amounts of fluid accumulating within the sac. The former is relieved by surgically splitting the sac, the latter by removal of the fluid.

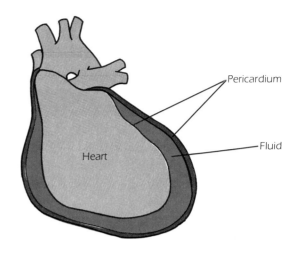

Pericarditis, with fluid filling the pericardial sac.

Congenital heart defects

The heart begins to develop about three weeks after conception, when it consists of a single pulsating tube. During the next five weeks it twists and divides, becoming a four-chambered organ. While undergoing this marvelous transformation, from a single tube to a four-chambered organ with four valves that control the inflow and outflow of blood, it is able to continuously pump blood!

Considering its complex plan of development, it is not surprising that mishaps occur from time to time that result in malformations of various structures of the heart and of the large connecting vessels. Almost one out of every 100 babies is born with some deformity of the heart or of the large vessels adjacent to it.

The deformities include defects or holes in the septa between the right and left atria and the right and left ventricles; narrowing of the valves

797

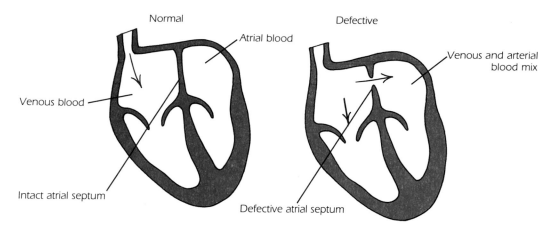

An atrial septal defect allowing returning venous blood to mix with arterial blood coming from the lungs.

due to fusing of the valve leaflets; and abnormalities of the large vessels adjacent to the heart. The more frequent defects are briefly described.

"Blue baby" or cyanotic heart disease

In this condition the skin and lips are dark blue rather than pink. A defect, usually of the septa, permits unoxygenated or venous blood (of bluish color) returning from the body to mix with blood coming from the lungs with its quota of oxygen, thus sending unoxygenated blood back through the body. Abnormal connections between vessels coming to and leaving the heart, or a failure of one or both chambers on the left side of the heart to develop, will also cause this problem.

Patent (open) ductus arteriosus

Because the fetus's lungs do not oxygenate its blood, it must receive its oxygen from the mother via the placental circulation, in which oxygen passes from the mother's blood to the fetus's blood. A special vessel causes the blood to bypass the infant's lungs and directs it instead into the aorta. This vessel closes when the newborn begins to breathe. When this fails to occur and the vessel remains open, the infant will suffer from shortness of breath on exertion and eventually become cyanotic.

The degree of handicap from the many types of congenital heart disease varies from person to person. The immediate treatment of severe cyanosis in a newborn is to add extra oxygen to the air that it breathes. The long-range treatment consists of discovering and treating the fundamental cause.

Modern diagnostic techniques and modern methods of performing heart surgery offer a great deal for correcting these and other malformations of the heart.

798

CHAPTER 3

Blood vessel diseases

Diseases of the arteries

Arteries are musculo-elastic tubes that carry blood from the heart to all parts of the body. The aorta, the largest artery, attaches to the heart. Its branching arteries become smaller and smaller until they become microscopic-size capillaries. When an artery becomes diseased, the part of the body that receives blood conveyed by this vessel will suffer accordingly. Diseases that affect arteries produce disorders in (1) the lining, obstructing the flow of blood; (2) the muscles, causing either dilatation or constriction; and (3) the wall, causing hardening or weakening that results in arteriosclerosis or an aneurysm.

Hardening of the arteries (arteriosclerosis)

Arteriosclerosis is a gradual loss of elasticity and an almost imperceptible but continuous hardening of the walls of arteries. This, in itself, may cause few if any problems. However, arteriosclerosis most often accompanies atherosclerosis (see page 779).

The two disorders together diminish the blood available to the area supplied by the arteries; the hardened vessels expand less easily, and the plaque formation decreases the flow of blood. This results in serious problems, such as coronary heart disease, stroke, and chronic kidney failure, depending on which arteries are involved.

The problems associated with arteriosclerosis and the steps you and your physician can take to avoid or correct the disorder are given in detail under the discussion of atherosclerosis.

Aneurysm

An aneurysm consists of a weak area in the wall of an artery, which, because of the pressure within the artery, bulges outward. The weakness in the wall usually occurs in the muscle layer. A person may be born with such a weakness, or he may acquire it, most commonly through atherosclerosis, but also from high blood pressure, an injury, or infection, such as endocarditis or syphilis. Acquired aneurysms occur most often between the ages of forty and seventy, and more often in men than in women.

Aneurysms occur most frequently in the aorta (the large artery that carries blood away from the heart) in both its thoracic (chest) and its abdominal portions. Aneurysms of the arteries within the skull rank second in frequency.

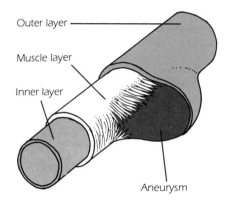

Outer layer

Muscle layer

Inner layer

Aneurysm

The aneurysm is the bulge in the weakened wall of the artery caused by the pressure within.

Aneurysms may not produce any symptoms, but when they do occur, symptoms depend on the location of the lesion. The pressure put on organs and structures adjacent to the aneurysm often causes the symptoms. An aneurysm in the chest (arch of the aorta) typically produces marked symptoms, including a peculiar brassy cough (not relieved by cough medicine), hoarseness, much pain, difficulty in breathing, and distended veins in the upper neck and chest. If lower down in the chest, the aneurysm may cause difficulty in swallowing. If in the abdominal aorta, no symptoms may occur; but if erosion of a vertebra occurs, it causes severe back pain. Aneurysms in the brain frequently go undetected. They may, on occasion, cause headache, especially on exertion. They also may interfere with the action of certain of the cranial nerves, a symptom that aids in the diagnosis. Rupture of a cerebral aneurysm is associated with severe headache, unconsciousness, and death.

What you can do. If you suspect an aneurysm, see your physician.

What your physician can do. A number of imaging methods are available to determine precisely the type, location, and extent of the aneurysm. Surgery is the treatment of choice, but even in skilled hands it carries a mortality rate of about 30 percent. If surgery cannot be tolerated for physical reasons, rupture of the aneurysm may possibly be delayed or prevented by reducing the blood pressure.

Stroke

A stroke results from damage to some part of the brain because of an interruption in its usual supply of blood. The interference in the blood supply may be due to (1) a thrombus or blood clot forming in one of the arteries; (2) an embolus or floating fragment of blood clot lodging in a brain artery; or (3) a brain hemorrhage caused by a rupture of the wall of an artery.

While the onset of a stroke is sudden, the underlying cause, typically atherosclerosis, has usually developed over a long period of time. Three conditions can interfere with

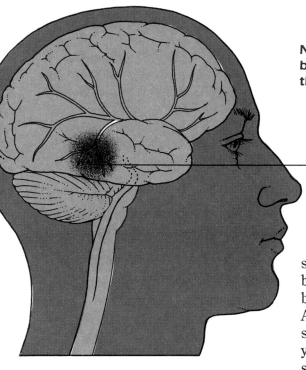

Note the area of the brain affected by the hemorrhaging of a branch of the middle cerebral artery.

Area of hemorrhage

the brain's blood supply. A clot or thrombus forming on the roughened lining of an artery, partially or completely blocking the flow of blood through the vessel, can cause a stroke. A fragment of a clot or embolus breaks off from some other roughened artery or from the inner surface of a diseased heart and, carried in the blood, plugs an artery in the brain. The third possible cause of a stroke occurs when a wall of an artery in the brain, weakened from atherosclerosis or from an aneurysm, bursts, causing seepage of blood into the tissues of the brain. This complication results from high blood pressure.

The demands of the brain for blood are so great that it receives one fifth of the blood pumped by the heart. A complete interruption of the supply of blood to any part of the brain causes permanent damage to brain cells within about five minutes. About 80 percent of deaths from stroke occur in people sixty to eighty years of age. Four out of five people survive their first attack, but many remain severely handicapped.

Often a major stroke is preceded by certain warning signs. These are called **ministrokes** or **transient ischemic attacks (TISs),** and are believed to be associated with vascular changes such as the formation of small clots **(thrombi)** or the constriction of blood vessels **(vasospasm).** Certain forms of migraine may also produce similar symptoms. Ministrokes develop suddenly and last from a few minutes to several hours (but never more than twenty-four hours), after which they completely disappear. Symptoms may include blurring or loss of vision, difficulty in speaking, weakness or paralysis in one side of the face or body, dizziness, and hearing loss.

Specific areas of the brain control specific functions, such as move-

801

ment, speech, sight, and memory. Loss of any specific function indicates which artery is affected. The symptoms of a stroke are extremely alarming, especially the outstanding symptom—paralysis of one side of the body, called hemiplegia. Loss of feeling (hemianesthesia) in the area of paralysis may often occur, along with difficulty in speaking (aphasia). The sufferer frequently loses control of the sphincter muscles of the bladder and rectum. Other symptoms include headache, vomiting, and altered consciousness.

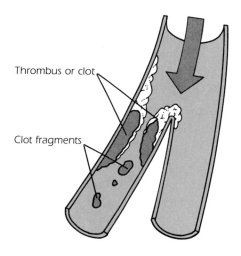

Thrombus or clot

Clot fragments

A clot breaks up, liberating its fragments, which are carried (as emboli) in the direction of blood flow until they encounter smaller vessels, which they occlude.

What you can do. When a stroke is suspected or has occurred, seek professional advice. Once brain cells are destroyed, they do not regenerate. Some improvement frequently occurs by learning to use other nerve circuits and also by a recovery from the tissue swelling at the margins of the destroyed area. Even

a mild stroke is a serious matter.

Prevention is of primary importance. To reduce your susceptibility to stroke, you should make every effort to minimize a number of risk factors, including: high blood pressure, smoking, overweight, uncontrolled diabetes, high blood cholesterol levels, sedentary living, and neglected phlebitis (inflammation of the veins).

What your physician can do. Immediate care depends on the severity of the stroke, but generally the sufferer is admitted to a hospital. If the victim is unconscious, circulation and breathing must be maintained. X-rays of the skull and brain scans can pinpoint the exact area of damage. Angiograms of the carotid arteries in the neck may aid diagnosis. Surgical removal of atheroma (from the carotids) which may be obstructing blood flow or contributing emboli usually proves successful. The physician may prescribe an anticoagulant (blood-thinner) unless a hemorrhage causes the stroke. Good nursing care, combined with appropriate rehabilitation to allow the sufferer to regain as much activity as possible, should be provided by trained personnel. Physical therapy and occupational therapy, a courageous outlook, along with mental and emotional support, aid recovery.

Shock

Shock develops when the major organs of the body fail to receive an adequate supply of blood and, due to lack of oxygen, are unable to function. The numerous causes of shock can essentially be placed in one of

802

the following groups: (1) the heart fails to pump sufficient blood (cardiogenic shock); (2) insufficient volume of blood or other body fluids (hypovolemic shock); and (3) collapse of the blood vessels of the body (anaphylactic or toxic shock).

Cardiogenic shock can result from a heart attack (10 percent of time), from heart failure, or from inability of the heart to function when the pericardial sac fills with fluid. Hypovolemic shock may follow the pain and trauma of a severe injury, or a profuse hemorrhage from a gunshot wound, a bleeding stomach, or a duodenal ulcer. It may also result from loss of body fluids caused by severe burns or prolonged diarrhea. Anaphylactic shock may follow an allergic reaction to an insect bite (bee, ant), or from an antibiotic (penicillin), from the poisons released from a snake bite, or a severe infection.

The symptoms include generalized weakness; sweating; pale, clammy skin; nausea with occasional vomiting; fast, weak pulse; rapid, shallow breathing; restlessness; mental confusion; and even unconsciousness. If untreated, the shock becomes progressively worse until death ensues. The kidneys and brain, deprived of blood, may sustain irreversible damage.

What you can do. For anyone in shock, get professional help immediately. The person in shock can do nothing for himself. Keep him warm and lying down with his feet elevated to drain blood to the heart (see page 512). As soon as possible, take the victim to a hospital.

What your physician can do. In severe shock, prompt diagnosis and treatment are crucial. The physician will direct immediate treatment toward restoring blood pressure by intravenous fluids, but preferably by giving plasma or a transfusion of whole blood. He will order oxygen and, in cases of anaphylactic shock, prescribe norepinephrine, cortisone, and antihistamines. Once the victim is stabilized, the cause of the shock can be treated. In toxic shock, the physician will prescribe antibiotics directed against the infection. In hemorrhagic shock, surgery may be required to stop the loss of blood. Shock from severe pain can be helped by relieving the pain.

Fainting

Fainting involves the temporary loss of consciousness resulting from a reduction in the blood supply to the brain, and thus loss of oxygen to the brain cells. Unpleasant emotions such as receiving bad news, panic (fear), the sight of blood, or torn flesh may also trigger a fainting spell.

Some people, especially if they suffer from arteriosclerosis, may faint if they stand up abruptly. Standing still in the sun for a long time may initiate fainting. Reduced capacity to carry oxygen, caused by anemia or carbon monoxide poisoning, and low blood sugar or hypoglycemia (from excess insulin), may cause one to faint.

When a person is found unconscious, one must consider several other possible conditions in addition to fainting, because the real cause should determine the method of han-

803

dling the problem. Unconsciousness may be caused by acute alcoholism, an overdose of sedatives or tranquilizers, head injury or stroke, epilepsy, diabetes.

Treat ordinary fainting by placing the individual flat on his back with the feet slightly elevated, which will encourage blood flow to the head. If someone seated is about to faint, have him place his head between his knees and push his head up against some resistance (someone pushing downward). This will force blood to the brain.

Low blood pressure

Modest degrees of low blood pressure, with the systolic pressure approximately 90, occur quite commonly in perfectly healthy people and cause no problems. The most common cause is standing abruptly from a lying or sitting position (postural hypotension). Normally an adjustment occurs automatically, increasing the tone in the blood vessel walls to maintain the blood pressure. If for any reason this does not happen, less blood reaches the brain, and dizziness or fainting result.

Low blood pressure may also result from an impoverished diet, some chronic, wasting disease, disturbances in the adrenal glands, defective autonomic control, pregnancy, and emotional shock. Medications taken for high blood pressure may also cause this problem.

What you can do. If standing suddenly causes your faintness, learn to stand slowly. If it occurs after lying down, first sit up slowly, and then gradually stand up. For other causes seek your physician's help. Should you be taking antihypertensive medicines, your doctor may advise you to decrease the dose.

Cold extremities (poor circulation)

Normal warmth in the hands and feet depends on an adequate circulation of blood through the extremities. For a number of reasons the flow of blood through these parts may be diminished. Insufficient physical exercise and simply not covering the limbs adequately during cold weather can cause cold hands and feet. Still other reasons exist: the body's need to conserve heat, a decline in the heart's ability to pump blood, a reduced capacity of the blood vessels to convey blood (atherosclerosis), the autonomic nerves restricting the size of the vessels and, therefore, the flow of blood through them, as in emotional tension or when studying intently.

More serious reasons for poor circulation of hands and feet include shock, heart disease, advanced atherosclerosis, thromboangiitis obliterans (Buerger's disease), and Raynaud's disease. If simple measures will not help, seek your physician's advice.

Buerger's disease (thromboangiitis obliterans)

Buerger's disease is a recurrent inflammation of the lining of the blood vessels. Occurring more commonly in the arteries than in the veins, and involving the legs more than the arms, the inflammation causes thrombosis (the forming of clots within the vessels), resulting in partial or complete closure. This decreases and may later entirely block the flow of blood through the vessels. This rare disease occurs most frequently in males aged twenty to forty, and almost always involves a cigarette smoker. The cause is not known, but there appears to be a heredity factor, and, possibly, a reaction to some component of cigarette smoke.

Although Buerger's disease involves all four extremities, it more commonly affects the legs. The limb feels cold, painful, and tender, and often has a mottled red appearance. Little or no pulse can be felt. In severe cases, ulcers and even gangrene develop. Exercise intensifies the pain, but "rest pain" may occur in severe cases, especially at night.

What you can do. Exercise only within tolerance, and protect against cold. Keep the limb scrupulously clean and dry, being careful when trimming toe and finger nails to avoid injury, in the hope of avoiding ulceration. The most important treatment is to give up cigarette smoking because the symptoms generally improve. In severe cases, keep the affected limb slightly lower in the bed to encourage circulation. If the disease affects only one limb, you can encourage circulation by applying heat (an electric light cradle) to the opposite limb (never to the affected limb).

What your physician can do. Your physician may prescribe medication to dilate the vessels in an attempt to improve circulation. Sometimes an operation is performed to sever the sympathetic nerves that cause the blood vessels to constrict. However, neither of these treatments may prove effective. When gangrene develops, amputation is usually necessary. Eventually the attacks may subside.

Raynaud's disease (Raynaud's phenomenon)

In Raynaud's disease nervous stimulation through the autonomic nerves causes reduced blood flow in the arteries. This stimulation causes the muscles in the walls of small arteries to contract, producing spasms. Cold, emotional upsets, and the intake of nicotine from tobacco commonly initiate constriction of the vessels. The disorder appears to affect people using vibrating equipment, such as pneumatic drills, dirt compactors, pianos, and typewriters. The disease affects the hands more commonly than the feet, and occurs more frequently in women than in men.

When the condition occurs as a complication of some other disease it is called "Raynaud's phenomenon." These diseases include Buerger's disease, rheumatoid arthritis, and scleroderma (hardening of the skin).

The attacks typically include numbness, tingling ("pins and needles"), blanching, and sometimes pain. In severe cases the skin and underlying tissue of the fingers become dry and shrunken, occasionally developing gangrenous spots. In the usual attack the discomfort may last from a few minutes to a few hours.

What you can do. You can relieve the discomfort of an attack by immersing the affected part in warm (not hot) water. Gently rubbing the fingers or toes may also help. If you are a smoker, discarding the habit is essential. Keep the extremities warm with appropriate clothing and by moving to a warm climate (if possible). Avoid nervous or emotional strain, or any activity which previous experience has shown will precipitate an attack.

What your physician can do. Medications which dilate the arteries may improve the circulation. Beverage alcohol has been suggested as a treatment. However, the observed beneficial effects in some may result from a mood change rather than a direct effect. Occasionally surgically cutting the nerves that control the arteries provides relief. If the problem is Raynaud's phenomenon, the underlying disorder should be determined and treated.

Varicose veins

Veins carry the blood from the capillaries back to the heart in ever enlarging vessels. When one is standing, the veins in the legs must work against gravity. Since the heart cannot force the blood through the capillaries back to the heart, the venous flow is aided by the pumping action of the muscles and a series of one-way valves within the veins that prevent back-flow.

Typically the term *varicose* applies to conspicuous, unsightly veins appearing just under the skin of the legs. These veins became dilated and tortuous from increased volume and the pressure of blood within them. Just why varicosities develop is not fully understood, but defective one-

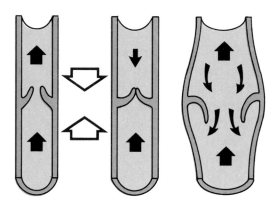

Normal valves open and close efficiently. Dilated valves allow back-flow.

way valves that allow back-flow, or an inherent weakness in the vein wall that allows stretching, or both, are probably basic to the problem.

While an estimated 10 percent of all adults have conspicuous varicose veins, the problem occurs twice as commonly in women as in men. Most varicosities develop before the age of forty and tend to persist thereafter. Pregnancy, overweight, the wearing of tight garters about the legs, and pelvic tumors predispose to the condition. In susceptible people, standing still for long hours may also contribute to varicose veins.

Usually varicose veins are a benign condition. However, aching in the leg, swelling of the foot and ankle, eczema of the skin with itching and scaling, and, if not properly cared for, a varicose ulcer just above the ankle may develop. Ulcers are hard to heal, and may recur. A serious problem, phlebitis, occurs occasionally when the vein lining becomes inflamed and a clot (thrombus) forms (see under "phlebitis").

Internal varicose veins may occur in the rectum or occasionally in the esophagus near the point it enters the stomach. Rectal varicosities, commonly called hemorrhoids, are readily detectable and effectively cured by surgery. The varicose veins in the lower end of the esophagus are neither easy to detect nor easy to treat. Their presence usually remains unknown until they rupture, causing a serious hemorrhage. They commonly develop as a complication of cirrhosis of the liver.

What you can do. For those with moderately severe varicose veins, some simple common-sense procedures will be helpful and may even prevent the development of an ulcer. Avoid stationary standing for long periods of time. Move your legs every few minutes to keep your leg muscles compressing the enlarged veins, and thus pumping blood. Several times a day lie down and raise your legs above the level of your heart. Wear elastic stockings to compress the veins and keep the blood from stagnating. Walk to improve the circulation in your legs. And do not sit with your legs crossed, as this tends to restrict the flow of blood through the superficial veins.

What your physician can do. Should your skin break down or an ulcer develop, consult your physician. He may suggest hot-and-cold foot and leg baths taken twice daily: two and a half minutes in the hot water alternating with half a minute in the cold water, repeated five times. After each treatment, dry the skin gently but thoroughly.

For varicose ulcers, apply a mild antiseptic ointment and cover with a

Varicose veins may occur (a) in the rectum (where they are called hemorrhoids) and (b) in the esophagus

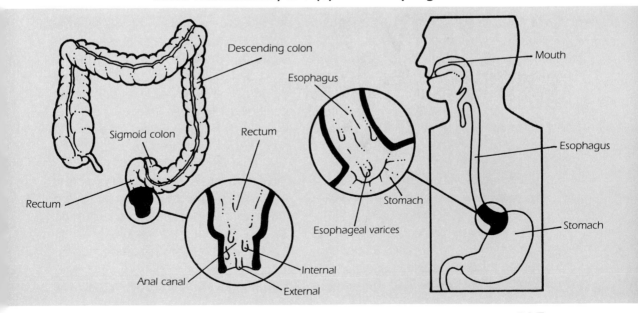

sterile but firm-fitting bandage. For troublesome cases, surgical removal of the varicose veins, called **stripping,** is the most satisfactory treatment. Another procedure is to inject a sclerosing agent into the veins and then to wrap the limb firmly for a few days. After a stripping or injection treatment, walk as much as possible to accelerate healing.

Phlebitis

Phlebitis is a condition in which a vein becomes inflamed. Usually, in the course of the inflammation, blood platelets adhere to the inflamed lining, and a blood clot or thrombus forms, constituting thrombophlebitis. The clot often completely obstructs the vein.

Two types of phlebitis occur: one that involves the superficial veins, the other the deep veins. Superficial phlebitis, which is not life-threatening, contrasts with deep-vein thrombosis, which is a dangerous condition. Thrombophlebitis occurs most commonly in the veins of the leg and thigh, and affects women more frequently than men.

Varicose veins increase susceptibility to superficial thrombophlebitis. Thrombophlebitis may develop following an injury to the leg, during or following pregnancy, during abdominal or pelvic surgery, or during acute infectious fevers.

In superficial thrombophlebitis the involved vein is red, swollen, and tender. Other symptoms include pain and a heavy feeling in the entire leg. The vein itself feels hard and unyielding. Deep-vein thrombophlebitis may exhibit no symptoms at all, or the entire limb may be swollen and painful.

What you can do. If you smoke, give it up, because nicotine accelerates the clotting of blood. Treat superficial thrombophlebitis with appropriate rest in bed with the leg elevated. Apply hot compresses to relieve the pain and swelling. An elastic stocking or bandage may be helpful. If the problem persists, seek a physician's advice. He may prescribe anti-inflammatory medication and possibly an antibiotic. For deep-vein thrombophlebitis, see your physician.

What your physician can do. With deep-vein thrombophlebitis, your physician will put you to bed and elevate your leg. He will prescribe anticoagulant medicine to prevent further clot formation and to try to dissolve the clots already formed. This medication may be maintained for several months to prevent recurrence. He may also prescribe antibiotics. Should a thrombus break loose, it will travel up the vein until it lodges in the heart, or, most commonly, in the lungs (pulmonary embolism). Because a large embolus will cause serious problems and may be fatal, resume activity under the direction of your physician.

Embolism

A blood clot, or thrombus, may form inside a vein, an artery, or the heart itself. When a portion of such a clot breaks off and is carried along the bloodstream, it is called an embolus. Pulmonary embolism occurs as a complication of pregnancy, surgical operations, and injuries, where prolonged inactivity enhances the possibility of blood clotting.

An embolus traveling in a vein moves toward the heart, then through the right side of that organ and out into the pulmonary artery, finally

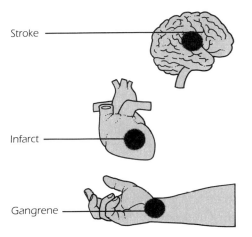

Stroke

Infarct

Gangrene

Emboli, or fragments of a clot, travel in the direction of blood flow, causing serious problems wherever they lodge: in the brain, a stroke; in the heart, an infarct; in the hand, gangrene.

lodging somewhere in a lung. This problem, known as **pulmonary embolism,** occurs more commonly in women than in men. Emboli from the heart are the most common cause, followed by those arising from deep-vein thrombosis in the lower limbs.

In cases of few and small emboli, no symptoms may appear. However, when a large embolus or multiple small ones occur, the classic symptoms include pain in the chest, difficulty in breathing, and the coughing up of blood-tinged sputum. If not treated immediately, unconsciousness and death may follow. Treatment consists of administering oxygen, the prompt use of an anticoagulant, or the

surgical removal of the embolus following an angiogram.

When an embolus originates in the left side of the heart or in an artery, it is carried in a direction away from the heart and may lodge in any one of the smaller arteries in any organ of the body. If it lodges in an artery in an extremity, severe pain suddenly develops, and the limb usually becomes cold, pale, and numb. The pain tends to increase, the limb becomes dark-colored and blotchy, and gangrene may develop. Immediate surgery to remove the clot from the artery may save both life and limb. When an arterial embolus lodges in the brain, one type of stroke occurs; should it lodge in a kidney, renal failure may develop; if in some artery of the trunk, a variety of distressing symptoms may result.

What you can do. Following surgery or accidents requiring prolonged bed rest, preventive measures such as early ambulation and as much exercise as possible reduce the risk of forming an embolus. Once an embolus has been discovered, seek immediate medical help.

What your physician can do. He can provide emergency aid. Hospitalization is essential. Depending on the location of the problem and extent of damage, treatments will vary; he will choose among oxygen, anticoagulants, and possibly surgery.

Edema (swelling of the tissues)

Edema consists of an accumulation of excess fluid in the tissues. The extra fluid accumulates outside of the capillaries in the spaces between

809

the cells, causing the tissues to become soggy and swollen.

Normally, a continual exchange of fluid takes place between the blood within the capillaries and the tissue spaces outside the capillaries. The walls of capillaries permit water and relatively small molecules of other substances to pass through. Larger protein molecules and blood cells do not normally penetrate the capillary wall. A certain amount of fluid in the tissue spaces enters the lymph vessels instead of reentering the blood capillaries.

Four factors control the balance of fluid which enters and leaves the capillaries and the tissue spaces: (1) The osmotic pressure of the blood plasma as compared with that of the tissue fluid. This pressure depends, in large part, upon the presence of protein molecules (primarily albumin) in the blood plasma. The higher osmotic pressure of the plasma retards the escape of fluid from the capillaries. (2) The level of blood pressure within the capillaries. High blood pressure within the capillaries favors the escape of fluid from the capillaries. (3) The condition of the capillary walls. Only an abnormal capillary wall permits the escape of protein molecules. (4) The capacity of the lymph vessels to carry fluid. When these are obstructed, the fluid which would normally follow this route tends to accumulate in the tissue spaces.

Edema in heart disease. When the heart fails to put out as much blood as the body's tissues require, the kidneys respond by decreasing the volume of fluid they excrete. This increases the volume of total body fluid, with a resulting rise of blood pressure within the capillaries (item two of the preceding paragraphs). The edema or swelling of the tissues is noticed first in the ankles of ambulatory people and in the sacral region (lower back) of those in bed, typically increasing in severity at the end of the day.

Edema in kidney disease. Certain forms of kidney disease allow the escape of albumin from the blood plasma into the urine. As the level of albumin drops in the plasma, so does the osmotic pressure. This permits an excess of fluid to escape through the capillary walls into the tissue spaces.

Edema in cirrhosis of the liver. In cirrhosis, the liver's production of protein declines, with a consequent lowering of the blood's osmotic pressure. This favors the development of edema. Also, cirrhosis hinders the flow of blood to the liver from other abdominal organs, causing an increase of blood pressure in the capillaries of these organs. Fluid (ascites) accumulates in the abdominal cavity.

Edema in malnutrition. Due to an inadequate intake of protein, the albumin level in the plasma drops. This, together with a weakening of the capillary walls, leads to edema in the lower limbs and abdomen.

Edema in allergy. The tissue swelling that occurs in various allergic manifestations (hives, hay fever, angioneurotic edema, etc.) is attributed to the effect of histamine, a chemical released in the allergic reaction, on the walls of the capillaries.

Edema in local inflammation. Blood tends to stagnate in an in-

810

flamed tissue area. The capillary walls are damaged, fluid from the blood leaks outward, and local swelling occurs.

Edema in local injury. When local injury, whether by mechanical force, heat, cold, or chemical contact, causes damage to the capillaries, fluid from the blood leaks outward, resulting in local swelling.

Edema in poisoning and toxemia. Poisonous substances containing arsenic, lead, antimony, gold, or mercury; toxins produced by microorganisms as in diphtheria and scarlet fever; and certain snake venoms damage the capillary walls, permitting the escape of fluid into the tissues.

Edema from obstruction of the veins. When the return of blood through a vein is impeded, the consequent increase of blood pressure within the capillaries results in a swelling of all tissues drained by this particular vein. In some cases tumors compress the large veins that enter the heart, and the resulting edema may involve large portions of the body.

Edema from obstruction of the lymph vessels. The lymph vessels may be obstructed when involved in a region of inflammation, when invaded by a tumor, or when affected by such a disease as filariasis. With lymph drainage obstructed, fluid accumulates in the tissue spaces, causing edema in the affected area.

Edema in anemia. When anemia becomes so severe as to cause the heart to fail, together with increasing oxygen deprivation, edema may develop.

Edema in pregnancy. Swelling of the ankles often occurs during the last three months of pregnancy. The enlarging uterus may compress the veins that drain the lower limbs as they pass through the pelvis, causing back pressure and swelling of the ankles. A more serious form of edema, affecting the face, hands, and ankles, is due to a toxemia that develops late in pregnancy (see page 395).

Edema from sitting and standing. Long hours of sitting, for example when traveling by plane or bus, or of standing still at work, will cause swelling around the ankles and lower leg. Poor venous circulation and increased pressure within the capillaries, together with lack of exercising the muscles of the lower limbs, cause fluid outflow and edema.

CHAPTER 4

Blood and blood diseases

Blood consists of blood cells and a watery liquid, called plasma, in which the cells float.

The **plasma** comprises a complex mixture of proteins and other nutrients, gases, hormones, waste products of metabolism, and many other substances required for the operation of the body. This section will consider the various blood diseases.

Blood cells are produced in special tissues and organs. Bone marrow, the largest blood-forming organ, supplies red cells, certain white cells called granulocytes, and platelets. The spleen, lymph nodes, and other lymphoid tissues manufacture other white cells called lymphocytes and plasma cells.

The diseases of blood may involve any constituent of the blood: red cells, white cells, platelets, or plasma. The effects of disease may result in too few or too many of any component. Here are some of the broad terms used to describe some of these disorders:

Anemia—too few red cells
Polycythemia—too many red cells
Leukocytosis—large increase in white cells
Leukopenia—marked decrease in white cells
Thrombocytopenia—too few platelets
Hemophilia—too little of a certain plasma protein

Other than preventive measures, the lay person can do little for himself in regard to blood diseases. Their diagnosis requires modern equipment in hospitals and clinical laboratories, and their treatment demands the services of a physician.

Diagnosing blood disorders

Examination of the blood provides, as it were, a picture of conditions within the organs and systems of the body. The state of health, as well as the presence and progress of many diseases, is reflected in the findings of blood analyses. Samples of blood are taken generally from a vein in the arm (venipuncture), but many tests can be performed from a drop of blood obtained by a pinprick of a finger. A few examples of some of the more common tests will illustrate the wide range of evaluations that are possible.

Blood counts—number, size, and shape of red blood cells (RBC); number and type of white blood cells (WBC); number of platelets (platelet count).

Hematocrit—amount of cells per given volume of blood.

Sedimentation rate—rate at which cells settle out of drawn blood.

Clotting time—rate at which blood will coagulate.

Chemical tests determine the amount of plasma proteins, cholesterol, fat (triglyceride), fatty acids, glucose (blood sugar), vitamins, minerals, hormones, enzymes, antibodies, urea, creatinine and other wastes in the blood.

Examination of the bone marrow reveals a number of conditions related to the blood. As already mentioned, it is within the bone marrow (especially of the flat bones—ribs, breastbone, pelvis) that many blood cells are manufactured. Both their production and release are closely monitored. For example, as the red cells wear out, two to three million new ones enter the circulation every second; or when an infection occurs, millions of white cells flood the circulation. Anemias, the evidence of infections, and the presence of cancers can be determined by bone marrow studies.

Disorders of red blood cells

Normally blood is 40 to 45 percent red cells and 55 to 60 percent plasma. Generally there are 12.5 to 15.5 grams of hemoglobin per 100 milliliters of blood. The normal number of red cells is 4.5 to 5.5 million per cubic millimeter in men and 10 percent lower in women. A person is considered anemic if his blood values are less than the lowest figures mentioned here.

The primary function of red cells is to carry oxygen from the lungs to the tissues, and carbon dioxide from the tissues back to the lungs. Each red cell is essentially a package of hemoglobin, the chemical substance which transports these gases.

The more active the cells, the greater their need for oxygen. Three factors determine the amount of oxygen the blood can bring to a tissue: the amount of hemoglobin in each red blood cell, the number of red blood cells in the blood, and the rate at which the blood is flowing.

In anemia there is either a reduced amount of hemoglobin in the red blood cells, or there is an inadequate number of red cells for a given volume of blood. In either case the oxygen-carrying capacity of the blood is reduced, and the tissues suffer on this account. Strangely, in the opposite condition of polycythemia, in which a great excess of red blood cells exists, the tissues may also suffer from a lack of oxygen. Because of the high population of red cells, the blood becomes syrupy and moves so slowly that oxygen cannot be delivered to the tissues cells fast enough.

The causes of anemia are related to the amount of hemoglobin in the blood and the number of red blood cells and result from problems of production, destruction, and loss of hemoglobin or red cells.

Production problems show up when there is too little iron to manufacture hemoglobin (iron-deficiency anemia), too little vitamin B12 or folic acid to produce red cells (pernicious anemia), or suppression of the bone marrow from cancer or drugs (aplastic anemia).

Destruction problems arise when the red blood cells break down prematurely (hemolytic anemia) or when, because of faulty formation of hemoglobin, the red cells are destroyed by the spleen (sickle-cell anemia). Problems of loss occur from hemorrhage or blood loss, as in injuries, excessive menses, and bleeding stomach ulcers (secondary anemia).

The common symptoms of anemia, regardless of the cause, consist of fatigue and weakness, along with faintness, palpitation, shortness of breath with exercise, and paleness of the skin, eyes, gums, and nailbeds (the nails in severe anemia may be deformed).

Anemias due to production problems

Iron-deficiency anemia

With a deficiency of iron, the production of hemoglobin, and to a lesser extent of red blood cells, is affected. The red cells produced are pale (hypochromic) and small (microcytic).

The most common cause for lack of iron is loss of blood. Iron-deficiency anemia is more common in women, due to excessive menstrual bleeding. Pregnancy and loss of blood at the time of delivery may deplete iron stores. Bleeding from the stomach or intestine, because of an ulcer, polyp, hemorrhoids, or cancer, may be another reason. Certain intestinal parasites, especially hookworm, may produce an iron deficiency anemia. In all these situations more iron is lost than the diet eaten can replace.

Another cause of iron-deficiency anemia is the faulty absorption of iron. A lack of hydrochloric acid in the stomach diminishes absorption. Surgical removal of a large part of the stomach or small intestine, or cancer of these areas, may also reduce absorption.

A third reason for iron deficiency is insufficient iron in the diet. This is especially seen in young malnourished children or the elderly on restricted diets.

Iron—generally stored in the liver, spleen and bone marrow—is used mostly to form hemoglobin. The stores are replenished by food iron and from recycled iron obtained from worn out red blood cells.

What you can do. Because iron-deficiency anemia always has a cause, see your physician to determine where the problem lies. Report to him all changes in bowel movements, color of your stools, and the amount of menstrual flow. If the problem is simple, eating green leafy vegetables and other foods rich in iron will increase your iron intake. Do not rely on selfdiagnosis.

What your physician can do. A number of laboratory tests can determine where the problem lies. Once the cause is removed, the problem is easily treated. A change in diet or the taking of an iron supplement will provide an abundance of iron.

B12 deficiency anemia (pernicious anemia; macrocytic anemia)

A lack of vitamin B12 results in an anemia in which the red blood cells are larger than normal. About 90 percent of macrocytic anemias in temperate climates are due to B12 or folic acid deficiencies. The production of red blood cells depends on these vitamins. Vitamin B12 is also essential for the maintenance of the brain and especially the spinal cord.

Microorganisms in the soil, gut, and mouth produce vitamin B12. Plant foods do not contain significant amounts, but it is present in meat, milk, eggs, and their products. The amount the body needs partially correlates with the protein intake. Thus the higher the intake of protein, the more B12 will be required. Complete vegetarians face a higher risk for B12 deficiency, but they have the same risk for pernicious anemia.

Vitamin B12 is absorbed from foods containing it and from amounts produced in the mouth and intestines. It is stored in the liver. If the stored B12 is depleted, a deficiency may occur. A protein produced in the wall of the stomach, called "intrinsic factor," greatly aids the vitamin's absorption. This factor combines with B12 and acts as a transfer agent, guiding the vitamin across the gut lining into the blood. "Pernicious anemia" results from a lack of intrinsic factor, not just from a lack of the vitamin entering the intestine. Lack of intrinsic factor may arise from an atrophy of the cells producing it or from extensive surgery in which large portions of the stomach wall or intestine have been removed. In certain areas of the world a tapeworm may deprive the person of B12.

The onset of the disease is often subtle, and in addition to the usual symptoms of anemia, frequent indigestion, poor appetite, and weight loss occur. The tongue may be smooth, sore, or swollen, and it may feel too big for the mouth. Tingling of the hands and feet, along with diminished coordination and balance, are common, making walking in the dark difficult. Changes in behavior, nervousness, depression, memory loss, irritability, and confusion may occur.

What you can do. B12 deficiency anemia is a serious problem and should be treated promptly. Permanent damage to the nervous system may develop. Should you have a true pernicious anemia (lacking intrinsic factor), you will have to take B12 for the rest of your life. Otherwise be sure to eat foods providing B12 or take a supplement.

What your physician can do. He

815

will call for laboratory tests to determine the severity of the anemia and the level of B12 in the blood. He will prescribe B12 injections (intramuscular), frequently to begin with, and then at monthly or quarterly intervals. A health professional may teach you to inject yourself. The anemia and many of the other symptoms should improve promptly, but problems caused by nerve degeneration may take months for recovery. Occasionally they are irreversible.

Folic acid deficiency anemia (acrocytic anemia)

Folic acid, a member of the B vitamins, is readily obtained in a nutritious diet. When the diet contains insufficient amounts or when it is poorly absorbed (due to cancer, celiac disease, or other disorder), an anemia identical to B12 deficiency anemia develops, but the neurological problems do not occur. Treatment consists of providing a diet abundant in folic acid (generous in fruits and vegetables), using folic acid tablets, or injections.

It is important to distinguish between a B12 deficiency and a folic acid deficiency. If a B12 deficiency is treated with folic acid, the anemia itself will improve but the damage to the nervous system will be worse.

Anemias due to destruction problems

Hemolytic anemia

With this problem the rate of destruction of red blood cells exceeds the rate of replacement. Red cells that "wear out" normally are removed from the circulation by the spleen, liver, and bone marrow and eliminated as bile pigments. The body then reuses the iron and protein for the production of new hemoglobin. In hemolytic anemias the bile pigments may overwhelm the body's ability to eliminate them. The pigments accumulate in the tissues, causing jaundice, a yellow coloration of the skin and the whites of the eyes.

Some people inherit a condition in which the bone marrow produces red cells that are of a poor quality. The cells may have peculiar shapes, they may even be round (spherocytic), and they are prematurely destroyed by the spleen. Occasionally the body will develop antibodies which, instead of protecting against infections, attack its own red blood cells. Hemolytic anemias may result from drugs, from toxins, from infections, from artificial heart valves, or from faulty transfusions.

The symptoms parallel anemias in general, with the addition of possible jaundice and dark urine, due to the excess of blood pigments.

What you can do. See your physician promptly.

What your physician can do. He will order a number of blood tests which will identify the precise problem. The removal of the spleen may help in inherited conditions. If drugs are being taken, he will carefully evaluate them, along with considering toxins from the infections or pesticides. Cortisone may be helpful if the person's own antibodies are causing the problem.

Sickle-cell anemia

Sickle-cell anemia is a common hereditary disorder occurring frequently among Blacks of African descent, and also in a few Caucasians of Mediterranean origin. An abnormal type of hemoglobin (hemoglobin S) is produced by the bone marrow. If a person inherits a sickle cell gene from both parents, he will have sickle-cell anemia. If, on the other hand, he has inherited only one gene from one of his parents, he has "sickle cell trait" and should not have a problem.

Red blood cells with this type of faulty hemoglobin, when subjected to lowered oxygen concentrations, form sickle or cresent shapes. This may occur at high altitudes (above 6,000 feet), in an unpressurized airplane, or when suffering from pneumonia. In some, exercise may precipitate an attack.

These abnormal cells are more likely to break down (hemolize) and have difficulty passing through the smallest blood vessels or capillaries. When the hemoglobin gives up the oxygen, the cells sickle. This blocks the capillary further, limiting the available oxygen. This results in more sickling. Any of the major organs, such as the kidneys, lungs, and brain, may be damaged.

Among the first symptoms to be observed are sudden, severe abdominal pain, followed by the appearance of dark-colored urine. This is called a "sickle-cell crisis." Severe leg

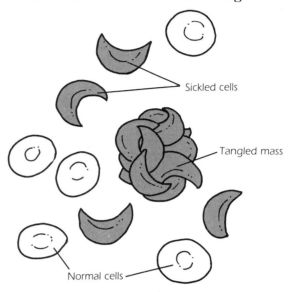

Sickled cells

Tangled mass

Normal cells

Note the normal and abnormal or sickle-shaped red blood cells. The sickled cells tangle with each other, forming clots.

cramps, repeated fevers, acute pain in the left side, and jaundice may also occur. Severe anemia, an enlarged liver, and chronic ulcers of the legs may characterize the severest cases.

Sickle-cell anemia is a serious disease for which there is no cure. The sufferer should be under the care of a physician who understands the disease. He should make every effort to maintain good health and deal promptly with infections, injuries, or other illnesses. Generally life expectancy is reduced, and death may occur during a crisis. Married couples who carry the defective gene should seek genetic counseling before deciding on a family.

817

Thalassemia

Thalassemia is one of a group of inherited problems in which abnormal hemoglobins are formed. The disease is fairly common among those of Mediterranean, Middle Eastern, and Far Eastern descent. The genetic defect inherited from one parent only is called a "trait," and is usually not serious. If, however, both parents pass on the defect, a serious anemia due to destruction of these atypical red blood cells occurs (called thalassemia major).

The symptoms parallel those of any severe anemia. However, because the treatment involves repeated blood transfusions, and there is a continuous destruction of red blood cells, the concentration of iron in the body increases. This may lead to liver damage, with resulting heart failure and death.

What you can do. See your physician. If you are aware that you or your spouse may carry the trait, your physician can advise you as to the possibility of your child being affected.

What your physician can do. Depending on the severity of the problem, the outcome will vary. Generally, repeated blood transfusions are necessary. Today chelating agents, chemicals which bind iron, make the elimination of excessive amounts of iron possible. The removal of the spleen may help. A nutritious diet, with generous amounts of green leafy vegetables providing folic acid, is important.

Hemolytic anemia of the newborn (Rh disease)

The blood of some people possesses the so-called Rh factor, while that of others does not. Individuals are said to be either Rh-positive or Rh-negative. About 85 percent of women have Rh-positive blood. When a woman with Rh-negative blood (15 percent of women) happens to marry a man whose blood is Rh-positive, the children of this union will usually have Rh-positive blood.

In such a case, during pregnancy, a few of the Rh-positive blood cells from the fetus may seep through the placenta and enter the mother's Rh-negative blood. When this occurs, her tissues build up antibodies capable of destroying the "unfriendly" Rh-positive blood cells of the fetus. Usually nothing happens during the first pregnancy. But with recurring pregnancies, sufficient antibodies may be present in the mother's blood, so that when they pass through the placenta to enter the fetal circulation, the antibodies begin to destroy the blood cells of the fetus. This results in a severe anemia, with a possible infant death.

What you can do. Before becoming pregnant consult with your physician to determine whether an Rh factor problem exists.

What your physician can do. By giving an Rh-negative mother an injection of "Rh immune globulin" at precisely seventy-two hours following the birth of every child, following an abortion, or following a miscarriage, her tendency to produce harmful antibodies is suppressed. If this preventive measure has not been taken, the infant's life may be saved by the prompt use of an exchange transfusion. In this procedure the blood of the baby is replaced by blood which does not contain the damaging antibodies.

Bleeding disorders

Blood circulates throughout the body through blood vessels. When these vessels are cut or injured, blood leaks out. This bleeding can occur internally or externally. Four mechanisms can stop bleeding: (1) the pressure of the surrounding tissues; (2) the retraction and contraction of the injured vessel; (3) platelets sticking to the injured site and to one another, forming a plug; (4) a network of fibrin forming at the point of bleeding, entrapping blood cells to form a clot. This congealed blood plugs vessel openings and pulls the end of the broken vessel together. It hangs on until the vessel heals; then it disappears, often without a trace.

Purpuras

Bleeding of tiny blood vessels just under the skin leave a purplish (purpura) blotch. Commonly seen in elderly people on the back of the hands, it occurs in the presence of normal levels of platelets, is not serious, and need not be treated.

Purpura also appears with vitamin C deficiency, following the administration of certain medicines, particularly cortisone, and in the presence of sugar diabetes or chronic kidney failure. It accompanies severe infections, such as erysipelas, plague, and sometimes measles and chicken pox. This is the cause of "black measles," "black pox," and "black plague." Purpuras which accompany infections are a serious disorder and require immediate attention by a physician.

Thrombocytopenia

Platelets help to stop bleeding. When their numbers are reduced, thrombocytopenia is present. The most common form of thrombocytopenic purpura is caused by the body's developing antibodies against its own platelets. These antibodies damage the platelets, which are then destroyed at a rapid rate. Bleeding into the skin and mucous membranes appears to be a rash of tiny bright red and dark red spots that are actually hemorrhages (petechiae).

The disorder may result from infections; from taking drugs such as quinine, quinidine, and cancer chemotherapy; from radiation therapy for cancer; and from disorders which depress the bone marrow, such as aplastic anemia or cancers such as leukemia or lymphoma. Frequent transfusions given over a short period may also be a cause.

The symptoms vary with the severity of the disease, from nosebleeds, small hemorrhages into the skin, and

819

prolonged bleeding from minor cuts, to fever, nausea, vomiting, abdominal and joint pains, prostration, bleeding from the bowel, bladder, or mouth, and hemorrhaging into the brain.

What you can do. If you observe the telltale skin hemorrhages or have prolonged bleeding from minor cuts, see your physician immediately.

What your physician can do. He will order laboratory tests to determine the level of platelets and the condition of your bone marrow. He will evaluate the drugs you may be taking, chemicals to which you might have been exposed, and the presence of some infection or other disease. If the cause can be determined, treatment will focus on attacking the problem. Discontinuing a drug, giving a transfusion of platelets, taking a steroid for an abnormal antibody, or sometimes removing the spleen may be indicated.

Clotting defects

Blood clotting depends on a complex series of chemical reactions involving proteins, enzymes, and minerals such as calcium and phosphorus that are present in the blood plasma and exuded from the damaged walls of the blood vessels. Many of these coagulation factors are made in the liver. In the case of liver damage, as in cirrhosis or hepatitis, or immaturity, as in some premature babies, adequate amounts of these factors are not synthesized to prevent bleeding. Some individuals are born with an inability to produce one or more of these factors.

Anticoagulants or "blood thinners" are given to lower these clotting factors. Patients who have suffered a heart attack or have developed thrombophlebitis are sometimes given anticoagulants to prevent a recurrence of a heart attack or the extension of the clot in thrombophlebitis. Excessive intake may cause serious hemorrhage, and anyone taking blood thinners should be under a physician's care.

Hemophilia

People with hemophilia, known as "bleeders," are unable to make factor VIII (antihemophiliac factor, AHF). This congenital defect is passed on by female "carriers," father to daughter to son. The males get the disease but must inherit it from their mothers. A man with hemophilia will have sons and daughters who are not bleeders unless the mother is a bleeder of the same type. The sons of his daughters, however, could be bleeders.

Hemophiliacs may have all degrees of bleeding, the more severe forms appearing in early childhood. The child will bruise easily, even from crawling. Slight cuts and even scratches will bleed for long periods. Any part or organ of the body may be involved, especially the large muscles of the back and buttocks, and the joints.

Depending where the hemorrhage has occurred, the symptoms can range from tender and swollen bumps and bruises to internal pain and distress. Repeated bleeding into

820

the joints will cause redness, swelling, and eventual stiffness.

What you can do. If you are a bleeder you should know of a center where factor VIII (AHF) concentrates are available in case of need. You must protect yourself as far as possible from any injury and should avoid taking aspirin. Your physician should be informed of your problem before any surgical procedure is undertaken, even the extraction of a tooth. You should carry an identification tag so that in an emergency the appropriate treatment can be given. Discuss with your physician your risk of acquiring AIDS from infected blood products.

What your physician can do. Treatment of bleeders generally requires concentrates of factor VIII or whole blood transfusions if the former is not available. Generally treatment should be continued for some eight to ten days. Your physician can determine the appropriate form of exercise for you.

Although there will always be some restrictions, most hemophiliacs today can lead relatively normal lives.

Vitamin K deficiency

Vitamin K is the parent substance from which the liver produces four of the blood clotting factors (II, VIII, IX, X). While the diet can provide vitamin K (especially green leafy vegetables), friendly bacteria present in the colon make most of the body's supply. When vitamin K levels drop below 10 to 15 percent of normal values, bleeding occurs from the bowel mucosa, gums, nose, throat, kidneys, and bladder.

A deficiency may result from a number of reasons: (1) Vitamin K, a fat-soluble vitamin, needs bile salts for its emulsification and absorption. If the flow of bile is blocked, say by gallstones, bile cannot reach the intestine, and a shortage develops. (2) Certain antibiotics, when taken by mouth, suppress the production of vitamin K by bacteria in the intestine. (3) In severe prolonged diarrheas, because of the rapid evacuation of the bowel contents, vitamin K absorption is greatly reduced.

What you can do. Alert your physician to any bleeding with no known cause.

What your physician can do. Some simple laboratory tests, such as the prothrombin time, can determine whether there is a shortage of vitamin K. The underlying cause can then be found and corrected. If the bleeding is severe, units (bags) of fresh, frozen plasma can be administered to restore coagulation levels.

Bone marrow failure

Aplastic anemia (pancytopenia)

Aplastic anemia exists when the bone marrow fails to produce the various blood cells customarily originating in the marrow bed: red cells, granulocytes, and platelets. Generally all types of cells are affected; hence the term pancytopenia is often used. The cause of primary aplasia is not known. Secondary aplastic anemia follows exposure to X-ray radiation; certain hair dyes; drugs, as chloramphenicol; and industrial chemicals, such as benzene, insecticides, and plant sprays.

Symptoms will depend on which type of cell is most affected. Depressed red cell production causes anemia. A decrease in the granulocytes (one kind of white cell that fights infections) will leave one unprotected against germ invasion. Platelets help blood to clot and prevent hemorrhages. When their production drops, spontaneous bleeding occurs from tiny cuts and bruises and from the nose, gums, and elsewhere. In women, menstrual flow greatly increases in duration and volume.

What you can do. If you have any of the above problems, see your

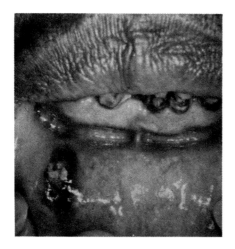

Canker sores around the mouth and tongue of a patient with aplastic anemia.

physician as soon as possible.

What your physician can do. He will determine the cause (if possible) and severity of your problem. If you are taking medications, he will carefully evaluate them and consider possible exposure to any toxic chemical. If you have anemia, blood transfusions are helpful. If infections, antibiotics may be lifesaving. If bleeding, whole blood or fresh frozen plasma may be administered. If the problem does not resolve spontaneously, the physician may recommend a bone marrow transplant from a close blood-relative. This serious condition has a high morality rate.

Agranulocytosis

In agranulocytosis a marked reduction in the white cells or neutrophils (granulocytes) in the blood stream occurs, due to decreased production by the bone marrow or increased destruction of the cells themselves. Several agents can suppress the production of granulocytes: certain drugs, the chemicals which cause aplastic anemia, and several cancers, as leukemia. Increased destruction may result from drugs, viral infections, or antibodies formed by the body.

The symptoms are associated with infection. An acute attack begins abruptly, with chills, fever, headache, severe sore throat, and prostration. Progression to pneumonia and death may be rapid. The mild form of the disease consists of a series of infections, followed by spontaneous recovery.

What you can do. See your physician immediately. Determine what drugs, prescription or nonprescription, you are taking and to what chemicals you might have been exposed.

What your physician can do. will order a biopsy of your bone marrow to indicate for a certainty whether agranulocytosis is present. The biopsy will also reveal whether a cancer, such as leukemia, is at work. Evaluation of any drugs you are taking might uncover the cause. He may prescribe an appropriate antibiotic to suppress the infection. Generally, the prognosis for complete recovery is good, unless a malignancy is present.

Multiple myeloma

This malignant disease of unknown cause produces abnormal plasma cells, one of the less common white blood cells of the bone marrow. Normally these cells produce antibodies in response to vaccinations and fight infections caused by microorganisms, such as bacteria and viruses. Once these malignant cells fill the bone marrow cavities, they suppress the production of other cells.

Multiple myeloma typically occurs only in persons above forty years of age, is twice as frequent in men, and disrupts the production of red cells, granulocytes and platelets. It erodes the bones, reduces the production of antibodies and gamma-globulin, and damages the kidneys. The initial signs—anemia and infections—are characteristically accompanied by severe bone pain, frequently leading to fractures, especially of the vertebrae. The progression of this fatal disease is slow in some cases and rapid in others. (See "aplastic anemia," page 821.)

What you can do. You should place yourself under the care of a physician.

What your physician can do. He will confirm the diagnosis by the presence of unusual proteins in the blood and urine. While there is no cure, the physician may suggest appropriate chemotherapy to prolong life for some years. Transfusions are given for anemia, antibiotics for infections, and X-ray therapy for bone pain.

Leukemia

Leukemia is cancer of the blood-forming tissues of the bone marrow and lymph nodes, affecting the white blood cells they produce, namely, the granulocytes and lymphocytes.

Normally, the bone marrow and lymph nodes produce white cells (leukocytes) at a rate sufficient to replace those that wear out in the circulation, thus keeping the total number of leukocytes constant. At first the young cells themselves can divide and redivide. As they mature they lose their ability to divide and develop their adult function of combating infection.

In leukemia the young leukocytes lose their ability to mature and become "juvenile delinquents," retaining their ability to divide but losing their ability to take up their adult duties. These leukemic cells not only multiply at a more rapid rate, they also live longer than normal white cells. As a result their numbers increase rapidly, filling the bone marrow and lymph nodes and spilling over into the circulating blood, affecting other organs, such as the spleen and liver. The normal white cells, the red blood cells, and the platelets are all affected, reducing their ability to fight infection, provide oxygen, and clot blood.

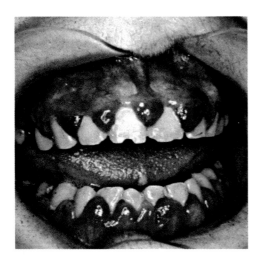

Infection of the mouth and gums in a patient with acute leukemia.

Two main types of leukemia occur: **granulocytic** (myelogenous), white cells of the bone marrow, and **lymphocytic,** white cells of the lymph nodes. Both can be **acute,** with rapid progression, or **chronic,** with the disease unfolding slowly. The more immature the cells, the more acute the leukemia; the more serious the disease, the less likely that treatment will be effective.

Acute leukemias

Acute leukemia occurs as commonly in adults as in children. However, children under the age of six typically suffer from lymphocytic leukemia, while adults tend to have granulocytic. There is no predilection as to race or sex.

The symptoms of either acute lymphocytic or acute granulocytic leukemia are indistinguishable except that lymph node enlargement occurs more commonly in the lymphocytic variety. The first indication consists of weight loss and anemia, with weakness, pallor, and fatigue. The symptoms arise suddenly, and become pronounced in a week or two. Symptoms commonly include infections of the mouth and throat, with fever and headache; easy bruising; and bleeding from the nose, gums, and rectum, and from minor cuts is frequent. An enlarged spleen and pain and tenderness in the bones and joints is typical. In the later stages, hemorrhage into the brain may occur.

What you can do. Should you have any of the symptoms outlined above, see your physician.

What your physician can do. He will diagnose leukemia by examination of the blood, where immature cells are seen, and further confirm the diagnosis by a biopsy of the bone marrow. Treatment is best given in a hospital by a specialist in cancer therapy. The physician will prescribe therapy with anticancer drugs to destroy all leukemic cells. This treatment also destroys normal cells. During this time antibiotics are given to prevent infections, transfusions of

824

blood for anemia, and transfusions of platelets for bleeding.

A remission occurs about 70 percent of the time, with normal cells reappearing. A remission may last five or more years, but ultimately leukemia reappears. Subsequent therapy brings poorer remissions with more frequent relapses. Bone marrow transplants at the time of the first remission appear to lengthen long-term survival and may, on occasion, produce a cure. Newer chemotherapeutic agents can also result in "cures."

Acute lymphocytic leukemia occurs most often in children. Therapy as described above, together with radiation and steroids, provides survival for five or more years in about half the cases. Improvement is almost always seen, and with regular checkups and recurring treatment, the child can live a fairly normal life. Parental support is essential.

Chronic leukemias

Chronic leukemias always have an insidious onset, symptoms commonly appearing only after several years of disease have elapsed. The cause is similar to that discussed under acute leukemia—the uncontrolled multiplication of cells—only the process is slower, and higher counts of cells are seen in the bloodstream. After a time there may be a hundred times the normal number of leukocytes. These extra cells infiltrate various organs, such as the spleen, the liver, and the bone marrow. The spleen may enlarge tenfold.

Invasion of the bone marrow suppresses normal red cell production with resulting anemia, white cell formation with greater liability to infections, and platelet reproduction with frequent bleeding. At times, particularly with chronic granulocytic leukemia, nearly as many white cells as red cells exist, hence the term "leukemia" or white blood.

Chronic leukemias progress slowly, with virtually no symptoms for years. Eventually the disease changes and resembles acute leukemia. The course then follows that outlined under acute leukemias.

What you can do. Regular medical checkups will reveal the onset of a leukemia.

What your physician can do. Tests on a blood sample or a biopsy from a lymph gland will make the diagnosis. Treatment will be determined by the stage of the disease. Therapy is similar to that for acute leukemias—chemotherapy and possibly radiation for the leukemia; antibiotics, blood transfusions, and platelet transfusions for infections, anemia, or bleeding.

CHAPTER 5

The lymphatic system

As blood flows through the capillaries, part of the blood plasma escapes into the minute spaces between the cells that make up the structures of the body and is then called **tissue fluid.** The lymphatic system provides an accessory route by which this tissue fluid can reenter the bloodstream. Blood cells and large protein molecules cannot pass through the capillary walls, so tissue fluid consists of water, nutrients, hormones, and other blood components.

Tissue fluid moves slowly, most of it seeping back into the blood capillaries. The rest, about 3 liters a day, enters a special system of channels called **lymph capillaries,** and is then called **lymph.** Thus lymph and tissue fluid are really the same. Lymph capillaries join each other to form small lymph vessels. These join to form larger lymph channels, just as small veins join to form larger veins.

Like veins, lymph vessels have valves that prevent back-flow and allow the lymph to flow in only one direction, toward the heart. This occurs every time a lymph vessel is compressed, for example by a contracting muscle. Again, whenever a lymph vessel is stretched by incoming lymph, the muscles in its wall act like a pump and automatically contract, squeezing the lymph to the next segment (the part of the lymph vessel between two valves). Each segment functions as an automatic pump, filling, stretching, and contracting, thus propelling the lymph through the lymphatic vessel.

Lymph from the viscera (organs) enters the **thoracic duct,** which empties into a large vein on the left side of the neck. Lymph from the left half of the head, neck, chest, and the left arm flows into the thoracic duct just before it joins the vein. The lymph from the right arm and the right half of the head, neck, and chest flows into a vein on the right side of the neck. In this way the lymph from the entire body returns to the bloodstream from which it came.

In their course toward the heart, many lymph vessels, rather than joining other lymphatics, empty into **lymph nodes.** These lymph nodes are tiny filtering organs, some as

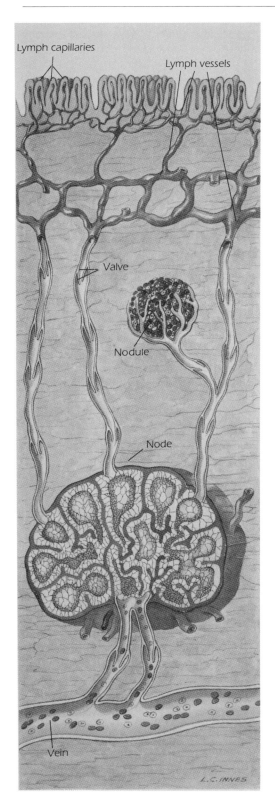

Lymph capillaries

Lymph vessels

Valve

Nodule

Node

Vein

L.C. INNES

small as a pinhead and some as large as a bean. A number of lymph vessels enter each lymph node. The lymph then percolates through the node, leaving through a single vessel. Within the lymph node are several kinds of cells which belong to the body's defense system. The phagocytes, or police-duty cells, swallow and destroy germs that might have entered the lymph. Many of the lymphocytes, the most numerous of cells, are produced in the lymph nodes themselves. Some stay in the lymph nodes, where they help to combat infection, while others travel in the lymph to enter the bloodstream, where they make up one third of the white blood cells. Some of the lymph cells produce antibodies.

Lymph nodes, with their various cell types, fight infection, and thus can be viewed as barriers to the spread of infections. You have probably noticed small, hard lumps (kernels) in the side of your neck when you have had a sore throat, or lumps under your arm when you have had an infection in your hand. These swollen, and often tender lymph nodes actively fight infection.

Lymph nodes play an important

Diagram showing channels through which the lymph passes on its way from the lymph capillaries to the blood (vein). The lymph flows through vessels of increasing size that contain valves. Some lymphocytes are added to the lymph by a solitary lymph nodule, others by a lymph node, through which the lymph filters.

827

role in the body. They swallow germs and small particles of foreign material that gain access to the tissues through an injury, into the lungs through the air we breathe, or from the food we eat. When smoke or coal dust is in the air, small particles of carbon enter the air passageways. These particles are swallowed by phagocitic cells, and the lymph carries them to nearby lymph nodes, where they are trapped. Over a lifetime these nodes become black, and are gritty when cut.

Cancer cells also travel in the lymph to the nearest lymph nodes, which may become involved as the cancer begins to spread. For example, cancer originating in the breast travels via lymph vessels to lymph nodes in the armpit. If neglected, the cancer may eventually enter the bloodstream and locate in distant parts of the body. To block possible spread, surgeons attempt to remove involved nodes, or they may be irradiated to kill the cancer cells.

Lymph nodes have important functions. The phagocytes swallow and thus remove foreign materials, germs, and cancer cells which enter the tissues. The lymphocytes form the body's second most numerous defense force, and they also trigger the plasma cells to produce antibodies. (See below.)

The lymphoid system

The body contains several organs and tissue masses composed of tissue practically identical to that which composes the lymph nodes. These include the spleen, thymus, tonsils, adenoids, appendix, and scattered collections of lymphoid tissue (Peyer's patches) in the wall of the lower small intestine and in the bone marrow. Some of these have specialized functions.

Lymphocytes, before ending up in lymphoid tissues, undergo processing. Some, called "T" lymphocytes, migrate to the thymus and are responsible for local or cellular immunity. Others, "processed" in bone marrow, are called "B" lymphocytes. These manufacture antibodies. The lymphoid system rejects certain poisons and injurious proteins and is responsible for the rejection of transplanted tissues and organs. Malfunction of this system appears responsible for certain so-called autoimmune diseases of the joints, skin, lungs, and kidneys, and susceptibility to infections and cancers.

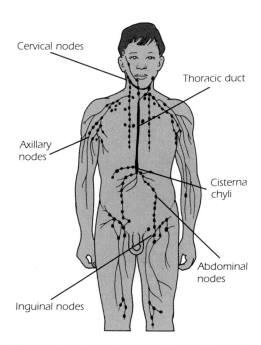

Cervical nodes

Thoracic duct

Axillary nodes

Cisterna chyli

Abdominal nodes

Inguinal nodes

The major lymph vessels and lymph nodes of the lymphatic system.

The spleen

The spleen is a large lymph node located in the upper left abdomen. But the spleen does not filter lymph; it filters blood. Its functions include: (1) destruction of germs and trapping of foreign particles, which escaped the lymph nodes and entered the bloodstream; (2) production of lymphocytes, and under certain circumstances, other types of blood cells; (3) storage of blood, and so acts as a small reservoir; (4) destruction of old red blood cells and recycling the salvaged iron and protein of the hemoglobin; (5) destruction of worn-out platelets; and (6) production of certain antibodies.

The tonsils

The tonsils, one on either side of the throat, are located between the

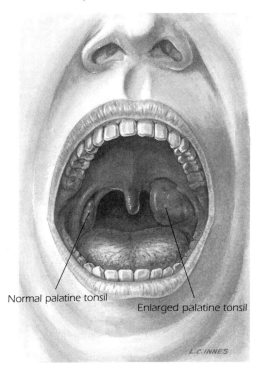

Normal palatine tonsil
Enlarged palatine tonsil

L.C.INNES

tongue and the pharynx. They filter neither lymph nor blood, but serve very effectively, especially during early childhood, as "barriers" because of phagocytes and lymphocytes in the tonsils that keep germs from entering the body. The surfaces of the tonsils have little pits in which germs are appraised and defenses, such as antibodies, activated. Sometimes the tonsils themselves become infected, swollen, and enlarged **(tonsillitis),** or they may become abscessed **(quinsy).** Before the days when penicillin and other antibiotics were available, tonsils were removed almost routinely. The present, more conservative attitude suggests that removal of the tonsils **(tonsillectomy)** be done only if tonsillitis develops repeatedly (three or more times in a year). Once they are removed, the tonsils should not grow back. During adolescence the tonsils shrink in size.

The pharyngeal tonsils **(adenoids)** are located on the upper part of the pharynx, back of the nasal cavity, partially surrounding the opening of the eustachian tube. Though they function similarly to tonsils, they do not atrophy as one gets older. They may become enlarged and block breathing through the nose. In children, mouth breathing may cause undesirable growth of the bones and tissues of the face. Should the eustachian tube leading to the middle ear be blocked, infections of the middle ear and even hearing loss may occur. Removal is never complete, and regrowth may occur.

The thymus

The thymus is located within the upper front part of the chest, just below the neck. Developing early during embryonic life, it attains its maximum development when the child reaches about eight years of age, but from then on it slowly decreases in size and regresses in function. The thymus plays an important role in the development of the lymphoid system, producing a hormone, **thymosin,** which stimulates the lymph nodes and spleen to produce the important "T" cell lymphocyte, a vital member of the body's defense force against infection.

The appendix

The appendix is a small, dead-end tube, about the diameter of a pencil and about 3 inches (7.5 centimeters) in length, attached to the first part of the large intestine (the cecum). Lymphoid tissue composes most of its wall. Probably its function is to sample the kinds of microorganisms that pass by and then to stimulate the body's defense mechanisms. Occasionally the appendix itself becomes infected, swollen, and inflamed **(appendicitis).** When this occurs it should be removed promptly **(appendectomy)** before it ruptures and spreads infection throughout the abdomen.

Disorders of the lymphoid system

The lymphoid tissues form a major part of the body's immune system. Certain chemicals and microorganisms can partially or completely suppress this immune system. Such drugs play a useful role in tissue and organ transplants, because they interfere with the body's efforts to reject the foreign tissues (the transplant). However, suppressing or blocking this system, either intentionally or by a disease organism, seriously weakens the body's defenses and makes the person liable to infections.

AIDS (acquired immune deficiency syndrome)

AIDS is a viral disease that impairs the lymphoid system in performing its usual function of protecting the body against infections. In this new and deadly disease, generally sexually transmitted, the immune system is suppressed.

Four population groups make up the majority of AIDS victims: (1) those who have had male/male sex with many partners, and (2) hemophiliac men and women (1 percent), who have received HIV-infected blood products; (3) in many parts of the world male/female sex with multiple partners spreads AIDS; (4) in the United States, the incidence of AIDS is three times higher among Blacks and Hispanics than among Whites.

Among the factors which play an important role in transmission of this blood-borne human retrovirus (HIV) are: sexual promiscuity; anal intercourse; venereal disease, such as syphilis; and intramuscular or intravenous drug abuse. The spread of the virus, isolated from blood, semen, and vaginal secretions, is more difficult than the transmission of syphilis. Most of those who have no symptoms, but have antibodies to the AIDS virus, develop the disease.

In the United States most AIDS presents as a secondary infection. This may be accompanied by shortness of breath developing gradually due to pneumonia, such as *Pneumocystis carinii.* A cancer of the skin, Kaposi's sarcoma, also occurs frequently. Other problems include diarrhea; meningitis; herpes simplex infections (cold sores) on the lips and in the mouth and anus; candidiasis of the mouth (thrush), esophagus, bronchus, and lung; and many other so-called "opportunistic" infections, such as tuberculosis. Secondary cancers, such as lymphomas and sarcomas, frequently occur as well. AIDS also presents as "Slim Disease" with weight loss, and diarrhea (without other cause) or as AIDS dementia.

Many of the infections, both common and rare, occurring because of the loss of immunity, can be treated successfully. However, the majority of sufferers become progressively worse, with increasing weight loss and weakness, ultimately dying from repeated infections.

The treatment of AIDS is directed toward the virus and toward secondary infections and cancers. AZT (azidothymidine), currently the only drug that attacks the virus, is, however, toxic, often causing anemia and granulocytopenia. Testing continues on other drugs; no vaccine is as yet available. Infections can be treated with antibiotics, and cancers, with chemotherapy, radiation, and surgery. Therapy, at best, attempts to keep the patient as comfortable as possible.

What you can do. Because no known cure exists at this time, preventive measures are all important. Avoid promiscuous sex; multiple sexual partners increase the risk of developing the disease. Avoid sexual contact with those known or suspected of having AIDS. Should you consider yourself at risk to develop AIDS or have positive antibodies to the virus, refrain from giving blood transfusions and from having sexual or other intimate contacts which might endanger others. Should you consider yourself at high risk and have a fever of unknown origin, with generalized swollen lymph nodes or other common symptoms listed above, see your physician immediately.

What your physician can do. Laboratory tests can determine whether you have positive antibodies to the AIDS virus. Lab tests can also isolate the virus from lesions. A prompt diagnosis and the initiation of therapy, which may be of indefinite duration, is essential.

We should emphasize that investigation of AIDS is so intense that today's knowledge regarding the disease and available treatment may tomorrow be drastically changed.

Swollen lymph nodes (lymphadenopathy)

A response to a local or systemic infection forms the most common reason for lymph nodes to be inflamed (lymphadenitis). It is the lymph nodes that attempt to prevent the spread of germs, toxins, and cancer cells within the tissues of the body. In the process of doing so, they themselves, as mentioned above, become infected, causing them to become enlarged, tender, and painful.

Infections of the scalp cause an enlargement of the nodes at the back of the neck. Those of the eyes, ears, teeth, mouth, and pharynx involve the nodes beneath the jaw and in the side and front of the neck, felt as tender lumps (kernels). Infections of the hand or foot activate the nodes in the axilla (armpit) or groin. Infections of the breast spread to nodes in the armpit or to nodes within the chest. Infections of the internal organs affect the nodes that lie in the path of the lymph as it flows toward the heart.

Infections affecting lymph nodes may be caused by bacteria, viruses, spirochetes, or fungi; streptococci and staphylococci are common offenders. A generalized infection, as in measles and infectious mononucleosis, can affect the lymph nodes of the entire body.

Lymph nodes become involved in the diseases of the lymphatic system such as leukemia and Hodgkin's disease. The lymph stream rather than the blood carries many types of cancer to other parts of the body. This explains why lymph nodes in the path of lymph drainage from a cancer often become cancerous. Lymph nodes so involved usually feel firmer than those activated by infection. Removal and microscopic examination of the nodes often provide valuable information on the spread of cancer.

Lymphomas

Lymphomas are a variety of lymph-gland cancers which may involve the spleen and bone marrow. These life-threatening cancers occur at any age, but more frequently in children and young adults, except for non-Hodgkin lymphoma, which increases with age. The symptoms vary, appearing late in some cases and early in others. The two main types are Hodgkin's disease and non-Hodgkin's lymphoma.

Hodgkin's disease

Some 6,000 new cases of Hodgkin's disease develop each year in the United States. Hodgkin's disease usually appears as a swelling of a lymph node in the neck, armpit, or groin. From here the condition spreads to lymph glands of the chest, abdomen, and pelvis; the spleen and often the liver are also affected, along with the lungs, bone, and bone marrow.

Besides the swollen nodes, the symptoms include persistent fever, night sweats, fatigue, loss of appetite, weight loss, itching, and anemia.

A number of diagnostic tests are available. A sample of the involved tissues will, under the microscope, reveal a unique cell structure (Reed-Sternberg cells) and specifically identify the problem. X-rays of the chest and abdomen (especially computerized tomography) and/or a biopsy of the bone marrow may be done.

What you can do. Report any lymph node that remains swollen for several weeks for no obvious cause, such as a local infection, to your physician.

What your physician can do. He will prescribe tests to enable a precise diagnosis. Therapy will vary, depending on the type and stage of the disease. Radiation therapy has a high success rate (80 to 90 percent) in treating disease that is localized. In advanced cases, chemotherapy with an anticancer drug alone, or combined with radiation, may be advised, but approximately only a third of such cases completely recover. Your physician will check you up two or three times a year for several years.

Non-Hodgkin's lymphomas

Non-Hodgkin's lymphomas occur more commonly than Hodgkin's disease and constitute a group of several separate forms of lymphomas. These are distinguished by differences in the cell types occurring in the affected tissues and occur more frequently as age advances.

The signs of these diseases parallel those of Hodgkin's disease, with weakness, weight loss, fever, night sweats, and anemia. In some cases, a persisting enlargement of the tonsils first calls attention to the illness, through involvement of abdominal organs and the bone marrow are more frequent. In **Burkitt's lymphoma**, for example, large abdominal masses cause kidney damage, and the disease may also affect the central nervous system.

Treatment is similar to that described under Hodgkin's disease, being tailored to the type and stage of the disease.

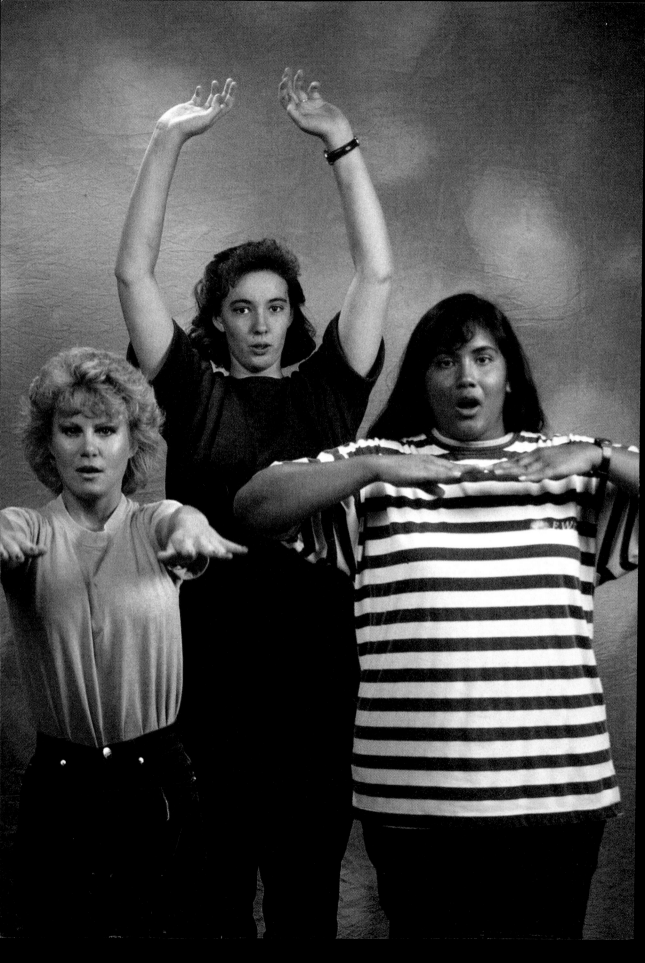

VOL. 3

SECTION 2

THE DIGESTIVE AND RESPIRATORY SYSTEMS

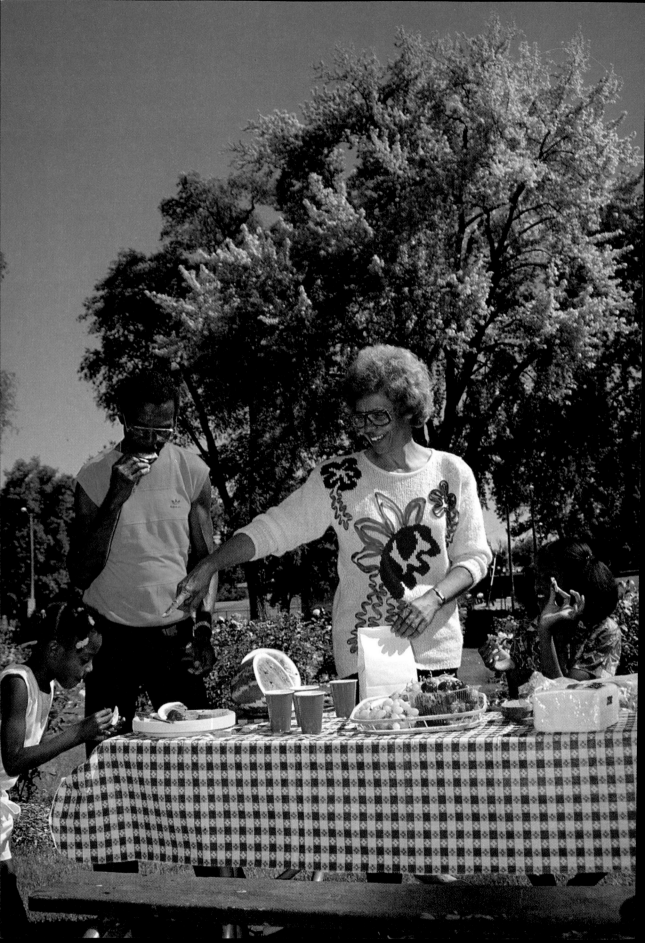

CHAPTER 6

The digestive system

The digestive system begins at the lips and ends at the anus. While continuous, it is divided into a number of parts because of changing structure and function. These are the lips, mouth, pharynx, esophagus (gullet), stomach, small intestine (duodenum, jejunum and ileum), large intestine (cecum and the ascending, transverse, descending, and sigmoid colon), rectum, anal canal, and anus. In addition, the liver and pancreas play important roles in digestion.

The purpose of the digestive system is to digest and absorb food and to eliminate undigested food and other wastes. The digestive process is extremely complex, requiring mechanical and chemical steps that are coordinated by nervous and hormonal control and affected by psychic influences.

The lips, mouth, pharynx, and esophagus

The lips form the opening of the mouth and are used for speaking, eating food, and drinking fluid.

The mouth has two sets of teeth (upper and lower), right and left cheeks, a hard and soft palate above, a tongue below, and it opens into the pharynx behind. Mucous membrane lines the entire cavity, except for the teeth. The teeth break and grind the food as it is manipulated between them by means of the tongue and cheeks. Saliva pours into the mouth from three pairs of **salivary glands:** two beneath the tongue (sublingual), two in the floor of the mouth (submandibular), and two at the angles of the mandible (parotid) below and in front of the ears. After the food has been pulverized and thoroughly mixed with saliva, it is swallowed.

The seven pairs of muscles in the **tongue** make it extremely maneuverable. It can twist and turn, protrude through the lips, and draw back into the mouth. On its upper surface are small projections called papillae, with groups of taste buds clustered around them. The **taste buds** can distinguish between sweet, salt, sour, and bitter. The flavor of foods brings pleasure to eating and may warn of spoiled food.

The pharynx—the back part of

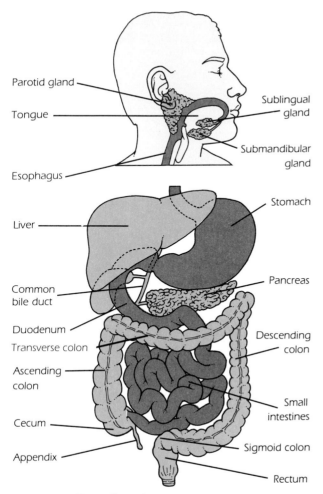

The digestive system.

the mouth—includes the area between the back of the nose and the entrances to the larynx and esophagus and contains the palatine tonsils. Its muscular walls are covered with mucous membrane.

The esophagus or gullet is a muscular tube approximately 10 inches (25 centimeters) long that conveys food and drink from the pharynx to the stomach. Located behind the larynx and trachea, it travels through the chest behind the heart. Just before it terminates in the

stomach, it passes through an opening (hiatus) in the diaphragm, a flat muscle that separates the chest and abdominal cavities. Its lining membrane contains mucus-secreting glands that lubricate and moisten its inner surface.

Chewing is accomplished by the teeth, aided by the lips, tongue, and cheeks. The teeth are embedded in the semicircular upper and lower jaws. The upper is fixed, while the lower moves. The mandible (lower jaw) resembles a horseshoe placed horizontally with its ends turned upward. The curving front gives form to the chin, while the rounded ends fit loosely into depressions on the underside of the skull, forming the **temporomandibular joints.** These joints permit the jaw to open and close, to move forward and backward, as well as from side to side. These movements allow food, as it is being positioned between the teeth by the lips, tongue, and cheeks, to be finely ground.

Swallowing is an intricate mechanism. The tongue first moves forward, then sweeps upward and backward along the palate, propelling the food into the pharynx, where it is molded into a ball. Now the soft palate closes the opening to the back of the nose, while the epiglottis bars the entrance to the larynx. The esophagus opens as the wavelike rhythmic contractions of the pharynx continue down the esophagus, carrying the bolus of food to the stomach in about six seconds. These coordinated muscular actions are such that a person can swallow both food and drink while standing on his head,

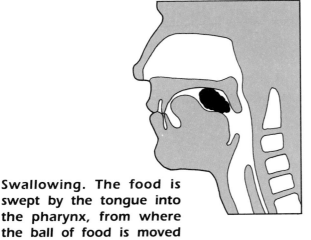
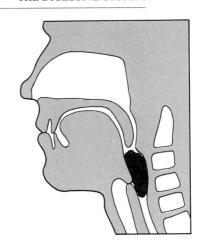

Swallowing. The food is swept by the tongue into the pharynx, from where the ball of food is moved down the esophagus.

and at the same time take periodic breaths of air.

The stomach

The pear-shaped stomach is located below the diaphragm in the upper left side of the abdomen. Not very large when empty, its muscular walls can stretch enormously. The larger section, the fundus and body, lies to the left, while the smaller antrum and pylorus are to the right. Two muscular gates or one-way valves open and close where the esophagus enters the stomach **(esophageal sphincter)** and where the stomach blends with the duodenum **(pyloric sphincter)**. A

membrane (the mucosa) containing glands that produce mucus, hydrochloric acid, pepsin, and a hormone gastrin, line its inner walls.

The stomach functions to store and process the food which has left the mouth and been swallowed. The rhythmic, back-and-forth wavelike contractions of the stomach wall, together with the added food-splitting acid and pepsin, further disintegrate the already pulverized food. It is now virtually liquefied and strongly acid. The acid destroys most germs that may enter with the food. Food begins to leave the stomach soon after entry, and continues for several hours to trickle into the duodenum,

The stomach and duodenum. Partially digested food moves from the stomach to the duodenum.

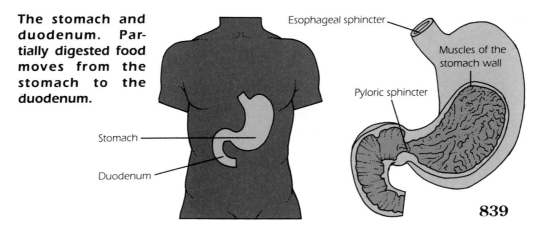

Esophageal sphincter

Muscles of the stomach wall

Pyloric sphincter

Stomach

Duodenum

839

the first part of the small intestine.

It is remarkable that the stomach does not digest itself. While some of the superficial layers of the stomach lining are constantly being eroded off and digested, a mucus layer, called the "mucus barrier," protects the stomach wall from damage. Over-production of acid, an inadequate supply of mucus, the taking of certain chemicals, such as aspirin and alcohol, or psychological pressures may allow the protective barrier to break, and so permit the lining mucous membrane to be injured. This may lead to symptoms described as indigestion, associated with gastritis, and ulcers of the stomach and duodenum.

The small intestine (duodenum, jejunum, and ileum)

The small intestine, apart from the duodenum, measures from 15 to 31 feet, averaging 22 feet (6.5 meters) in length. The duodenum is 10 inches (25 centimeters) long, while the jejunum is two-fifths and the ileum three-fifths of their combined length. Their many coils—extending from the stomach to the cecum—lie in the central abdomen, held in place by a broad fan-shaped, ribbon-like structure **(the mesentery).** In general, the digestive organs are partially or entirely covered with **peritoneum,** a smooth, moist, glistening membrane, which also lines the walls of the abdominal and pelvic cavities and allows for movement of the intestines without friction. The muscular walls of the small intestine churn the food with their back-and-forth wavelike move-

ments (peristalsis), mixing it with the digestive juices (enzymes), and gradually moving the food residue (chyme) toward the large bowel.

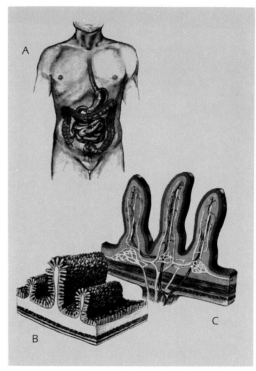

A. Coils of the small intestine. B. A section of the small intestine enlarged to reveal the fingerlike villi of its lining. C. Three villi magnified to show capillaries and lymph vessels.

The small intestine is the main organ for digesting and absorbing food. Its lining membrane (mucosa) consists of millions of microscopic, fingerlike projections (villi). Each villus contains a network of blood capillaries and a small lymph vessel. Their number gradually decreases from the beginning of the jejunum to the end of the ileum, as noted by the thinning of the wall. The villi greatly increase the surface area of the mucosa, facilitating the digestion of food and the absorption of released nutrients.

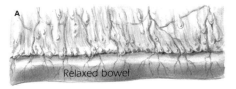

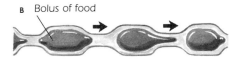

Diagram of segmental contractions

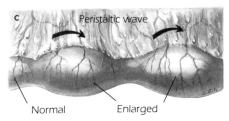

Normal   Enlarged

A section of the small intestine showing how wavelike muscle contractions (peristalsis) move the food along.

The large intestine

The horseshoe-shaped large intestine is about 4.5 feet (1.5 meters) long. It begins where the ileum joins the cecum in the lower right side of the abdomen. It then extends upward (the ascending colon) toward the liver, across (the transverse colon) toward the spleen, downward (the descending colon) to the left lower abdomen, where it bends back on itself (the sigmoid colon), to terminate in the rectum.

The cecum, the first part of the large intestine, is a large pouch which continues to the beginning of the ascending colon. From its lower

end projects a fingerlike, pencil-sized smaller pouch about 3 inches (7.5 centimeters) long called the appendix (for details see page 830). The appendix, while usually located in the lower right side of the abdomen, may be found at various positions along the right side, and occasionally even on the left side.

The lining membrane of the large intestine differs from that of the small intestine in that it has no villi.

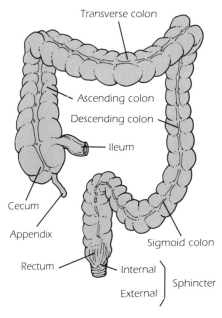

The large intestine, made up of the cecum; ascending, transverse, descending, and sigmoid colons; and the rectum, anal canal, and anus.

Also, digestive enzymes are not produced in the colon. Instead, its mucus-secreting glands provide large amounts of mucus, which not only lubricate its walls but provide adhesive to give form to its contents. Contractions of the colon walls provide some mixing of the contents (slow peristalsis), while periodic mass-propulsive movements help evacuate the bowels. Large numbers of a variety of bacteria inhabit the colon and further break down indigestible fiber and other food residues, synthesize vitamin K, and actually make up part of the stool mass.

The two functions of the large intestine are to absorb water, minerals, and certain vitamins from the liquid residue leaving the small intestine, and to prepare and store the fecal wastes until expelled in the stool. As water is absorbed, the once liquid chyme becomes mushy, then semisolid, and finally solid before being expelled.

Rectum, anal canal, and anus

The rectum, which is about 5 inches (12.5 centimeters) long, extends downward to the one-inch (2.5 centimeters) long anal canal, which opens to the outside at the anus. The rectum provides a temporary storage area for feces. The walls of the anal canal contain two sphincters, the internal (automatic) and the external (voluntary). The voluntary sphincter helps to control the moment of defecation. The lining membrane also contains sensors that enable one to distinguish whether the content of the rectum is liquid, solid, or gas.

Bowel movement (defecation)

The descending and sigmoid colon serve as a reservoir for retaining fecal material until bowel movement occurs. At the junction of the sigmoid colon and rectum is a weak sphincter. When feces enters the rectum, the desire to have a bowel movement is initiated. A mass contraction of the lower colon drives feces into the rectum, which, in turn, contracts as the **anal sphincters** relax, allowing the stool to be extruded.

The external anal sphincter can stifle this desire if the occasion is inconvenient and the urge not too compelling. However, done too frequently, a habit of ignoring the desire may develop and may contribute to the problem of constipation.

Between the time food is eaten and the waste residue eliminated in the stool some fourteen to twenty-four hours later, a beautifully orchestrated series of the most complex physical, chemical, hormonal, and nervous activities dissemble the food and provide the body with the raw materials essential to life itself. How wondrously have we been engineered!

The liver, gallbladder, and pancreas

The liver, the gallbladder, and the pancreas are indispensable parts of the digestive system.

The **liver,** the largest organ, weighing about 3 pounds (1.4 kilograms), or one fiftieth of the entire weight of the body, lies below the diaphragm, sheltered by the right lower ribs. It is unique in that it receives blood from two sources: The hepatic artery brings blood from the general circulation; the portal vein drains the entire digestive system, carrying to the liver the components derived from the food we eat.

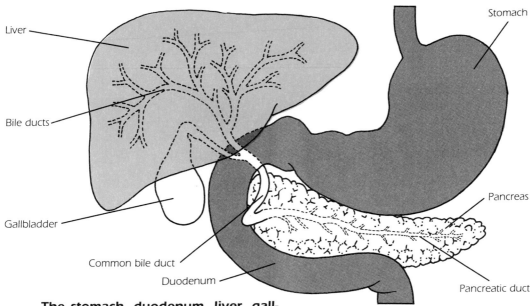

The stomach, duodenum, liver, gall-bladder, and pancreas, showing their interconnections.

The functions of the liver, in a sense a "gigantic" chemical factory, are too intricate and too numerous to detail. We will briefly mention only a few of its main activities.

1. Regulates the concentration of sugar in the blood. It removes excess sugar from the blood and stores it as **glycogen,** which it later releases as the level of blood sugar drops. It holds about 500 calories of energy for emergency use.

2. Plays a major role in processing fat, even though this can be done elsewhere in the body. It converts carbohydrates and proteins to fat, and synthesizes lipoproteins, cholesterol, and lecithin.

3. Continually produces bile, about 1 liter each day, synthesizes cholesterol, and also converts some cholesterol to bile salts.

4. Forms the plasma proteins of the blood and the protein globin which attaches to heme to make hemoglobin. It converts excess and discarded proteins to urea, which can then be eliminated by the kidneys. When needed, it can synthesize the so-called non-essential amino acids.

5. Actively stores vitamins, especially A, D, and B_{12}. Stores of A may last as long as two years, while those of D and B_{12} last many months.

6. Acts as a blood reservoir, storing up to 400 ml of blood.

7. Stores the largest amount of iron (apart from the blood) and releases it as needed.

8. Manufactures many of the substances required for the clotting of blood, such as prothrombin, and fibrinogen.

843

9. Inactivates, makes less harmful, or destroys many poisonous substances which enter the body (antibiotics, alcohol), and also alters or excretes in the bile excesses of many hormones (cortisone, thyroid hormone, estrogens), and other substances (bilirubin, bile pigments).

10. Manufactures blood cells during fetal life and during emergencies when the bone marrow is suppressed for various reasons (pancytopenia).

The **gallbladder** is a sac attached to the underside of the liver, designed for storing, concentrating, and releasing bile formed by the liver. While the liver manufactures up to 1,000 milliliters of bile each day, the gallbladder has a capacity of only about 60 milliliters. Water, salt, and other minerals are actively absorbed by the mucosa lining the gallbladder. In this way the bile coming from the liver, and shunted into the gallbladder, is concentrated five to fifteenfold, thus enabling the gallbladder to store the bile which is secreted over a twelve-hour period.

When the partially digested food leaves the stomach, the gallbladder is triggered to release the concentrated bile into the duodenum. The bile (bile salts and bile acids) then emulsifies the fat, facilitating its digestion, and aids in the absorption of fatty acids, cholesterol, and other fatlike substances.

The **pancreas** is a gland which

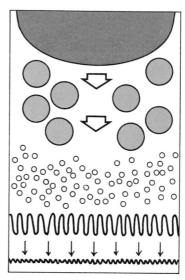

Bile emulsifies fat

Micelles form and are digested

Fatty acids enter blood

Steps in fat digestion. Fat droplets are emulsified by bile. The emulsion is further broken down to micelles by bile and fat-digesting enzymes, which are further reduced to fatty acids and glycerides for absorption.

lies transversely in front of the vertebrae, behind the stomach. Its head fits into the curve of the duodenum while its tail extends to the left kidney. The body and head manufacture (1) the digestive juices (enzymes), which are poured into the duodenum for the digestion of carbohydrates, fats, and proteins, and (2) sodium bicarbonate for neutralizing the acid coming from the stomach. The tail has specialized cells which synthesize and release **insulin** and **glucagon** into the blood. These hormones aid in regulating blood sugar.

844

CHAPTER 7

Diseases of the digestive system

Diseases of the digestive organs affect almost 20 million Americans and are the leading cause of hospitalization in the United States. They are second only to the cardiovascular diseases as a cause of days lost from work and as a reason for visits to physicians. The problems affect skin, moist membranes, bone, muscle, and glands.

The lips, mouth, tongue, and salivary glands

Harelip (cleft lip) and cleft palate

Harelip and cleft palate are developmental defects in which a gap or fissure occurs in either or both sides of the upper lip, in the palate, or in both the lip and palate. If these problems go uncorrected, defective speech and psychological problems from disfigurement occur. Harelip, and especially cleft palate, interfere with the infant's ability to nurse. The care of a physician is essential.

What your physician can do. Since the infant is growing rapidly, it is important that your physician decide the best time for surgery.

Harelip repair usually comes early at about three months of age. Cleft palate correction generally occurs later, when the child begins to talk. More than a single surgical procedure may be required.

Depending on the severity of the defect, the infant may experience problems in nursing. Since the baby has difficulty sucking, the milk should flow easily through the nipple. Sometimes the infant may have to be spoon-fed. A removable plate may be needed to cover the gap in the palate. A speech therapist can help the child to overcome difficulties in speaking correctly.

Temporomandibular joint problems (TMJ)

The right and left temporomandibular joints are the two joints on which the lower jaw hinges; you can feel them if you place your fingers in front of your ears as you open and close your mouth. These joints permit up and down, forward and backward, and side to side motions. These movements, produced by the attached muscles, allow for chewing, speaking, and facial expression.

Difficulties which arise include: limited and often irregular motion of the lower jaw; grinding and clicking when the jaw is moved; pain, frequently appearing to originate in the ear, radiating to the temple, side of the face, neck, and angle of the jaw; and muscle spasms that "lock" the jaw.

Problems result from habits related to emotional tension (such as grinding or clenching the teeth) or from malocclusion (the teeth failing to meet properly when closed). The remedy lies in learning to cope with stress-producing situations, or in correction, by a dentist, of problems of malocclusion. Heat, moist (fomentation) or dry (heating pad), with gentle massage, may provide considerable relief.

Cracking of the lips (cheilosis)

Vertical cracks or fissures appear in the lips due to excessive licking of the lips, too much exposure to sunlight (ultraviolet), drying of the lips, and a deficiency of vitamin B2 (riboflavin). Occasionally certain drugs may induce the problem. Removal of the cause and the use of lip creams should alleviate the condition.

Angular cheilosis (fissures at angles of mouth)

Fissures at the corners of the mouth result from the presence of excessive saliva due to malocclusion or poorly fitting dentures. A deficiency of the B vitamins may also cause the disorder. Germs may invade the fissure and cause infection. Treatment consists of removing the cause and providing good oral hygiene.

Cold sores or fever blisters (oral herpes simplex)

Cold sores are blisters caused by a herpes simplex virus that develop on the lips or inside the mouth. The initial infection, a systemic disease, spreads by intimate contact with an infected person. Generally occurring in childhood but occasionally developing at any age, the disease produces painful blisters on the lips, mouth, and skin; swelling of the adjoining lymph nodes; and fever. The symptoms may persist up to three weeks.

Viruses remain present for life. Recurrent infections consist of blisters, usually on a lip. One may feel a tingling at the site several hours before swelling and blistering occur. The sores, which heal spontaneously in five to ten days, are triggered by overexposure to sunlight, drying of the lips, periods of reduced resistance (such as fever, some other infection, menstruation, or fatigue), stretching the tissues around the mouth (such as during dental work), and undue emotional stress.

Treatment should be directed toward preventing causative factors. Once developed, cold sores cannot be cured. Should the blister cause extreme pain, your physician may prescribe a medication (acyclovir) for local application or to be taken by mouth. (See page 979.)

Canker sores (mouth ulcers, aphthous ulcers)

Canker sores are usually small red swellings or tiny blisters that occur on the membrane which lines the mouth, on the under surface of the tongue, on the gums, and on the soft palate. Occasionally numerous, they may fuse together and become large. The pain may make eating and speaking difficult.

A number of conditions may initiate canker sores. These include: injury due to a jagged tooth; lowered resistance due to some illness or from fatigue; emotional stress; nutritional deficiencies of vitamin B12, folic acid, and iron; a virus infection such as herpes simplex (cold sores); or a menstrual period. Canker sores affect girls and women more than boys and men. This usually self-limiting disease appears once or twice a year and causes little inconvenience except soreness of the mouth. A mouth ulcer may indicate a more serious problem, such as leukemia or a local malignancy.

What you can do. Rinsing the mouth with warm salt water or with an antiseptic mouthwash will relieve the pain. Ointments and lozenges may also provide relief. Avoid any

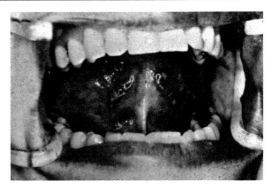

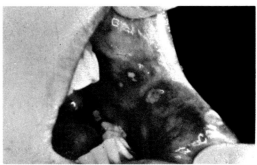

Canker sores in the mouth and on the tongue.

foods that produce discomfort, such as spicy or highly acid foods.

What your physician can do. If the ulcers do not heal within ten to fourteen days, your physician may recommend a steroid preparation or check for a more serious problem.

Tongue disorders (glossitis, and geographical, hairy, and furred tongue)

Disorders of the tongue may be due to a local problem or result from a systemic disease. Thus while the appearance of the tongue may differ widely from one person to another, changes in its color and texture may indicate some underlying disease.

Glossitis or inflammation of the tongue may occur from local damage or from certain systemic dis-

847

eases. Biting, burning, and repeated exposure to irritants such as alcohol, tobacco, and hot foods or drinks, cause injury, allowing germs, already present in the mouth, to inflame the tongue. Systemic diseases, such as certain anemias, nutritional deficiencies of iron, folic acid, vitamin B12, and allergies may induce glossitis. Usually the tongue becomes swollen, ulcerated, and sore. In severe cases, the lymph nodes in the neck become enlarged and tender, accompanied by fever.

In **geographic tongue** irregular red patches of inflamed mucosa, sur-

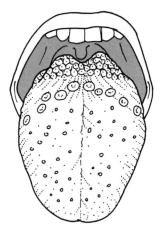

The tongue covered with circular papillae around which are clustered the taste buds.

rounded by a white margin, migrate over the surface of the tongue. The various shapes suggest islands and continents, hence the name. This benign but untreatable condition occasionally causes burning and pain.

In **hairy tongue** the papillae on the tongue's surface become discolored (from yellow-white to brown-black) and grow long and hairlike, giving it a furry appearance. No

cause is known, but it frequently follows antibiotic treatment. Exposure to irritant foods and tobacco may also allow germs to multiply, which causes the discoloration. Removing the dead material from the surface of the tongue with a brush or scraper improves the sense of taste and smell. No treatment exists, but when the underlying problem is removed, the condition disappears.

Furred tongue is a whitish coating on the surface, commonly accompanying some illness or fever. It results from an accumulation of dead cells, food, and bacteria which are not removed by the usual activity of eating and drinking. The tongue may be gently scraped, but the problem will disappear of itself.

What you can do. As mentioned above, you can use some simple procedures to give relief from any discomfort or pain. Should any of these conditions persist, seek a physician's advice.

What your physician can do. He will ascertain the underlying problem. When this is treated, the disorder of the tongue should disappear.

Thrush (oral candidiasis)

This painful infection is caused by a fungus *Candida albicans*, a normal inhabitant of the mouth. It usually affects babies and the elderly rather than the average adult, and follows a debilitating illness or antibiotic therapy in which the microbial balance is upset. A cheesy-white, velvetlike growth covers the tongue, the roof of the mouth, the inside of the cheeks and lips, and the pharynx. The lesions resemble milk curd but are difficult to remove. The symptoms include fever, poor appetite which, in an infant involves refusal to nurse, restlessness, and often diarrhea. If untreated in an infant, it may be life-threatening, spreading throughout the respiratory and digestive systems.

What you can do. If the infant is breast-fed, the mother's breasts and nipples should be cleansed with a saturated solution of boric acid and then rinsed with cooled boiled water, before and after nursing. If bottle-fed, nursing bottles should be sterilized (boiled) before use.

What your physician can do. A smear and culture of the exudate will reveal the organism. He may prescribe the antibiotic nystatin, given by mouth or, in adults, as lozenges.

Trench mouth (acute ulcerative gingivitis, Vincent's infection)

This is a severe inflammation and ulceration of the gums, caused by both a bacillus and a spirochete. This infection does not appear to be contagious, but occurs after a debilitating illness, poor dental hygiene, smoking, and throat infections. The disease makes talking and swallowing painful.

What you can do. A mouthwash every thirty to sixty minutes of half-strength hydrogen peroxide is effective, as is painting the affected areas with a paste prepared by adding a few drops of water to sodium perborate powder. Adequate rest, a nourishing diet of soft foods, and plenty of water will aid in recovery. Smoking should be eliminated.

What your dentist or physician can do. Although local therapy usually proves effective, in severe cases an antibiotic may be recommended. Following recovery a dentist should advise as to appropriate care to avoid recurrence.

Inflammation of the salivary glands

Mumps, the most common infection (viral) of the salivary glands, causes tenderness and swelling of one or both of the parotid glands (see page 729). Bacteria may also reach the glands through their ducts, especially if previously injured by a stone. The resulting infection causes a painful swelling. The lymph glands in the sides of the neck may become enlarged and tender. If untreated, the infection may destroy the gland. See your physician.

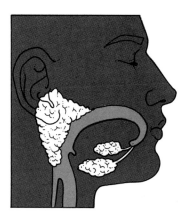

The salivary glands consist of three pairs: parotid, submandibular, and sublingual.

What your physician can do. He will generally prescribe an antibiotic. If he suspects destruction of a gland, he may ask a radiologist to do an X-ray examination, using a dye introduced into the gland (sialography) to

849

determine its functional capacity. Severely damaged glands are surgically removed, since the remaining glands will provide adequate saliva.

Stone in salivary duct

Sometimes a stone forms in a duct of a salivary gland, most frequently in the submandibular gland ducts (probably because of the uphill course of the ducts). The gland may become inflamed. As saliva is dammed back, especially at mealtime, swelling occurs in the floor of the mouth at one side of the tongue. The stone is easily removed by a minor surgical procedure.

Leukoplakia

Leukoplakia is a patchy hardening of the membrane lining the mouth and tongue. Cracks, fissures, and even ulcers develop in the yellowish-white, thickened, leathery areas. Occurring most frequently in men over forty, leukoplakia appears to be caused by prolonged irritation of the

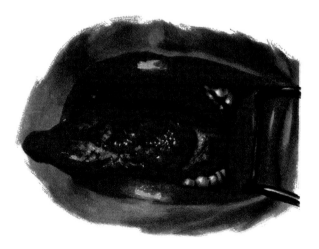

Carcinoma of the tongue (or leukoplakia).

membranes of the oral cavity, resulting from jagged teeth or rough dental restorations; the use of highly seasoned foods; the habitual drinking of hot beverages; and—most important of all—smoking and chewing tobacco.

Leukoplakia is considered a precancerous condition. Removing the causes of irritation should clear up the problem. Should it persist, a physician should do a biopsy.

Ptyalism (salivation)

Ptyalism is an excessive flow of saliva stimulated by food or even the thought of eating; by pain or the thought of pain in the mouth area (as when in a dental chair); and by some interference with swallowing. It is not a disease. Ptyalism also occurs in cases of poisoning by mercury or by one of the iodides.

Dry mouth (xerostomia)

The mouth may become dry from a stone obstructing a major duct of a salivary gland. It may also occur with destruction from a disease process of the salivary gland. Again, the mouth may become dry when one is anxious or under emotional stress, as in the case of a public speaker. Dehydration and the taking of medications that contain atropine or atropinelike compounds will dry the mouth.

Tumors of the salivary glands

Salivary gland tumors occur 80 percent of the time in only one of the parotid glands. The tumor usually develops slowly, producing a firm, round, painless swelling at the angle of the jaw. Since occasionally the growth may be malignant, it should be checked by a physician. He may recommend an X-ray (sialogram) or a biopsy. If malignant, the tumor should be removed promptly and probably followed by radiation therapy.

Cancer of the mouth (oral cavity)

Cancer in the region of the mouth accounts for about 2 percent of all cancers. Since the early stages of these cancers do not produce symptoms, any ulcer which does not heal within two weeks should be investigated by a physician. While cancer of the lower lip is the most common, cancer can develop in the gums, palate, tongue, cheek, and floor of the mouth.

Factors which predispose to cancer of the mouth include longtime exposure to the sun, as in sailors and farmers, the use of chewing tobacco and snuff, chronic drinking of alcoholic beverages, and the smoking of tobacco and marijuana. Examination

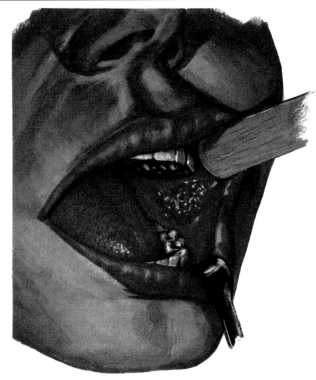

Carcinoma of the cheek.

of a sample of tissue removed by biopsy is the most reliable test. Surgical removal should be done as soon as possible. If the cancer has spread, radiation therapy may help. Early detection gives the highest success rate.

The esophagus (gullet)

Heartburn (reflux esophagitis)

Heartburn is a burning sensation felt behind the lower portion of the breastbone or just below the ribs in the upper part of the abdomen, sometimes extending upward to the throat and mouth. The discomfort occurs when the acid stomach contents or other digestive juices flow backward into the lower esophagus through the esophageal sphincter. While not related to the heart, at times of severe discomfort or pain the condition is sometimes mistaken for a heart attack. If the problem occurs repeatedly, it causes an inflammation of the lining (mucosa) called reflux esophagitis.

At the point where the esophagus joins the stomach, the circular

851

muscle fibers of the esophagus are strengthened to form a sphincter or valve. This valve opens to allow food or drink to enter the stomach, but it also acts to prevent stomach contents from backflowing into the esophagus. Factors which contribute to backflow include an inefficient sphincter, obesity, overeating (overfilling the stomach), high-fat meals, cigarette smoking, increased pressure in the abdomen due to straining or pregnancy, bending forward soon after eating, lying down soon after a meal, and wearing a tight belt or corset. A hiatus hernia at times allows reflex and so may also contribute to heartburn.

What you can do. Try a number of common-sense actions which will counter those factors that contribute to backflow. Avoid overloading the stomach. This requires eating less at each meal and refraining from food three hours before bedtime. Reduce the fat in your diet, and give up smoking or chewing. Lose weight if necessary. Elevate the head of your bed by using six-inch blocks under the legs. The use of a nonsodium antacid a half hour after meals may help. If despite the changes you make the situation does not improve, see your physician.

What your physician can do. He may have tests done to demonstrate reflux or the presence of inflammation. If medication does not ease the problem, surgical intervention may be necessary.

Narrowing of the esophagus

When the esophagus is narrowed, swallowing causes discomfort, and

even pain, deep in the chest. **Tumors** (possibly cancer) within the esophagus or pressing on it from surrounding areas may cause the narrowing. Due to loss of nervous control, the lower end of the esophagus may become narrowed and twisted, a condition called **achalasia.** Severe narrowing (stenosis or stricture) can result from scarring caused by the accidental drinking of acid or alkali (lye) or by longstanding esophagitis. Occasionally temporary spasm of the esophagus may occur.

The symptoms include fullness and pain deep to the breastbone, especially when swallowing. At first, eating slowly proves helpful. As the condition worsens, food is regurgi-

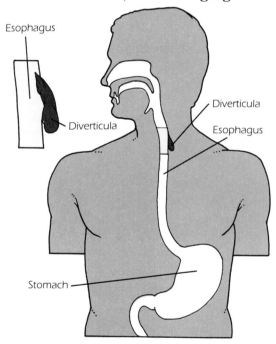

Esophagus

Diverticula

Diverticula

Esophagus

Stomach

An esophageal diverticulum (plural = diverticula) is an outpouching through a weak area of the muscular wall. It is most commonly seen in the upper one-third.

852

tated (returned to the mouth), but it is not acid, as it has not reached the stomach. The individual risks lung infection from inhaling regurgitated food, especially during sleep.

What your physician can do. A fluoroscopic examination using a barium meal and an endoscope passed down the gullet, allowing for a visual appraisal, will enable a precise appraisal of the problem. Periodic stretching of a contracting scar by inserting a special tube may help. Surgery is necessary for the removal of tumors and may be needed to alleviate narrowing from other causes.

Hiatus hernia

In hiatus hernia the abdominal part of the esophagus and part of the stomach are pushed or pulled upward through the opening (hiatus) in the diaphragm through which the esophagus normally passes. This occurs because of weakness of the muscles around the hiatus. The hernia consists of a pouch of the stomach which has pushed through the hiatus. Because of the acid reflux into the esophagus, inflammation or an actual ulcer may develop at the junction of the esophagus and stomach. Many people have no symptoms at all; when symptoms are present, they are those of heartburn and are aggravated by the same things.

What you can do. The treatment parallels that of heartburn. If the problem cannot be avoided and antacid therapy becomes constant or fails to provide relief, check with your physician.

What your physician can do. If additional medication fails to alleviate the distress, surgical repair may be the answer.

The stomach

Indigestion (dyspepsia)

Indigestion is a symptom of problems of the upper gastrointestinal tract—esophagus, stomach, duodenum, gallbladder and pancreas. These symptoms involve vague feelings of distress after eating or drinking. The symptoms vary from person to person and from time to time. They include a sense of discomfort in the upper abdomen, heartburn, belching, distention or bloating, a sick feeling (nausea), and even pain. Gas formation and intestinal irritation may cause diarrhea. There may be headache and a sensation of mental dullness.

The causes of indigestion vary widely. They include eating certain foods, such as peppers, onions, cucumbers; eating rich foods, as cakes and gravies; eating too rapidly, too much, or when under emotional stress. Caffeine-containing beverages, alcohol, and carbonated drinks may also trigger a bout of indigestion. Another cause of indigestion is malabsorption due to lactose intolerance. Indigestion sometimes signals a more serious problem, such as stomach or duodenal ulcer, gallbladder disease, or even cancer.

What you can do. Avoid as far as possible the factors enumerated above which cause indigestion. Eating leisurely of appropriate kinds and amounts of food, at regular intervals (no eating between meals), in a relaxed atmosphere are wise preventives. The use of an appropriate antacid at times will give relief. Should a change develop in the conditions provoking indigestion or should there occur a sudden increase in the severity of attacks, immediately consult with your physician.

What your physician can do. A number of diagnostic tests can determine whether any serious underlying problem exists. If any are found, your physician can institute appropriate treatment. He may recommend a different antacid or suggest certain changes in lifestyle after carefully evaluating your history of indigestion.

Gastritis

Gastritis is an inflammation of the membrane which lines the stomach and can be both acute or chronic.

The causes of **acute gastritis** include infections, most commonly viral but also bacterial or parasistic (termed gastroenteritis); drugs, especially aspirin and other anti-inflammatory agents; swallowing corrosive acids or alkalis; heavy drinking; unintentional consumption of a variety of poisonous mushrooms; allergic responses to certain foods; and stress-induced gastritis occurring in cases of severe burns, multiple injuries, or major surgical operations.

Chronic gastritis may be due to a variety of poorly understood causes, including certain infections, perni-

cious anemia, and the heavy use of tobacco and alcohol.

Acute gastritis typically causes an uncomfortable feeling in the stomach, distention of the abdomen, headache, nausea, a coated tongue, and a bad taste in the mouth. Severe cases may include pain and tenderness in the upper abdomen, vomiting, fever, and sometimes bleeding from the stomach or black, tarry stools.

The symptoms of chronic gastritis are similar to those of acute gastritis, with the possible addition of discomfort in the upper abdomen after meals, tenderness over the stomach, and a general feeling of debility.

What you can do. During the acute stage, abstain from food for one or two days. Repeated doses of a liquid, nonabsorbable antacid may provide some relief. Avoid dehydration (especially in cases of vomiting and diarrhea) by taking sips of water every ten to fifteen minutes or by sucking ice. Applying heat over the abdomen with fomentations or a heating pad may relieve the discomfort. When tolerated, take small amounts of food, with a gradual return to a normal diet. When the gastritis persists or hemorrhage occurs, or when a corrosive poison has been swallowed (after instituting emergency first aid), see your physician immediately.

For chronic gastritis you should review your habits of eating and drinking and determine to correct unhealthful ones. Eating less, eating at regular times (no in-between snacking), avoiding foods and drinks which aggravate the condition, and discontinuing alcohol and tobacco will be beneficial. Avoid factors which cause worry, anger, and other emotional upsets.

What your physician can do. He can help determine the underlying cause and then institute appropriate therapy. If a drug appears responsible, he can change or discontinue the agent temporarily. When vomiting and diarrhea continue, he will suggest medication to remedy the situation. In case of dehydration, intravenous fluids will help, as will a transfusion if blood loss has been extensive.

Peptic ulcer (stomach or duodenal ulcer)

The term *peptic ulcer* includes gastric ulcers that occur in the stomach; duodenal ulcers that develop in the first part of the duodenum just beyond the stomach's outlet; and occasionally ulcers in the terminal esophagus.

The ulcer is a raw, inflamed crater in which the mucous membrane lining (mucosa) appears to have been punched out. While the exact cause of such ulcers is not known, they can develop where gastric juice is present. This juice contains hydrochloric acid and a protein-splitting enzyme called pepsin (hence the name "peptic"), designed to digest or break down proteins. Fortunately, a marvelous protective mechanism—the mucous barrier—appears to shield the cells forming the mucosa from being digested.

It is thought that when this barrier is broken, the corrosive juices attack the mucosa. However, a number of

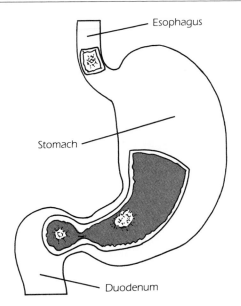

Esophagus

Stomach

Duodenum

Peptic ulcers form in the proximal duodenum (duodenal ulcers), the stomach wall (gastric ulcers), and in the terminal esophagus (esophageal ulcers).

factors predispose to ulcers. Drugs such as aspirin, and emotional stress with accompanying anxiety, affect both acid and mucus production. Should their balance be sufficiently altered, erosion of the mucosa may occur. Coffee, tea, maté, soft drinks, and alcohol increase acid production and thus favor ulcer formation. Tobacco increases gastric ulcers in ways not understood.

Ulcers may develop at any age. While the incidence of stomach ulcers is about the same for men and women, duodenal ulcers occur more frequently in men than in women. Women have fewer ulcers than men during their menstrual life.

The principal symptom of ulcers is a burning, gnawing pain in the upper part of the abdomen, but in some duodenal ulcers the pain may be felt in the back. Other symptoms include heartburn, belching of acid, bloating, nausca, loss of appetite, and loss of weight. The pain of a duodenal ulcer typically appears two or three hours after a meal, and is quickly relieved by food (milk) or an antacid. On the other hand, food often aggravates the pain of a stomach ulcer. However many people do not experience pain and may not realize they even have an ulcer until some complication develops, such as bleeding.

A number of diagnostic procedures can evaluate the state of an ulcer. Samples of digestive juice can be analyzed to determine the amount of acid being secreted. A barium meal allows the radiologist to show (by contrast) the outlines of the stomach and duodenum and the location, extent, and depth of the ulcers. An endoscope (a fiber-optic device) inserted into the stomach and duodenum can visually examine these organs. Samples of tissues from an ulcer can be taken and examined under a microscope.

Four serious complications may result from ulcers: cancer, hemorrhage, obstruction, and perforation.

Cancer. Stomach cancer occurs frequently. Gastric ulcers do not become cancerous, but gastric cancers may ulcerate. For this reason every stomach ulcer should be evaluated by a physician.

Hemorrhage. As erosion by the digestive juices continues within an ulcer, an artery may be encountered. When its wall breaks down, bleeding occurs. A modest but persistent hemorrhage may cause anemia to develop in time. In heavy bleeding, fresh blood may be vomited or blood passing down the intestinal tract may emerge as black, tarry stools. Rapid loss of blood may induce shock. Such a hemorrhage poses a life-threatening problem and constitutes an emergency to control the bleeding. A transfusion may be necessary to replace lost blood.

Obstruction. Ulcers in the pylorus of the stomach near the duodenum or in the duodenum may, because of swelling, scarring, and adhesions, partially or completely block the emptying of the stomach. Such an obstruction is known as **pyloric stenosis.** Since the stomach fails to empty, it becomes dilated. Belching and profuse vomiting (foul smelling) are the main symptoms. If medical means fail to relieve the condition, surgery will be essential.

Perforation. Sometimes the erosion of the floor of an ulcer continues through the muscle wall of the stomach or duodenum, causing a perforation. The contents of the stomach and duodenum can now escape into the general abdominal cavity, causing **peritonitis** (inflammation and infection of the membrane lining of the abdomen). This is a surgical emergency that requires prompt treatment to prevent shock, infection, and death.

What you can do. Many ulcers heal by themselves. First, you must try to help the ulcer heal and then prevent its reappearance. Attempt to correct those factors causing indigestion (see page 853) and ulcers (see page 855). Regularity in eating is extremely important. While many advocate multiple small meals, others find that three meals, widely spaced to allow the stomach to complete its work and rest, are beneficial. Drinking warm water or taking an antacid two to three hours following a meal may help. Avoid troublesome foods that provoke indigestion, such as hot, spicy dishes. Give up smoking, drinking, and the use of all caffeine-containing beverages. Consult with your physician if you are taking aspirin or a similar drug, so he can prescribe a substitute. If you are under emotional stress, study what changes you can make to reduce the pressures of life.

What your physician can do. He may recommend a more appropriate antacid than the one you are using. If excessive production of hydrochloric acid causes your problem, he may suggest a new medication which reduces the production of this acid. Since ulcers tend to recur, your physician should periodically give you a careful examination. Ulcers which refuse to heal after all possible measures have been employed may require surgical removal.

Cancer of the stomach

Cancer of the stomach often starts in an ulcer of the lining of the stomach wall. Stomach cancer occurs twice as often in men as in women, usually occurring in those who are middle aged or older. The risk of gastric cancer increases if blood relatives have had a stomach cancer. Deaths from stomach cancer have greatly decreased in the past fifty years in the United States, from 25 percent of all cancer deaths in 1930 to 2 percent at the present time. Some countries have a much higher

Note the chronic gastric ulcer in the center of the stomach near the top edge.

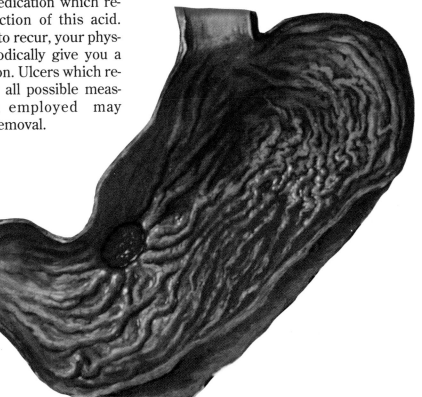

death rate than others. Japan has one of the highest.

At an early stage, stomach cancers may cause few if any symptoms. One may experience vague feelings of discomfort, indigestion, and loss of appetite. Later, vomiting of blood or the passing of blood in the stool, weight loss, anemia, and pain over the upper abdomen may occur.

Cancer can be detected by visual examination of the interior of the stomach by means of a gastroscope, by samples of tissue (biopsy) taken for microscopic examination, and by a fluoroscopic examination using a barium meal.

What you can do. Should you have persistent indigestion and other feelings of distress in the upper abdomen, or should indigestion suddenly develop for no apparent reason, consult with your physician.

What your physician can do. He can make the appropriate examinations and institute immediate therapy. Even after treatment, periodic examinations are mandatory.

Early diagnosis and removal of the cancer usually prevents a recurrence. However, frequently the malignancy, prior to its detection, has already spread to other organs, such as the liver and the lungs. Chemotherapy and radiation may prove helpful. The survival rate depends on the stage of the cancer at the time of diagnosis. Caught early, 90 percent may recover. If late, the cancer may be inoperable.

The small intestine

The small intestine is designed to complete the digestion of the food leaving the stomach and entering the duodenum, and to absorb the released nutrients.

Malabsorption syndromes

This category includes a number of conditions in which food nutrients fail to be absorbed into the bloodstream. The causes for such failure include: (1) faulty digestion of food due to lack of a chemical or enzyme to break apart a food (such as lactose intolerance); (2) faulty absorption of nutrients resulting from damage to the intestinal lining, which is caused by inflammation (Crohn's disease), intestinal infection (tropical sprue), congenital defects (celiac disease),

and radiation therapy; (3) nutrient deficiencies (iron, B12); and (4) miscellaneous problems arising from bacterial overgrowth, intestinal tumors, diseases of the pancreas, and surgical removal of portions of the intestine.

While the symptoms vary, depending on the specific disorder, those usually seen include weakness, pallor, poor appetite, weight loss, distension of the abdomen, diarrhea, sore tongue, nutritional deficiencies, and anemia. Stools change color and consistency and may be foul smelling and float on water.

Lactose intolerance

Lactose intolerance—the inability to digest lactose, (milk sugar)—results from the congenital lack of the digestive enzyme lactase, or from its loss as a child matures. It occurs most commonly in certain ethnic groups such as Blacks and Asians, although many adults have degrees of intolerance.

Since the lactose is not digested, it passes into the colon, where it is acted on by bacteria, causing diarrhea, gas, and cramps.

What you can do. Should symptoms develop after drinking milk or using milk products, lactose intolerance probably exists. Avoid such products or use cultured milk, where the lactose has been broken down. Infants with the disorder should be given soya milk or a product from which lactose has been removed.

What your physician can do. He can order a lactose tolerance test, in which one takes a dose of lactose. Cramps, diarrhea, and no rise in blood sugar confirm intolerance.

Crohn's disease (regional ileitis)

This disease is a chronic inflammation of the various layers of the intestinal wall, generally near the junction of the small and large intestines (ileum), that causes the walls to become thick and firm. It tends to affect segments of the intestine, in some cases remaining local, in others, spreading to other areas. The cause of the disorder is not known, but it usually begins before age forty and seems to run in families. Its incidence is increasing.

The main symptoms include diarrhea, with pus and sometimes blood in the stool, usually accompanied by a mild fever with abdominal pain, anemia, and weight loss. The condition becomes better or worse by spells and may disappear after one or two episodes, but often persists for years. Abscesses may develop, with serious complications of perforation or obstruction.

What you can do. Since no known specific treatment exists, try to maintain your general health in the best possible condition. Eat the best diet possible, exercise to tolerance, avoid fatigue, and work closely with your physician.

What your physician can do. He can make a precise diagnosis by means of X-rays following a barium meal, or by means of an endoscopic examination, together with the symptoms. He may prescribe steroids, especially during severe attacks. Antibiotics and surgery may be necessary should perforation occur. Scarring may narrow the intestine and require surgery. Even after surgical removal of a localized lesion, the disorder may recur.

Tropical sprue

Tropical sprue is a lesion of the small intestine in which some flattening of the mucosal villi occurs. While its cause is not known, researchers link its occurrence to vitamin deficiencies due to infectious organisms. It occurs most freqently in the West Indies, India, and Southeast Asia. Severe loss of appetite may account for some of the weight loss. Symptoms include profound fatigue, severe anemia, and diarrhea with bulky, foul-smelling, fatty stools. Without treatment, permanent changes develop in the mucosa.

What your physician can do. He can make the diagnosis by microscopic examination of the intestinal lining which shows deformed villi. Treatment with folic acid and antibiotics is curative. Treatment should be maintained until all signs of the disease have disappeared. Celiac disease, with symptoms somewhat like tropical sprue, does not respond to folic acids or antibiotics.

Celiac disease (nontropical sprue)

Celiac disease is an inherited sensitivity or intolerance of the intestinal lining to gluten, a protein found in wheat, rye, barley, and oats. In the presence of gluten, the fingerlike villi shrink, and the lining becomes smooth, hindering the absorption of nutrients. Onset generally begins in infancy, but sometimes the condition is not recognized until childhood or later. The disease may disappear, only to reappear later.

The consumption of a gluten-containing cereal or food will elicit the symptoms of abdominal discomfort, weight loss, anemia, and greasy, foul-smelling stools which float. Should an infant, after cereals are included in the diet, lose its appetite, fail to gain weight, and have foul-smelling stools, suspect celiac disease.

What you can do. Should you have celiac disease, you will have to avoid those cereals (wheat, rye, barley, oats) which contain gluten, and any products to which gluten has been added. Apart from these restrictions, your diet can be wholesome,

and you should remain healthy.

What your physician can do. He will do tests to determine whether you have anemia or any nutritional deficiencies. A sample of tissue from the intestinal lining examined by a pathologist will confirm the presence of celiac disease. The only treatment is to avoid foods that contain gluten.

Intestinal obstruction

Intestinal obstruction, which may be partial or complete, prevents the normal movement of intestinal contents. Obstruction results from two major causes. One is **mechanical blockage** as from strangulated hernia, adhesions, twisting of the intestine (volvulus), telescoping of a portion of the bowel (intussusception), fecal impaction, tumors, a foreign object such as a coin, and large worms in the small intestine. Another cause of intestinal obstruction is **adynamic ileus,** or paralysis of the intestine due to loss of nervous control. This condition occurs most often after abdominal surgery, but also from injuries (of vertebrae or spinal cord), infections (pneumonia or other severe infection), uremia, or diabetes.

The symptoms vary, depending on the site of the obstruction and whether it is partial or complete. Pain generally occurs in the midline of the abdomen, especially if the small intestine is involved. Vomiting, frequent and profuse, at first resembles ordinary vomitus, but soon becomes green with bile. It then becomes brown and has a fecal odor, especially in the case of total obstruction in the lower colon.

Complete constipation is the rule.

Because the obstruction dams up the intestinal contents, gas accumulates and increasingly painful distention occurs. Mild fever and severe thirst accompany dehydration due to loss of fluids. A strangulated hernia may become gangrenous and perforate. In infants, young children, and sometimes in the elderly, the intestine telescopes or infolds within itself (intussusception). Along with the usual symptoms of blockage, bleeding usually occurs.

What you can do. Intestinal obstruction always constitutes an emergency. See your physician if your symptoms suggest obstruction.

What your physician can do. He will have you hospitalized and start intravenous fluids to replace the fluids and salts you have lost and to prevent shock. If you are already in shock, a blood transfusion may be necessary. The symptoms, together with X-rays, will confirm the diagnosis. Most cases require surgical intervention, especially when a tumor blocks the passage or a strangulated hernia becomes gangrenous. If a perforation has occurred, an antibiotic will be administered to treat the resulting infection.

Intestinal infarction

An intestinal infarction occurs when a segment of the intestine is deprived of its blood supply. Due to atherosclerosis, blood clots (thrombi) form in a vessel, obstructing the flow of blood, or an embolus (a floating part of a blood clot) coming from some other part of the body lodges in an intestinal artery. When blood flow stops, the portion of intestine deprived of blood becomes engorged with stagnant blood, ultimately dies, and becomes gangrenous.

The symptoms parallel those of intestinal obstruction. Surgery should be performed as soon as possible to remove the infarcted area and to rejoin the severed ends. To prevent or

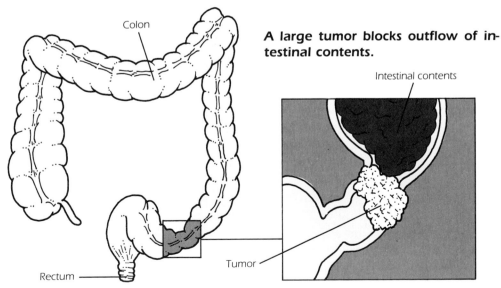

Colon

Rectum

Tumor

A large tumor blocks outflow of intestinal contents.

Intestinal contents

treat shock, intravenous fluids or a blood transfusion may be given. Recovery should be complete, unless the infarction involves a very large section of the small intestine, in which case malabsorption problems may arise.

Hernias

In an intestinal hernia a loop of intestine protrudes through a weak area of the muscle forming the abdominal wall. A person may be born with a weakness at certain sites or may develop a weakness through disuse or injury (healed surgical incision). The common sites occur where structures enter or leave the abdomen, such as the navel, the right and left inguinal areas where the testicles descend into the scrotum, where the femoral arteries leave the pelvis, where the esophagus passes through the diaphragm, and in the epigastrium (area just above the navel in the midline).

Conditions which increase the pressure within the abdominal and pelvic cavities favor the development of a hernia. These include lifting weights, persistent cough, chronic constipation, marked obesity, pregnancy, and an injury or incision through the abdominal wall which has healed poorly. Unless properly treated, a hernia tends to progressively enlarge.

The symptoms usually consist of a slightly tender lump or swelling which appears gradually, or suddenly after some vigorous exertion, sometimes accompanied by a feeling of heaviness in the area. An untreated hernia carries the danger of

becoming incarcerated, that is, the loop of intestine cannot be pushed or drawn back into the abdomen (irreducible). The intestinal contents may not be able to pass through the loop and become obstructed, causing nausea, vomiting, and pain. Should the hernia enlarge and cut off its blood supply, the hernia is then said to be strangulated, the intestinal loop will die and become gangrenous, and life will be threatened. The enlarged hernia will become very painful.

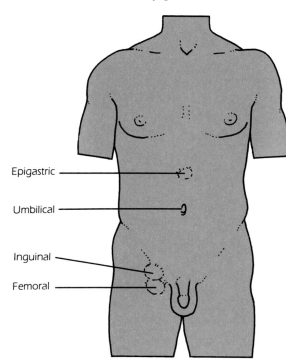

Epigastric
Umbilical
Inguinal
Femoral

Common areas where hernias develop: epigastric, umbilical, inguinal (above groin), and femoral (below groin).

What you can do. Generally you can push a hernia back into the abdomen (reduce) by applying pressure with the fingers over the protrusion. You should report the problem to your physician in any case. A hernia that will not push back in is a medical emergency that should be reported to your physician immediately. Remember, a small or newly developed hernia is easier to repair than an enlarged or old one.

What your physician can do. By examination, your physician can determine the presence of a hernia and ascertain its size and extent. Surgical repair, the only truly satisfactory remedy, usually is considered a simple procedure.

The large intestine

The 4-foot-long large intestine or colon mainly absorbs salt and water and prepares liquid waste, entering from the small intestine, for discharge in semisolid form.

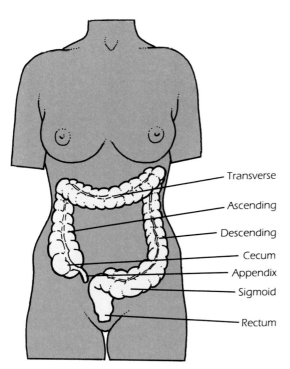

Transverse

Ascending

Descending

Cecum

Appendix

Sigmoid

Rectum

The large intestine or colon.

Appendicitis

Appendicitis is the inflammation of the appendix, a 2- to 4-inch (5 to 10 centimeters) long pencil-shaped ex-

tension of the cecum, the first part of the ascending colon. It may develop at any age but occurs most frequently between the ages of ten and twenty-five. Its function is not fully understood (see page 830), nor the reason why it becomes inflamed or when it will occur. Appendicitis is probably the most frequent surgical emergency.

Severe pain, starting in mid-abdomen, gradually shifts to the lower right side of the abdomen. Acute tenderness on pressure over the painful site accompanies a low fever, nausea, vomiting, and constipation (rarely diarrhea). The sufferer often draws up his right leg to relieve the tension on the sore spot. Coughing and breathing deeply make the pain worse.

If removal of the pus-filled appendix is delayed, the appendix may rupture or perforate, spreading germs in the abdomen. Rupturing relieves the pressure within the appendix, and for a time the pain subsides. Actually this may be a danger sign. Should the infection localize, an abscess forms.

A number of other disorders of the lower abdomen may give similar symptoms, such as, inflammation of the oviducts, rupture of an ovarian cyst, and Crohn's disease. Besides, the appendix is not always located in the right lower abdomen (see page 841), so, should you have the above symptoms, see a physician immediately.

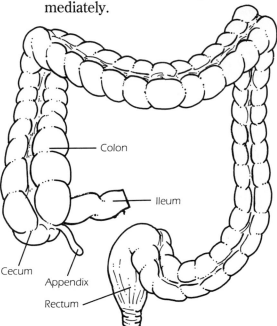

The appendix, continuous with the cecum, near the junction of the small and large intestine.

What you can do. Do not take an enema or a laxative. This may cause the appendix to rupture, scattering infected material in the abdominal cavity. Placing an ice bag over the most tender spot, fifteen minutes on and then fifteen minutes off, will temporarily relieve the pain and slow the inflammation. Go to a hospital as soon as possible because delay may cause a rupture.

What your physician can do. A blood test will usually show a rise in the number of white cells (indicating an infection). He will evaluate your symptoms and determine the course

of treatment. Prompt surgical removal is the treatment of choice. If rupture has already occurred, he will prescribe antibiotics in an attempt to prevent peritonitis or abscess formation.

Irritable colon (mucous colitis, spastic colon)

Irritable colon is a condition in which the contractions of the muscular walls of the colon no longer occur rhythmically but become irregular and uncoordinated. The contents of the bowel cannot move along smoothly, resulting in either diarrhea or constipation. Symptoms, ranging from abdominal discomfort to cramplike pain, generally are relieved by belching or a bowel movement, although bowel movements themselves may be painful. Appetite may vary, and gas, headache, sleeplessness, and fatigue may be present.

While the precise cause is not known, emotional stress appears to play a major role in many cases, with more occurrences among women than men.

What you can do. Try to determine what triggers an attack or makes the problem worse. You may find that you tolerate certain foods better than others. Many find that a diet high in fiber provides relief. Others do better on a low-fiber or bland diet. Since emotional stress may cause irritable colon, you should make every effort to reduce the pace of life and avoid stress-provoking situations.

What your physician can do. Your physician will consider other disorders which may be confused with irritable colon. A barium meal or barium enema, or a sigmoidoscopic or colonoscopic examination may prove helpful. Lactose intolerance should be ruled out. He may recommend taking a fiber supplement, such as ground psyllium seed (available under various names). In severe cases an antispasmodic medication may provide relief.

Ulcerative colitis

In this condition the tissues lining part or all of the colon become inflamed and ulcerated. It is seen more often in women than in men and appears about the third decade in life. The condition may come on suddenly, but its onset is usually gradual. While the cause is not known, family predisposition, infection by bacteria and viruses, and emotional tension may play a role.

The symptoms of this noncontagious condition include pain with bowel movements, which are watery and filled with pus and bloody mucous. Severe attacks may include fever, loss of appetite, nausea, and anemia. Recovery may be followed later with a relapse. Those suffering from ulcerative colitis for ten or more years have a higher risk of developing cancer of the bowel.

What you can do. Evaluate your diet to determine what foods you tolerate best. A diet high in fiber appears to give the best relief. Reduce the intake of foods devoid of fiber, such as milk, eggs, and meat. Relief from emotional problems may prove beneficial. Work closely with your physician.

What your physician can do. He may do a number of diagnostic tests which may include analysis of blood, evaluation of stool specimens for bacteria and parasites, visual examination of the rectum and colon using a sigmoidoscope or colonoscope, a barium meal or enema, and a microscopic study of a specimen of the bowel lining. Severe attacks are treated in a hospital. The physician may prescribe steroids, given orally or by enema, transfusions if large amounts of blood have been lost, or fluids given by vein to relieve dehydration. Sometimes surgical removal of the diseased area of bowel becomes necessary. Milder cases are effectively treated with long-term medication.

Diverticular disease (diverticulosis, diverticulitis)

Diverticula or pouches (diverticulosis) sometimes develop in the walls of the terminal portion of the descending colon. They occur more frequently in older people, contributing factors being an inherent weakness of the muscle coat of the colon, a low-fiber diet such as is commonly consumed in the Western world, and psychological stress. One rarely sees the condition in peoples of Africa, India, and Southeast Asia.

Diverticula may be present without any symptoms, discovered only when X-rays are taken for some other purpose. Depending on the degree of inflammation, the symptoms may range from mild discomfort with alternating diarrhea and constipation, to severe pain with

865

nausea and fever. Blood may appear in the stools. As in appendicitis, the pouch might rupture, producing a localized abscess or generalized peritonitis.

The diagnosis of diverticular disease is made by a barium meal and direct visual inspection using a sigmoidoscope or colonoscope.

What you can do. With acute diverticulitis you should be under the care of your physician. For mild inflammation, a diet high in fiber proves beneficial, and generally prevents the development of the disorder. Choose a diet containing whole-grain cereals and whole-grain breads, the moderate use of wheat and oat bran, and extensive use of fruits and vegetables. Avoid highly refined foods and food products, such as white bread and foods made largely of refined flour, sugar, and fat (cakes, cookies, pies), along with any food which has hard, indigestible parts, such as seeds of berries, grapes, corn, and nuts. Finely ground psyllium seed (sold under various names) will soften and form the stools.

What your physician can do. He will probably hospitalize you during an acute attack and diagnose your condition with a barium meal and direct visual inspection, using a sigmoidoscope or colonoscope. He may prescribe antibiotics to check infection. Recurrent attacks, associated with bleeding and possible perforation, will require surgical removal of the involved area.

Polyps (benign growths)

Polyps, growths of the lining membrane of the colon, may have a stalk (like a mushroom) or be flat. They range in size from tiny (1 millimeter) to large (5 centimeters), and more than one usually develops. Why polyps develop is not known, but the condition appears to run in families. Polyps sometimes bleed, and the larger the polyp, the more likely it is to become cancerous.

Polyps may cause no symptoms and may be discovered only during examinations for other reasons. Whenever a polyp is found, additional polyps should be searched for. Blood in the stool should be followed up with a barium enema and a sigmoidoscopic or colonoscopic examination to confirm the diagnosis. Polyps may be removed endos-

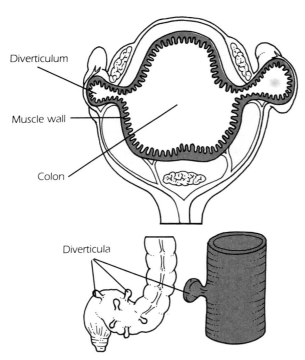

Diverticulum

Muscle wall

Colon

Diverticula

Diverticula (singular = diverticulum): saclike swellings that protrude outward from the colon.

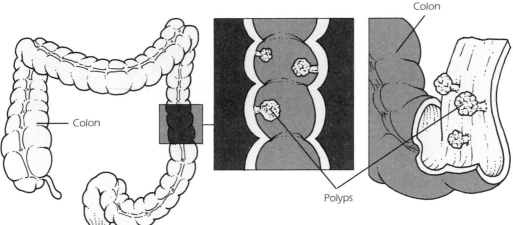

Polyps: mushroomlike growths on the inner lining of the colon.

copically. All polyps should be removed to reduce the risk of malignancy.

Colorectal cancer (cancer of the colon and rectum)

Cancer of the terminal colon and rectum—the third most common cancer, exceeded only by lung cancer in men and lung and breast cancer in women—strikes some 120,000 victims each year, half of whom will die. It seldom develops before the age of forty, and affects both men and women equally.

While the cause for colorectal cancer is not known, it occurs infrequently in countries with a high intake of dietary fiber. It seems that fiber accelerates the passage of waste through the bowels, allowing little opportunity for cancer-producing agents (carcinogens)—either ingested in the food or formed in the colon—to remain in contact with the lining of the intestine.

Cancer may not produce symptoms, or it may cause bleeding from the rectum, changes in bowel habits with alternating constipation and diarrhea, and persisting discomfort and even pain in the lower abdomen. The finding of blood in the stool, X-rays using a barium meal, with sigmoidoscopic and colonoscopic examinations will make the diagnosis. A scan may be used to determine if the cancer has spread to other organs, such as the liver.

What you can do. Should you have any change in bowel habits, such as constipation or diarrhea, or notice blood in your stools, see your physician immediately. Also, you should adopt a diet high in fiber, similar to that described above. For more information, see page 92.

What your physician can do. He will do the necessary tests to determine the cause of your problem. Surgical removal of the cancer is the treatment of choice. Should the cancer have already spread, the prognosis worsens, but chemotherapy may prove helpful.

867

The rectum and anus

The rectum and anus are the terminal, non-absorptive portions of the large intestine, designed for the elimination of preformed waste.

Hemorrhoids (piles)

Hemorrhoids or piles are dilated or varicosed veins located in the membrane lining the anal area. They enlarge because of increased pressure within the veins. Constipation with straining at stool, straining at childbirth, back pressure arising from pregnancy, obesity, and cirrhosis of the liver contribute to the pressure. Hemorrhoids, depending on their location, are termed **internal** if they are located well within the anal canal, or **external** if they are at the anal opening.

Hemorrhoids cause mild discomfort, a heavy feeling, and most commonly bleeding. Bright red blood is seen on the toilet paper. Sometimes a hemorrhoid pushes out through the anus, or the blood within it clots, producing pain.

What you can do. Any bleeding from the intestinal tract should be checked by your physician, as it may indicate a serious problem such as ulcerative colitis, a bleeding polyp, or cancer. After being assured you have hemorrhoids, you can do a number of helpful things. Avoid constipation by drinking plenty of water and by eating more fruits, vegetables, and whole-grain products. Taking some bran or psyllium seed powder or stool softener provides relief, as does sitting in a tub of hot water. Soothing suppositories are also available.

What your physician can do. He can confirm the presence of hemorrhoids by a manual examination or by visual observation through a proctoscope. He may wish to have a barium enema done to rule out other problems, and he may recommend cortisone-containing suppositories or

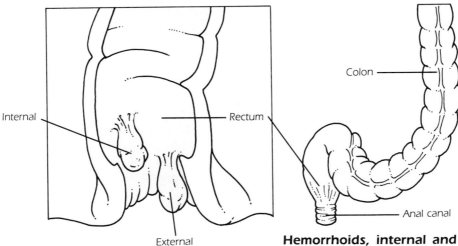

Internal

Rectum

External

Colon

Anal canal

Hemorrhoids, internal and external, in anal area.

868

creams. Should medical management be ineffective, the hemorrhoid can be destroyed by freezing or removed surgically (hemorrhoidectomy).

Anal fissure

An anal fissure is a narrow tear or ulcer extending up the lining of the anal canal, generally resulting from the passing of a large hard stool, from rectal surgery, or from the presence of hemorrhoids. The outstanding symptom consists of severe pain at the time of defecation. During healing, an analgesic ointment or suppository will relieve pain, but curing the constipation is essential. A generous intake of water, a diet high in fiber (see page 92), and the use of a stool softener or psyllium-seed powder should bring about complete healing. Severe cases may require surgical repair to prevent possible abscess formation.

Anal fistula

An anal fistula is a tiny passageway extending from the anal canal or an underlying abscess to the surface of the skin near the anal opening, through which a watery pus drains. This causes skin irritation with itching and burning. Usually caused by an extension of an anal abscess, the disorder may result from Crohn's disease, ulcerative colitis, or colon cancer. Your physician can by appropriate examination exclude more serious disorders. Surgical repair is usually curative. To prevent a recurrence see recommendations under "anal fissure."

Disorders of the liver

Although the liver has a remarkable capacity for self-healing, serious problems do affect this organ.

Jaundice (icterus)

Jaundice is a yellow coloration of the skin and the whites of the eyes caused by excess bile pigment (bilirubin) in the system. The breakdown of hemoglobin from red blood cells forms bilirubin, which is excreted by the liver in the bile, passes into the intestine, and is eliminated in the stool. When bile cannot leave the liver or cannot be eliminated fast enough, the concentration of bilirubin builds up in the blood and liver, and jaundice results.

Liver diseases such as hepatitis and cirrhosis, as well as the blockage of the bile ducts with a gallstone or cancer, hamper or block the excretion of bilirubin, causing jaundice. When large numbers of red cells break down rapidly (hemolytic anemia), bilirubin overwhelms the eliminative capacity of the liver, resulting in jaundice.

What your physician can do. Since jaundice is not a disease in itself, but a symptom of some other disorder, your physician will determine the underlying cause and prescribe the appropriate therapy.

Hepatitis

Hepatitis is an inflammation, and often destruction, of liver tissue.

Hepatitis is most commonly caused by virus infections, but it may be caused by bacteria and certain other organisms and also by alcohol and certain drugs.

The time of exposure to the virus and the onset of the disease vary widely, depending on the particular virus involved. Type A may take from two to six weeks, while the other forms may take from four weeks to six months. The symptoms also differ, from a mild influenzalike illness to liver failure and even death. The usual symptoms include loss of appetite, nausea, vomiting, fatigue, and fever, with the liver becoming enlarged and tender. The appearance of jaundice (lasting a week or two) causes itching, dark-colored urine, and light-colored, loose stools. The gradual disappearance of jaundice and other symptoms indicate recovery, but complete recuperation may require several weeks.

Type A (infectious hepatitis) occurs most commonly among children. The virus is spread by contaminated food or water, and, during the illness, is present in the blood and bowel movements of the patient. The disease is less severe than is Type B, the mortality rate being extremely small.

What you can do. To prevent the spread of the virus, wash your hands and those of the patient. Disinfect all articles that might be contaminated with blood or feces by laundering or by using a disinfectant. Provide a nutritious diet and plenty of bed rest. Alcohol, which will further injure the liver, must be avoided.

What your physician can do.

The disease, even after contact with an ill person, can be prevented or modified by pooled gamma globulin. The protection afforded lasts up to six months. Recovery from Type A hepatitis gives lasting immunity.

Type B (serum hepatitis) typically affects adolescents and adults. The virus is carried in the blood, saliva, nasal secretions, and sperm. Transmittal usually involves accidental injection by means of some contaminated instrument (such as a hypodermic needle used in drug abuse, a tattooing needle, or an awl for piercing ear lobes) a blood transfusion, or sexual contact. The disease is more severe than Type A; 10 percent of those with Type B do not recover completely but develop chronic hepatitis. People with chronic hepatitis have a high risk to develop cirrhosis or cancer of the liver.

What you can do. Follow the procedures suggested for Type A. Avoid contact with any discharge that may carry the virus or use of any contaminated article that cannot be sterilized. A nutritious diet and exercise when tolerated are beneficial.

What your physician can do. Since liver failure can develop suddenly (resulting in hepatic coma and death), the patient should be under the care of a physician, and, depending on how ill the patient is, in a hospital. The administration of a hepatitis B immune globulin can reduce the severity of the hepatitis. Since no cure exists, the treatment is symptomatic. A vaccine (Heptavax-B) has proved effective in protecting 90 percent of persons at high risk of contracting Type B hepatitis.

870

Non-A, Non-B hepatitis (post-transfusion hepatitis). This form of hepatitis is not caused by the Type A or Type B viruses, but possibly by a retrovirus not as yet identified. Usually occurring after a contaminated blood transfusion (the virus cannot be detected in advance), its symptoms parallel those of Type A and Type B hepatitis. It frequently becomes chronic and terminates in cirrhosis of the liver or chronic active hepatitis.

Chronic active hepatitis is a serious disease that persists over a period of years, and appears to occur in those who have had Type B, Non-A, or Non-B hepatitis. In some it progresses to cirrhosis of the liver with symptoms of fatigue, abdominal pain, jaundice, ascites (fluid in the abdomen), and enlargement of the liver. Others exhibit few if any symptoms.

In some it may also be an autoimmune disease in which the body forms antibodies which, rather than protecting it, attack and destroy its own liver cells. The diagnosis requires a liver biopsy for confirmation, especially when suspected by persistently positive liver tests. Many respond favorably to steroid medications which reduce the inflammation, and the majority recover completely.

Other types of acute hepatitis

Hepatitis or inflammation of the liver cells can result from **a sensitivity to certain drugs.** The treatment is, of course, to withdraw the drug and provide supportive therapy.

Certain types of **wild mushrooms** contain a specific poison which attacks and destroys liver cells. Even small amounts can cause serious damage, and the mortality rate is high. Because no antidote exists, supportive treatment is all that can be given.

Cirrhosis of the liver

In cirrhosis the functioning cells of the liver are gradually destroyed and are replaced by fibrous tissue. Patches of damaged cells exist beside islands of regeneration, but gradually the architecture of the liver becomes distorted with scarring and deposits

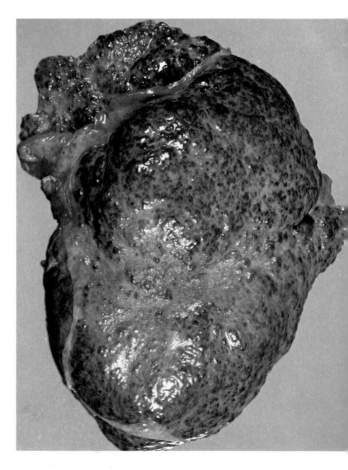

Cirrhosis of the liver.

871

of fat. Eventually the liver becomes shrunken, rock-hard, and irregular.

While cirrhosis can result from a number of causes including specific types of hepatitis and poisoning from certain chemicals and drugs, the most common cause in America and the Western world is drinking large amounts of alcohol **(alcoholic cirrhosis).** Although alcohol is directly toxic to the liver, the organ can destroy small amounts of alcohol, but larger amounts over time damage the functioning cells.

As the liver shrinks and hardens, its normal functions decline, and the flow of blood through the liver becomes increasingly difficult. This back pressure in the portal vein results in the accumulation of fluid in the abdomen **(ascites)** with distention. Other symptoms of liver failure include loss of appetite, loss of weight, nausea, vomiting, anemia, loss of vitality, and jaundice. In an effort to bypass the liver, some of the portal blood flows through the veins of the lower esophagus, causing them to enlarge (varices). These tend to rupture and hemorrhage.

What you can do. Should you have cirrhosis, place yourself under the care of a physician. The prognosis for alcohol cirrhosis, unlike other forms of the disease, is good if detected at an early stage. However, you must discontinue the use of alcohol. If you are an alcoholic, you should by all means seek the aid of Alcoholics Anonymous or enter an alcohol rehabilitation program. A good nutritious diet is also essential.

What your physician can do. By means of laboratory tests and a bi-

opsy, he can make a specific diagnosis. Since no remedy exists, therapy will depend on the problems as they develop. Supplements or transfusions may be needed for anemia, diuretics for edema, and surgery for ruptured esophageal veins.

Biliary cirrhosis

Biliary cirrhosis results from the destruction of the tiny ductules that normally carry bile toward the hepatic duct. As a consequence, the bile produced by the functioning cells has no route of escape. It typically affects women between thirty-five and fifty-five years of age.

Primary biliary cirrhosis develops for no known cause. Some suspect that an autoimmune response may be present. It also occurs as a secondary symptom of chronic disease in the gallbladder and bile ducts, such as blockage of the common bile duct by a stricture, stone, or cancer (of duct or pancreas), or infection in the biliary tree. The disease progresses slowly over a period of ten to twenty years.

Itching is usually the first symptom, followed by jaundiced skin that often shows fat deposits (xanthomas) and brown pigmentation. Additional symptoms include high cholesterol levels, light-colored stools, and dark urine. Commonly, sufferers develop osteoporosis due to an alteration in vitamin D metabolism and lack of calcium absorption.

Since no known treatment for primary biliary cirrhosis exists, the therapy is supportive. If the cause of secondary biliary cirrhosis can be removed, the disease will be arrested.

A wholesome diet, exercise to toleration, sunbaths, and supplements of vitamin D and calcium are helpful.

Liver abscess

A liver abscess is a pus-filled cavity caused by bacteria or parasities. The germs commonly reach the liver from an infection in the common bile duct (resulting from a gallstone), from an infection in the intestines (carried by the blood), or from peritonitis (as from a ruptured appendix). A complication of amebic dysentery is the spread of the organism *Entamoeba histolytica* via the bloodstream to the liver, where it forms a solitary **amebic abscess.**

The usual symptoms include chills, fever, loss of appetite, vomiting, and weight loss. Additional symptoms consist of pain over the right abdomen and even in the right shoulder, with a tender, enlarged liver.

Blood tests and stool analyses, together with a CT scan, will enable a precise diagnosis. Treatment will involve the appropriate antiinfective medications (antibiotics or anti-amebic agents), and drainage of the abscess, with a needle or by surgery.

Cancer of the liver

Primary cancer of the liver is common in developing countries where chronic hepatitis B is widespread. Elsewhere it is rarely seen.

Metastic cancers develop elsewhere in the body and are carried to the liver by the blood. Common sources are the gastrointestinal tract (the stomach, colon, pancreas, gallbladder, etc.), the lung, the breast, and the blood itself (leukemia).

As the metastatic tumors grow, the condition becomes worse. Sometimes no symptoms appear until the late stages of the disease. Weakness with loss of appetite and weight, an enlarged, tender liver, and jaundice with ascites (accumulation of fluid in the abdomen) eventually develop.

Your physician may recommend chemotherapy, and possibly radiation, but generally temporary benefit is all that can be expected.

Disorders of the gallbladder and bile ducts

Gallstones

Gallstones, as the term suggests, are stonelike objects that form within the gallbladder. They start as tiny granules and gradually enlarge. In the Western world some 10 percent of people suffer from the disease, and 30 percent of those over sixty-five. Gallstones occur twice as frequently in women as in men. Obesity, high levels of cholesterol or bilirubin (a breakdown product of hemoglobin) in the bile, and the presence of estrogen favor the formation of stones.

The majority of those with gallstones have no symptoms, or the symptoms are "silent." Difficulties arise when the stone or stones move out of the gallbladder and become

873

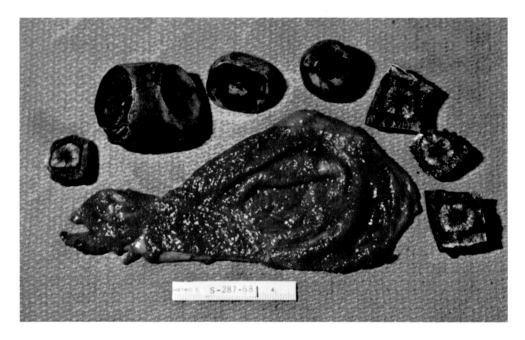

Gallbladder, showing inner lining and a variety of gallstones.

lodged in a bile duct. The bile duct goes into spasm, causing excruciating pain, chills, and fever. The pain may be felt in the right shoulder. The consumption of alcohol and meals high in fat may trigger an attack.

Should the stone move on down the duct into the intestine, the symptoms immediately subside. However, when the stone prevents the flow of bile into the duodenum, jaundice results. Backed-up bile may also cause an inflammation in the gallbladder (cholecystitis). Should the blockage occur beyond where the duct of the pancreas joins the common bile duct, the pancreas may become inflamed (pancreatitis).

What you can do. You can do little or nothing to prevent gallstones. Dietary procedures are uncertain. If you are overweight, this should be corrected.

What your physician can do. He will order certain blood tests and an X-ray study of the gallbladder and bile ducts using a dye which concentrates in the bile (cholecystogram). Most gallstones cast shadows on the film. Other tests include visual appraisal using ultrasound. While some cholesterol stones can be dissolved using bile acid medications (chenodeoxycholic acid), the procedure takes months to years, and the stones may recur. Following surgical removal—the most common treatment—recovery is prompt, and residual handicaps rare.

Inflammation of the gallbladder (cholecystitis)

Inflammation of the gallbladder, called cholecystitis, is usually caused by a gallstone lodging in the gallblad-

874

der (cystic) duct, but may, on occasion, result from an infection traveling up the bile duct from the duodenum.

The symptoms of acute inflammation of the gallbladder include nausea, vomiting, severe pain in the right upper abdomen, and possibly jaundice. It may subside in a few days or may become chronic. Chronic cholecystitis may cause feelings of indigestion, bloating, gas formation, and mild discomfort to severe pain. A severely inflamed gallbladder sometimes ruptures. This is a serious complication, that causes peritonitis.

What you can do. If you have had gallbladder problems or develop any of the above symptoms, see your physician.

What your physician can do. He will make the diagnosis, following procedures described under "gallstones." Either immediate surgical removal or a course of antibiotic therapy is usually the treatment of choice. A chronically inflamed gallbladder may become malignant.

Disorders of the pancreas

Pancreatitis is an inflammation of the pancreas, a gland which provides digestive enzymes to the upper small intestine, and the hormones insulin and glucagon to control blood sugar levels.

Acute pancreatitis

Acute pancreatitis is a complication of gallstones, alcoholism, mechanical injury, a perforating peptic ulcer, the mumps virus, and many medications. The symptoms include severe pain in the upper abdomen and back, nausea, vomiting, fever, and jaundice if the bile ducts are involved. The sufferer may have a drop in blood pressure and lapse into shock.

What you can do. Should you suspect this problem, seek medical help immediately. Discontinue all beverage alcohol.

What your physician can do. Blood tests will reveal certain changes in the levels of pancreatic enzymes. X-rays may aid in diagnosis. The treatment requires immediate hospitalization, with the relief of pain, intravenous fluids to prevent shock, and antibiotics if an infection is suspected. The activity of the pancreas is reduced to a minimum by giving certain medications, prohibiting food, and removing gastric fluids. Complications such as kidney failure must be treated. If the physician suspects gallbladder disease, the gallbladder is removed as soon as practical. An abscess in the pancreas requires surgical intervention.

Chronic pancreatitis

Chronic pancreatitis is commonly associated with chronic alcoholism. It may also result from repeated attacks of acute pancreatitis, gallbladder disease, obstruction of the pancreatic duct, injury, familial pancreatitis, medications, and unknown causes. Portions of the pancreatic tissue may be destroyed in this slowly developing disease. Symp-

875

toms include an inability to handle fatty foods, stools that are fat filled and float on water, and usually a dull, boring pain deep in the mid-abdomen. Alcohol and fatty meals often precipitate an attack.

What you can do. Abstain completely from alcohol and follow a diet low in fat and high in fiber.

What your physician can do. Sometimes surgical removal of damaged tissue proves helpful. In a few cases total removal of the pancreas has been beneficial. Enzymes and hormones produced by the pancreas must be taken to make up the loss.

Cancer of the pancreas

Cancer of the pancreas has been increasing during the past fifty years, and now accounts for 3 percent of all cancers and about 5 percent of all cancer deaths. It is one of the least favorable forms of cancer, for its survival rate, even after treatment, is less than 1 percent. Recent evidence suggests that cancer of the pancreas is more common among coffee drinkers than among non-users, although this has not been fully confirmed.

The usual symptoms include loss of appetite, nausea, vomiting, weight loss, pain, and frequently jaundice. Unfortunately, by the time the tumor is discovered 80 to 90 percent of cancers have already spread (metastasized) to other organs. Surgical removal of the cancer improves prognosis only when it is performed early. Chemotherapy and irradiation therapy seldom extend survival.

General disorders of the digestive system

Gas

Gas formed within the digestive tract is expelled either through the mouth by belching or through the passing of gas through the rectum (flatus). The gas trapped in between may cause distention, discomfort, and even pain.

Without realizing it, some people develop the habit of swallowing air, especially when they are nervous, anxious, or chewing gum. This air accumulates in the stomach, giving a feeling of fullness, and is relieved by belching. Unless the individual corrects the habit of air swallowing, relief will be temporary.

Air formed in the small and large intestines passes out through the rectum and is termed **flatulence.** Foods especially prone to cause flatulence include cabbage, celery, cucumbers, onions, peppers, beans, and broccoli. Carbonated or alcoholic drinks may have the same effect. Those who lack the enzyme lactase are unable to digest milk sugar or lactose, which produces much gas (see page 858). Avoiding those foods which by experience are found to produce gas can provide relief.

Because a number of serious disorders, such as gastritis, celiac disease, sprue, ileus, ulcerative colitis, and intestinal obstruction cause gas and distension, see your physician if you are troubled with gas, especially if you have other symptoms.

Constipation

Constipation is a condition in which bowel movements are poorly timed and infrequent, inadequate, being hard and small, or are difficult to pass.

The term means different things to different people. Some feel they need several stools a day, while others are content with one every few days. When the individual pattern of evacuation is less frequent than usual, becomes harder, and passes with greater difficulty, the person is constipated.

While a number of factors may result in constipation, without a doubt the most common is simply ignoring the urge to defecate, the so-called "call of nature." Generally the urge is strongest on arising or soon after breakfast, but people may find this an inconvenient time and suppress the urge. Suppressed repeatedly, the natural desire declines and eventually is lost.

Other causes include an inadequate intake of water, lack of physical exercise, a decreased intake of food, a diet low in fiber or roughage (refined foods and foods of animal origin), emotional tension, and confinement in bed. Still other reasons, some more serious, consist of fear of pain (due to hemorrhoids or anal fissure), hypothyroidism, the use of pain killers (codeine, etc.), aluminum antacids, and obstruction or stricture of the bowel (from polyps, cancer, etc.).

What you can do. Try to determine which cause fits your situation and then take corrective action. Establish a specific time for going to stool and do not be rushed. Drink generously of water, eat a diet high in fiber (see page 92), and take some extra fiber (ground psyllium seed). Exercise regularly and check your medications. Taking laxatives regularly may establish a laxative habit. If the above suggestions do not help, discuss your problem with your physician. If you have experienced a sudden change in your bowel habits, see him immediately.

What your physician can do. A thorough physical examination will relieve your mind that no serious problem exists. If you suspect your medications, consult with your physician.

Diarrhea

Diarrhea, an increase in the frequency and fluidity (looseness) of the stools, is caused by too much water in the intestine. Normally the intestine processes an estimated 10 quarts (9.5 liters) of water daily, allowing only 3 to 4 ounces (90 to 120 milliliters) to reach the rectum. When water fails to be absorbed from the intestine or is drawn into the intestine, diarrhea results. Several causes for this problem exist.

1. Failure of digestion. An example consists of a lack of lactase, which inhibits the digestion of lactose (milk sugar), draws water into the intestine, and causes diarrhea. Diseases of the pancreas and malnutrition are the underlying causes.

2. Food sensitivities. As an example, the gliadin found in the gluten

877

of certain grains (wheat, rye) has a toxic action on the villi of the intestinal mucosa, leading to, among other problems, diarrhea.

3. Infections of the digestive tract. So-called stomach flu or **gastroenteritis** may be due to viruses and bacteria **(enteritis)** in children, and usually to bacteria or parasites in adults. In enteritis the inflamed mucosa pours out fluid, and intestinal contractions increase, propelling the fluid mass downward for evacuation. Diarrhea results from the body's attempt to rid itself of the infection. Salmonella and Shigella frequently cause food poisoning, and Giardia and ameba may be involved. Pathogenic colon bacilli and other organisms bring on **"traveller's diarrhea."** In some parts of the world cholera and typhoid fever cause diarrhea.

4. Toxic substances. The ingestion of poisonous mushrooms, or other toxic substances may cause severe gastroenteritis and diarrhea.

5. Medications. A number of medications act on the bowel wall. Antibiotics are among the most common. They frequently kill off susceptible microorganisms in the intestine, thus upsetting the balance of organisms and causing diarrhea.

6. Emotional diarrhea. Anxiety and emotional stress excite the muscles and mucous glands in the lower colon, causing increased mucus and strong contractions that result in severe diarrhea.

7. Diseases of the digestive tract. Numerous diseases cause diarrhea, including ulcerative colitis, Crohn's disease, celiac disease, sprue, irritable colon, pancreatitis, and cancer of the large intestine.

Symptoms of diarrhea may vary from mildly loose stools to violent purges, accompanied with cramping and abdominal pain, vomiting, fever, and blood-tinged stools.

What you can do. Usually one should not treat a mild diarrhea because the diarrhea is the body's attempt to rid itself of the infection or irritation. If the diarrhea is accompanied with vomiting, abdominal pain, blood in the stools, and fever, see your physician. If these symptoms are not present, preparations of kaolin with pectin or bismuth often bring prompt relief.

What your physician can do. He may order a culture of the stool and do a rectal (sigmoidoscopic) examination should he suspect some serious disorder.

Depending on the severity of the problem, he may advise intravenous fluids, an antibiotic, or medication which will prevent the diarrhea. If an antibiotic causes the diarrhea, he may change or discontinue it, and he may recommend that you take yogurt, cultured milk, or a powder of Lactobacillus acidophilus to restore balance among the bowel microflora.

Abdominal pain

The abdominal and pelvic cavities form a single unit. Within them are found the digestive, urinary, and reproductive systems, and large blood vessels, lymphatics, and nerves pass through them. Thus abdominal pain may be a symptom of many different disorders. Therefore a physician finds it difficult to differentiate the types of pain and to pinpoint a specific problem.

The person who has pain can greatly facilitate the work of the physician by keeping a detailed record of the type of pain (aching, boring, burning, cutting, dull, gripping, stabbing, sharp, or throbbing) and whether it is continuous or comes and goes, when it was first noticed, and how it began—suddenly or gradually.

You should also try to give the physician answers to these questions: Is the pain general or localized in some particular area? If localized, where is it most noticeable? Has its location changed since it began? If so, from where to where? Has it become more intense or less intense? Has it been relieved by lying down, change of position, or by other activity?

How does food intake affect the pain? Does it increase it or relieve it? Does the type of food make a difference? Is it influenced by a bowel movement? Has the pattern of bowel movements changed recently? Do you belch or pass rectal gas? Is your abdomen distended? Does exercise have any effect? Is it worse at certain times of the day, or does it wake you at night? Have you experienced recent weight change—gain or loss? If the problem is with an infant or small child, has the growth rate been affected? Has the pain been accompanied by other symptoms such as nausea, vomiting, diarrhea, constipation, or blood in the vomit or stool? Have you taken any medications, and what has been their effect?

Information such as the above will help your physician assess your problem and speed an early diagnosis so that appropriate treatment can be instituted.

Peritonitis

Peritonitis is an inflammation of the peritoneum, the smooth membrane that lines the abdominal cavity and covers the organs within it. Generally it is a complication of a disorder in the abdomen or pelvis, such as a ruptured appendix or diverticulum, a perforated stomach or duodenal ulcer, an infection carried through the Fallopian tubes, a penetrating wound from the outside into the abdominal cavity, and abdominal surgery.

When peritonitis develops, the underlying condition suddenly worsens. The new symptoms include severe pain in the abdomen or pelvis, rigidity of the abdominal muscles, progressive distention (bloating), nausea, vomiting, fever, and pain on breathing.

What you can do. Peritonitis is generally a surgical emergency, so see your physician immediately or go to a hospital.

What your physician can do. He will order blood tests and possibly X-rays and then schedule surgical repair of the underlying problem as soon as possible. He may prescribe intravenous fluids for dehydration and shock, and antibiotics to help quell the infection. The contents of the stomach or intestines may be removed by suction.

CHAPTER 8

The mouth and teeth

The term *mouth* is used loosely to refer to the lower part of the face, and especially to the space behind the lips in which the teeth and tongue are located.

The external mouth

Just beneath the skin of the face are many small muscles that control facial expression. These respond to moods and emotions and enable the face to convey unspoken feelings of joy, delight, amusement, perplexity, disapproval, or sorrow. The portions of the face around the mouth, as well as those around the eyes, cooperate in forming smiles, frowns, and grimaces.

The upper and lower lips form a *door* that can open and close, revealing the teeth and the entrance to an inner chamber. The framework of the mouth consists of a lower jaw **(mandible)** that is movable and an upper jaw **(maxilla),** that is stationary.

The lower jaw is shaped like a flattened horseshoe with upturned ends. You can feel the round shape of your jaw by placing your thumb and index

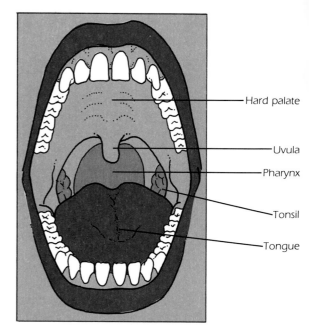

Diagram of open mouth showing major structures.

— Hard palate

— Uvula

— Pharynx

— Tonsil

— Tongue

finger at the center of your chin just under your mouth and moving them back on either side of your face. You can feel the movement of the upturned, rounded ends of your mandible by placing your fingers just in front of your ears and opening and closing your mouth. As you continue opening and closing your mouth you will discover that the lower jaw is the only bone of your face that moves.

The right and left rounded ends

of the mandible, called **condyles,** fit into two shallow depressions on the underside of the right and left temporal bones. These bones make up a part of the skull. The two joints, the **temporomandibular,** are unique because they not only permit the mandible to be hinged so that the mouth can be opened and closed, but also allow the jaw to slide forward and backward and from side to side. Since the teeth are anchored in the upper and lower jaws, this wide range of motion aids in the grinding of food. These movements are accomplished by the specifically located muscles of mastication.

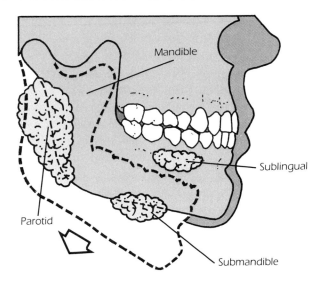

The salivary glands as related to the mandible.

The internal mouth (oral cavity)

Like a room, the mouth has walls, a roof and a floor, and an entrance and an exit. Its walls are formed by the cheeks and lips. Its roof, which also forms the floor of the nose, consists of a hard palate in front that continues on to become a soft palate in the back (see accompanying diagram). The tongue makes up part of the floor. The front entrance is opened by parting the lips. At the back of the mouth is the pharynx that opens two ways: above into the nasal cavity, and below into the larynx and esophagus. The upper and lower jaws have embedded in their opposing surfaces the upper and lower sets of teeth.

The salivary glands

The entire inside of the mouth is lined with a membrane (the mucosa) that is embedded with glands that secrete mucus. This mucus membrane is smooth and slippery, and it is especially designed to reduce the friction from the movement of food in the mouth. The food is moved about in the mouth and placed between the teeth by the tongue, lips, and cheeks so that it can be crushed and ground.

The saliva, pouring from three sets of salivary glands, further moistens the mucosa, and at the same time mixes with the food as it is ground between the teeth. Without saliva it would be almost impossible to swallow food.

The largest of the salivary glands, called parotids, are located below and in front of each ear. The saliva is conveyed from each gland by a tiny duct within the cheek. These ducts open just opposite the second molar teeth

881

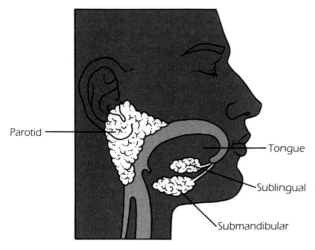

The salivary glands as related to the tongue and cheek.

on the upper right and left sides of the mouth. Two salivary glands are located on the right and left sides underneath the tongue. Their secretions enter the mouth by a number of very small ducts. Two submandibular glands lie on the floor of the mouth at the tip of the tongue, their two ducts opening on the right and left side of the midline just behind the lower front teeth.

The tongue

The tongue is a marvelous organ, especially designed for precise movements. It is the primary means by which food is moved about in the mouth for chewing and swallowing. It also helps to shape the sounds of words. The tongue is made up of seven pairs of muscles whose fibers interlace and run vertically, longitudinally, and sideways. This permits the tongue to be extended out of the mouth or drawn back, and moved in just about any direction.

The tongue is covered on its sides

and undersurface by the same membrane that lines other parts of the mouth. However, this covering is modified on the tongue's upper surface by many tiny papillae that make the surface rough enough to move food from place to place as it is being chewed. Although it is a small organ, the tongue is supplied by three sets of nerves. One set activates the tongue's muscles and controls its movements. Another set provides the sensations of temperature, touch, pressure, and pain. The fibers of the third set terminate in **taste buds** that are embedded in the surface of the tongue and make it possible for us to taste food that is sweet, sour, bitter, and salty. (For further discussion, see page 1155.)

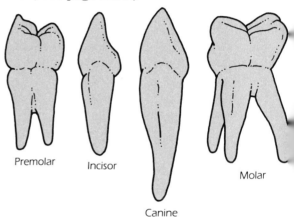

The teeth

The teeth are set in the upper and lower jaws (mandibles) and help to shape the face. During his lifetime, each person is provided with two sets of teeth. The first set consists of twenty "primary teeth," also called deciduous, milk, or baby teeth. A secondary set of thirty-two teeth appears later and gradually replaces the primary teeth.

The individual teeth of these two sets make their appearance in the mouth according to a fairly precise schedule (see figure at right) that begins when an infant is about seven and a half months old and continues throughout childhood to about age twenty-one. The ages given in the diagram are approximately those at which the teeth erupt through the soft tissues of the gums and become available for chewing.

However, the teeth are in the process of formation long before that event—some for many months and others for many years. Each tooth, both primary and secondary, begins developing before birth as a group of cells or **"tooth buds"** in the upper and lower mandible. The primary teeth begin to develop about seven weeks after conception and are already well formed at the time of birth. Several months after birth they make their appearance by pushing through the soft tissues of the gums, as indicated in the diagram.

The permanent teeth begin their development about five months after conception. Thus a preschool child has two sets of teeth present in the mouth: the primary teeth, already in place by the time he is three, and the permanent teeth, still hidden within the deeper tissues of the jaws awaiting their respective times for erupting.

The body provides two successive sets of teeth during the life cycle to accommodate growth. The smaller primary set is adapted to the smaller jaw of a young child, but as the jaws become larger they are replaced by the permanent teeth.

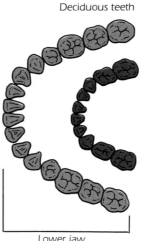

Deciduous teeth   Permanent teeth

Lower jaw   Upper jaw

1. Central incisor (7-9 yrs.)   8. Wisdom tooth (17+ yrs.)

2. Lateral incisor (7-9 yrs.)   9. Central incisor (6-8 mos.)

3. Canine (9-12 yrs.)   10. Lateral incisor (8-10 mos.)

4. First premolar (10-12 yrs.)   11. Canine (16-20 mos.)

5. Second premolar (10-12 yrs.)   12. Anterior molar (12-16 mos.)

6. First molar (6-7 yrs.)   13. Posterior molar (20-40 mos.)

7. Second molar (11-13 yrs.)

The deciduous and permanent teeth with approximate times of eruption.

Eruption of the permanent teeth. The thirty-two permanent—twelve more than in the primary set—include three molar teeth on each side of the upper and lower jaws, just behind the last tooth of the baby set. The first molars of the permanent set come into the mouth at approximately age six ("six-year molars"), about the same time that the central incisors of the primary set are being replaced by the central incisors of the permanent set. The replacement of these central incisors attracts special attention, because children notice that their front teeth start to get loose and are soon ready to drop out or be pulled out. The slightly larger central incisors of the permanent set emerge into the space that is left.

The eruption of the first molar tooth of the permanent set is often unnoticed, and even after it has erupted it is sometimes mistaken for a baby tooth. This is unfortunate, for this first permanent tooth is designed to remain throughout life unless it is destroyed by disease. If the child and his parents fail to take care of this first molar tooth, it will become the most susceptible of all the teeth to dental decay.

The permanent teeth make their appearance in the mouth during the childhood and early teen years, while the jaws are still growing. That is why the third permanent molars, called "wisdom teeth," do not erupt until after the seventeenth year. There isn't enough room in the jaw for all thirty-two teeth until that age. Since we all have just two sets of teeth during our lifetime, adequate care is important, especially proper brushing and regular visits to the dentist.

Impacted and crowded teeth. Occasionally the jaws do not grow enough to provide room for the third molars, even by adulthood. When this happens, the third molars move into abnormal positions, sometimes being directed toward the second molars and preventing them from erupting. Teeth that cannot erupt are said to be impacted. Your dentist will advise you as to whether an impacted tooth should be removed.

A jaw that is not large enough to accommodate all thirty-two permanent teeth may also cause some teeth to be misplaced, overlapping one another and coming in crooked. Children who have this problem should be taken to

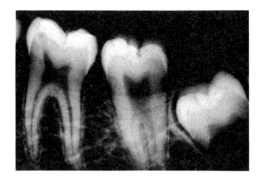

X-ray of the third molar prior to eruption.

an orthodontist—a dentist who is especially trained to treat misaligned teeth. The orthodontist may recommend removing certain teeth to make room for others. He may also fasten braces to the teeth—temporary mechanical devices that apply a constant, gentle pressure to the misplaced teeth, guiding them into more favorable positions.

Care of the primary teeth. Because the primary teeth serve as space retainers for the permanent teeth, the premature loss of a baby tooth allows adjacent primary teeth to crowd into the space that should be reserved for a later permanent tooth.

For this reason, a child's primary teeth should be given adequate care (proper brushing and hygiene) to preserve them in a healthy state. This will encourage proper alignment of the permanent teeth.

If a primary tooth is knocked out of your child's mouth accidentally, or if it must be removed for some reason, your dentist will advise you whether a false tooth or a dental retainer would be the best way to maintain

A tooth: its structure and surroundings

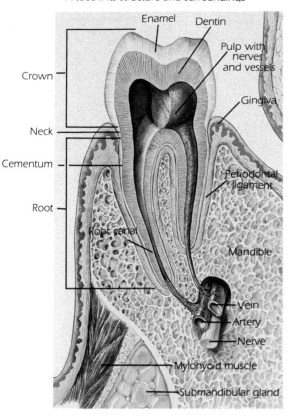

Cutaway showing the internal structures of a tooth, gum, and mandible.

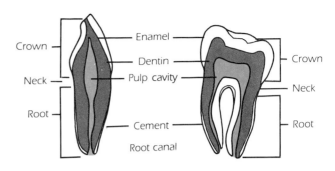

Section through an incisor and a molar tooth.

the space into which the permanent tooth will grow.

Some children develop habits such as thumb sucking, nail biting, lip biting, tongue thrusting, and pencil biting that exert pressure against their teeth while the tissues of their jaws are still pliable. These practices may adversely affect the positioning of their teeth. Helping a child to break these habits requires that the parents be firm, yet wise and understanding. Consistent direction should be accompanied by warmth and affection. Your dentist may be very helpful during this time.

Tooth shape and structure. The teeth are designed for a variety of functions. The chisel-shaped incisors cut and bite. The canines tear food and shred it. The premolars tear and grind, while the heavy-faceted molars, with their rounded prominences, crush and grind.

All teeth, both primary and secondary, are constructed of the same basic materials. A layer of **enamel** covering the tooth above the gum line forms the visible portion of the tooth called the **crown.** Dental enamel, made largely of slats of calcium and phosphorus, is the hardest substance in the body. Fully formed enamel is inert and incapable of repairing itself. Once it is damaged by decay or chemically or physically eroded (by acid-containing drinks or by excessive brushing), it must be replaced by materials selected by your dentist.

Underneath the enamel, the body of a tooth consists mostly of **dentin,** a substance softer than enamel but slightly harder than bone. The dentin

885

is made of thousands of tiny tubes radiating from the pulp chamber (see above) to the enamel. The fluid that flows through these tubes is an internal defense mechanism that protects the tooth from decay. The dentin, rather than the enamel, is the part of the tooth that is sensitive to pain, pressure, heat, and cold.

The hollow within the dentin, called the **pulp cavity,** extends into the **root** or roots (root canals) of each tooth. The pulp chamber and root canal are filled with blood vessels and nerves that enter at the tip of each root and provide nourishment and life to the tooth. The dentin of each root is covered by a hard, bone-like substance called cementum. A **periodontal ligament** (see illustration on page 885) attaches the cementum-covered root to its bony socket. The incisors and canines usually have a single root, the premolars or bicuspids one or two, while the molars have two or three and sometimes four.

Each tooth is embedded in a **socket** lined with a dense tissue called the periodontal ligament. This tissue, which is very strong, acts as a cushion that allows slight movement of the tooth and helps to prevent fracture when something very hard is bitten.

The gums (gingiva)

The gums or gingiva firmly surround the tooth between the crown and the root. The gingival crevice is a tiny space above the place where the gum attaches to the periodontal ligament. The periodontal ligament securely fastens the gum to the tooth, and it also fastens the teeth to one another.

Preventive tooth care

Germs are constantly present in the mouth. These germs can be reduced by keeping the teeth clean, but the mouth will never be germ free, regardless of the claims made for certain toothpastes or antiseptic mouthwashes. Food particles remain in the mouth after a person eats, and fragments of food cling to the surfaces of the teeth, especially in the fissures of the grinding surfaces and in the spaces between the teeth and between the teeth and the gums. Unless they are removed, these food particles, along with bacteria and mucus, form a gelatinous film called **plaque** that adheres to the surface of the tooth.

If the teeth are neglected, additional layers of plaque are added to the film day after day. If it is not removed, this plaque will eventually calcify into a hard, rough surface called **calculus.** Plaque especially tends to form in areas that are hard to reach with a toothbrush—between the teeth and at the gum margin. The bacteria in plaque break down food particles, especially sugar, producing an acid that erodes the enamel and initiates decay. The rough edges of the plaque irritate the gum margins, which become red and swollen and bleed easily **(gingivitis).** If the problem is neglected, the site becomes infected and eventually results in **periodontitis.**

Regular **brushing** of the teeth, especially after meals and before bedtime, will reduce the presence of food remnants and help prevent the formation of plaque. It is best to use a soft-bristle brush with a gentle, vibrating motion, allowing the bristles to work from the gums to the spaces between the teeth. This should be done on both the outer and inner surfaces of all teeth. Fluoride toothpaste is helpful but not essential. Brushing the gums will also help to prevent gingivitis.

Also important is the use of **dental floss** to clean the spaces between the teeth. Floss removes both food particles and developing plaque. The floss should be rubbed against the side of the tooth with both a back-and-forth and up-and-down movement. Care should be taken to avoid snapping the floss through the space between the teeth, as this can injure the gums. One of the best safeguards for the teeth is regular cleaning by a dentist or dental hygienist. They will be happy to show you how to brush and how to use floss. Both procedures are simple, but they must be done correctly in order to avoid damage to your gums and teeth.

Diet plays a very important role in preventing tooth decay. Refined cereals (white flour, degerminated corn meal, white rice) and foods to which large amounts of refined sugar have been added, should seldom be eaten. These include many breakfast cereals, cakes, pies, cookies, candy, soft drinks, and ice cream. Refined sugar produces acid and gives bacteria a ready source of energy. Damage may occur within twenty minutes, and repeated exposure can weaken the enamel.

Sugar also has a systemic effect on the teeth. A large amount of sugar raises the blood sugar level, causing the fluid flowing through the tubes in the dentin to slow and perhaps even to stop. Since the fluid flows from the pulp cavity outward, the invading bacteria are not resisted.

During World War II, refined cereals and sugar were highly rationed in England and other countries of Europe. After the war it was found that the children of parents who ate this less refined diet prior to and during pregnancy were less susceptible to tooth decay. The longer the mother had been on this unrefined diet before becoming pregnant, the greater was her children's resistance to tooth decay.

By altering its crystalline structure, **fluoride** plays an important part in the formation of enamel. Because the enamel is more resistant to the acids produced by bacteria, the tooth is less susceptible to decay. The resistance of the teeth to decay is increased whenever fluoride constitutes one part per million (0.7 to 1.2) of drinking water, whether the fluoride is naturally present in the water or added by the municipal water supply. Despite the fact that dietary habits have changed little and caries-producing bacteria still inhabit the mouth, there has been a significant drop in tooth decay in children since the addition of fluoride to many of the city water supplies across the country.

Some people are bitterly opposed to adding fluoride to drinking water. However, large numbers of cities have more natural fluoride in their drinking water than is added to water supplies that lack this element. About half the cities in the United States now have fluoride in their water supplies, either naturally or added. It is true that excessive amounts of fluoride are harmful to the teeth, causing them to develop white spots called **fluorosis.** However, appropriate amounts cause no side effects.

Toothpastes and mouth washes containing fluoride appear to have a protective effect at any time of life. However, fluoride's greatest benefit is seen before and for about one year after the tooth erupts. Children especially need fluoride during the period of tooth formation, from soon after birth till about fourteen years of age. Your dentist can recommend a fluoride supplement if the water in your area lacks this mineral.

See your dentist regularly and catch problems early.

CHAPTER 9

Disorders of the teeth

The story of dentistry dates back to very early times. Egyptian records depict "dentists" extracting teeth. During the following centuries, history records that teeth were wired into place to protect the facial appearance, gold was used for restoration, and bridge work was attempted, as was the transplanting of teeth!

Two hundred years ago there were less than 100 dentists in the United States. Dentistry was performed by surgeons, pharmacists, barbers, and any layperson who had the courage to undertake the procedures. The "dentist" was required to be both a mechanic and an innovator. His instruments were crude but oft times ingenious. He worked in a shop, required a good chair, steady hands, and a brave heart. But little progress could be made until pain could safely be relieved.

It finally happened in 1844. A dentist by the name of Horace Wells and a friend were attending a circus. In one of the sideshows volunteers were asked to inhale nitrous oxide

(NO_2) or laughing gas. Wells' friend did so, and forthwith fell into a fight with the attendant. During the scuffle his friend gashed his leg. When asked about his injury he was surprised to find he was hurt, for he had felt no pain.

Wells put it together. Later he inhaled the nitrous oxide gas while a dentist friend painlessly extracted a tooth. About the same time, another dentist by the name of William Morton used ether as an anesthetic. In this way two American dentists introduced pain-free dentistry to the world.

Until the early part of the nineteenth century, no formal course in dentistry existed. Each man stood on his own, learning what he could from what he heard and read. Then, in 1840, in Baltimore, Maryland, the Baltimore College of Dental Surgery was established, the first school of dentistry in the world, and America became the leader in training quality dentists.

Dentists quickly adapted new discoveries to their professional needs.

For example, Charles Goodyear invented vulcanizing, and for many years vulcanite was used for holding teeth in partial and complete dentures. Casting techniques improved, and the drill and other specially crafted instruments became commonplace tools in the dentist's office. The invention of the X-ray as a diagnostic instrument and the discovery and use of local anesthetics enabled dentists to accomplish otherwise impossible tasks.

Dentistry today is a highly specialized discipline. As a result, teeth are rarely lost. High-speed drills prepare teeth to be filled with a spectrum of materials—amalgams, plastic resins, and ceramics. Misaligned teeth are moved into place (orthodontics). Infected root canals are restored (endodontics). Infected gums are treated and preserved (periodontics).

Preventive measures are now in the forefront. Better nutrition, fluoridation of drinking water, improved hygiene of teeth and gums, and early treatment have greatly reduced tooth decay and gum disease in the United States and other countries.

Modern dentistry is indeed a science and an art. The once-feared visit to the dentist's office has given way to painless procedures that protect and restore the structures of the teeth, the mouth, and even the face.

Dental problems

Malocclusion

Ideally the teeth of each jaw are straight and regularly spaced. The ones above mesh with those below, except for the front upper teeth, which slightly overlap those below. Unfortunately, this ideal is not commonly seen.

One usually sees crowding (too many teeth for the space available), gaping (too few teeth), crooked teeth (sloping forward, backward, or sideways), excessive tooth wear, loose teeth, offset jaws (either protruding or one poorly aligned to the other), pain in the joints of the jaw, or an assortment of these problems. Depending on the degree of the malocclusion, one may have difficulty in chewing; trouble keeping the teeth clean, thus making them more susceptible to tooth decay and inflammation of the gums around the teeth (periodontitis); and adversely affected appearance.

Malocclusion occurs for a number of reasons. Many are born with one or more of these problems, inherited from their parents. The loss of baby teeth from tooth decay or from an accident causes gaping. Because of the gaps, the spacial relationships between the primary and permanent teeth are disturbed, and as the latter erupt, the teeth may come in crooked or crowded.

What you can do. Your main concerns should be to keep your teeth clean and the gums healthy by careful brushing and flossing and to seek appropriate help from your dentist. Guard against premature loss of baby teeth, and if such should occur, seek dental advice.

What your dentist can do. In minor cases of crowding, gaping, or malalignment, your dentist may be able to handle the problem. Generally you will seek the care of an **orthodontist,** one who specializes in these conditions. In children, X-rays will reveal the condition of the primary and permanent teeth. Sometimes, to provide more space, it may be necessary to remove one or more teeth. By the use of metal, plastic, or rubber appliances, crooked or out-of-line teeth can be slowly moved and positioned in proper relationship to the other teeth, resolving the problems of malocclusion. In adults, severe malocclusion may require corrective surgery, in which portions of the mandibles are removed or repositioned. With less severe problems, bridges and crowns can improve the situation.

Tooth decay (dental caries)

Tooth decay is the erosion of the enamel and underlying dentin to form a cavity of varying size.

Ninety-five percent of Americans suffer some tooth decay at one time or another, and it ranks as the second most common disease in the United States, exceeded only by the common cold. Fifty percent of three-year-olds have one or more decayed teeth. Grade school children have three or more, while those in high school (sixteen years of age) have seven decayed or missing teeth. By high school graduation, nine out of ten have some decay problem.

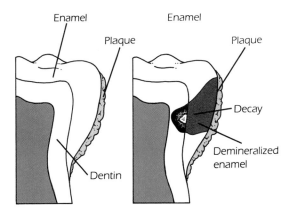

Diagram showing plaque, demineralized enamel, and decay.

The factors which combine to produce caries include bacteria in the mouth, food particles left in contact with the teeth, a generous intake of refined sugar, and an inherent susceptibility of the tooth to caries.

Bacteria (especially *Streptococcus mutans*), mucus, and food particles stick together to form a gelatinous film called plaque. Plaque adheres to the surface of the tooth, most frequently between the teeth and at the gum margin. The bacteria derive most of their energy from sugar. As the bacteria break down the sugar, acid is formed, eroding the enamel and forming a cavity. In time the dentin also erodes, and, if unchecked, the bacteria may travel via the tubules to the pulp cavity.

As the cavity in the dentin deepens, the tooth becomes sensitive to heat and cold. When the cavity reaches the pulp, it becomes inflamed and engorged with blood. The dilated vessels put pressure on the nerves, and the tooth becomes

891

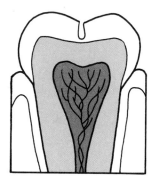
Acid attacks enamel

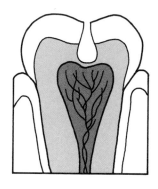
Acid erodes dentin

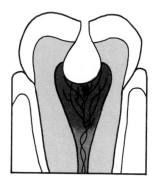
Decay enters pulp cavity

Stages of tooth decay: acid erodes enamel and dentin, and decay enters pulp chamber.

extremely painful. If the pressure is not relieved, the nerve may die. This decay process may extend down the root canal, causing an abscess in the depths of the socket.

Eating refined sugar gives bacteria a ready source of energy and produces acid. Damage occurs within twenty minutes, and repeated exposures weaken the enamel. However, sugar also has a systemic effect. When one eats generous amounts of sugar, blood sugar rises. This rise in blood sugar interferes with the regulation of the fluid flow through the dentinal canals, causing the fluid flow to slow and even stop. Because the fluid flows from the pulp cavity outward, the invading bacteria are not resisted.

During World War II the diet of people in England and on the Continent was greatly reduced in refined sugar and refined cereals. Mothers who ate this less-refined diet prior to and during pregnancy gave birth to children whose teeth were less susceptible to tooth decay. The longer the mother had been on this unrefined diet before becoming pregnant, the greater was the resistance of the teeth of her offspring.

The symptoms of tooth decay vary widely. Frequently you first realize you have a cavity when your tongue feels the rough edge or a portion of your tooth breaks. Sometimes eating very hot, very cold, or very sweet foods causes discomfort. Decaying food in a cavity may cause an unpleasant odor and taste. When the pulp is affected, one usually feels severe throbbing pain.

What you can do. If you have tooth decay, you should promptly see your dentist. However, you can do a number of things to lower the risk of, or even prevent, developing caries.

Brushing your teeth regularly after meals (especially before bedtime) will reduce the presence of food remnants and, in turn, hinder the formation of bacterial plaque.

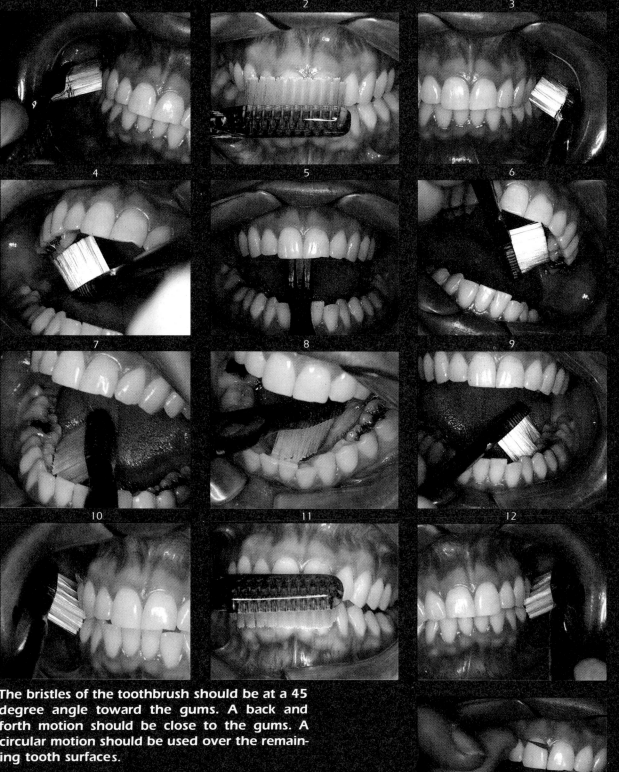

The bristles of the toothbrush should be at a 45 degree angle toward the gums. A back and forth motion should be close to the gums. A circular motion should be used over the remaining tooth surfaces.

Place the floss between the teeth and wrap it against the tooth. Move the floss up and down five to ten times. Repeat the process between all the teeth and behind the last tooth.

Use a soft-bristle brush and gently, using a rotating motion, allow the bristles to work downward from your gums to the spaces between your teeth. Do this both on the outside and inside of all your teeth. The use of toothpaste is not essential. Brushing your gums also helps to prevent gingivitis.

Flossing with either waxed or plain dental floss cleans the spaces between the teeth, removing food particles and developing plaque. The floss should be rubbed against the side of the tooth with a back and forth and up and down movement. Do not injure your gums by allowing the floss to snap through the space between your teeth. Safeguard your teeth by having them periodically **cleaned** by your dentist or a dental hygienist.

Your **diet** should include only small amounts of foods high in refined sugar and refined cereals. These include any food or drink to which a significant amount of sugar has been added. Certain breakfast cereals, cakes, pies, candy, soft drinks, and ice cream fall into this class.

See your dentist regularly so as to catch any problem early.

What your dentist can do. Should you have a cavity, your dentist will do his best to save your tooth. After removing the decayed material he will likely fill the cavity with amalgams, composites (plastic materials), cast inlays, or gold foil. If the destruction of your tooth is extensive, he may cover the tooth with a cap or crown. He will shape the good parts of the tooth, make a mold, and after the crown has been cast, anchor it to the stub. Sometimes the crown is faced with porcelain to match the color of the teeth.

As a preventive, especially for developing teeth, your dentist may recommend a fluoride supplement if your water supply is naturally deficient in fluoride. Painting the teeth with a fluoride solution has also been found to reduce caries. Even though excessive intakes of fluoride are harmful, the long use of fluorides in amounts naturally present in most drinking water supplies has shown no harmful effects.

Pulpitis

Pulpitis, an inflammation of the pulp (the most central tissue of a tooth), is the most common cause of toothache. Usually caused by neglecting to treat a cavity, infection inflames the pulp tissues, which beome swollen and put pressure on the nerves. Because the throbbing, shooting, or intermittent pain radiates, it may be difficult to identify the involved tooth.

What you can do. See your dentist. In the interim, thoroughly rinse your mouth and then place a pledget of cotton dipped in clove oil in the cavity. Mixing a few drops of clove oil in zinc oxide ointment forms a paste which may be applied to the cavity. This should provide relief for a few hours.

What your dentist can do. Your dentist (or **endodontist**) will remove the infected pulp tissue, clean the pulp cavity and root canal, and fill both. It will take more than a single visit to accomplish this. Sometimes the tooth may have to be removed. When the pulp (blood vessels and nerve) are destroyed, the tooth dies, but a dead tooth may function for years.

Abscess

A tooth abscess is a pocket of infection at the apex or tip of a root. The infection travels via the pulp down a root canal, as an extension of pulpitis, causing the bone to erode, the gums to swell, and the lymph glands in the neck to enlarge and become tender. The gum swelling or boil may burst and pus exude from the opening. The intense pain is increased by chewing and by hot and cold foods or drinks.

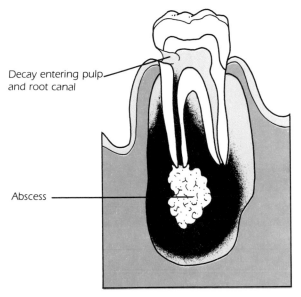

Decay entering pulp and root canal

Abscess

Diagram showing abscess at the apex of the root canal.

What you can do. Holding a mouthful of hot salt water in the area of the abscess may help bring it to a head. One teaspoonful of salt to a glass of water, held in place for a minute, done three or four times at intervals of a half hour, may be helpful.

What your dentist can do. Your dentist or orthodontist will treat the abscess in a way similar to the treatment of pulpitis.

Periodontal disease (gingivitis and periodontitis)

Periodontal disease is a bacterial infection of the tissues which surround and support the teeth, namely, the gums or gingiva, the periodontal ligament, and the bone into which the teeth fit. It is the principal cause of tooth loss after age thirty.

The disease process starts with inflammation of the gums **(gingivitis)** due to irritation caused by the products of bacterial plaque. The gums become swollen, bleed easily, and if the problem is neglected, the gum and other supporting tissues gradually separate from the teeth. Deepening pockets filled with plaque, food debris, and pus destroy the cementum and erode the bone **(periodontitis or pyorrhea)**. Pressure on the gum will cause pus to exude from the tooth margins and will be accompanied by a bad taste in the mouth and foul-smelling breath. The teeth become sensitive, eventually loosen, and may fall out.

The disease results from both local and sometimes systemic factors, most commonly poor dental hygiene. Inadequate brushing and flossing allows for plaque formation, which may mineralize to form calculus **(tartar).** As plaque builds up, irritation and infection increase. Poor dentistry

895

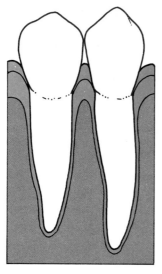
Normal

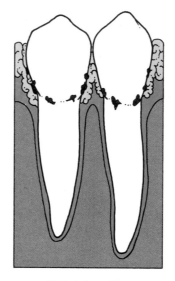
Plaque formation

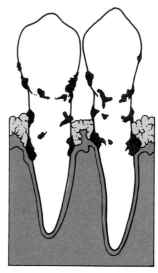
Gum retraction

with rough margins on the fillings or crowns encourages plaque development. Malocclusion, teeth grinding during sleep, and smoking also enhance the condition. Other factors that foster periodontal disease include the taking of certain drugs, vitamin C and folic acid deficiencies, diabetes, thyroid disorders, and the periods of pregnancy and puberty.

What you can do. The practice of good dental hygiene is essential (see under "dental caries"). Using a water-pick may help. However, the removal of calculus must be done by a professional.

What your dentist can do. Your dentist will employ X-rays to determine whether bone is involved, and by means of a pick measure the depths of the pockets of inflammation. Scaling will remove calculus, and a curette will remove the inflamed tissue and pus from the pockets. He may need to do surgery to open up deep pockets and decrease their depth (gingivoplasty). A

Plaque formation, gingivitis, and gum retraction.

dressing will protect the area for a week or two until the healthy tissue has reattached itself to the tooth. He can recement loose teeth and anchor them in place. Your dentist will advise you as to the best procedures.

Bridges and dentures (prosthodontics)

When a permanent tooth is lost, the missing tooth leaves a space that can, in time, produce a number of problems. The tooth above or below the gap will move downward or upward, causing trouble as the jaws move one on the other. The offending tooth will have to be ground shorter or removed. Teeth adjacent to the gap will tilt toward the space. Therefore, any missing tooth should be replaced as soon as possible.

What your dentist can do. Your

896

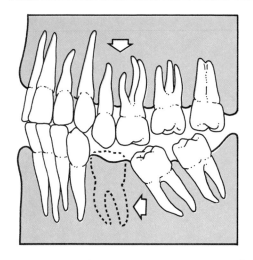

Migration of upper and lower teeth due to a missing tooth.

dentist has a number of options. He may provide you with a fixed or removable bridge. These devices hold an artificial tooth or teeth in a metal frame, either permanently fixed with crowns to the teeth on either side of the gap, or held in place with clasps and braces to adjacent teeth, to be removed as needed. He may fit you with partial or complete dentures—artificial teeth embedded in plastic material—when many or all the teeth are missing. A partial denture is held in place with clasps. A full upper denture is held in place by suction to the hard palate; a lower denture rides on the gum ridge.

The use of dentures. Even the best fitting prosthesis (bridge or denture) is less efficient and requires more care than do natural teeth. They should be kept clean at all times because food particles tend to lodge under them. Removable appliances should be carefully brushed and periodically soaked in a germ-killing solution. Because pressure placed on them during chewing is not evenly distributed on the jaws, pressure points become sore and painful, sometimes forming ulcers. See your dentist periodically for guidance and help. Because of bone shrinkage in the jaws, dentures become loose and may have to be replaced. Applying dental adhesives to the undersurface of dentures helps hold them more securely in place and prevents food from becoming lodged underneath. Metal implants are sometimes used to stabilize dentures and to replace missing teeth. Your dentist can advise as to what is best in your case.

Accidents involving teeth (fractured or dislodged)

If your tooth is accidently fractured or dislodged, act promptly. Your dentist can place a protective covering over the fracture until he can do permanent repair. If the tooth is extremely loose, do not remove it. Even a tooth moved out of place may gradually shift back into its normal position. If the tooth has fallen out, wrap it in a damp cloth (or place it in a salt solution) and go immediately to your dentist. A tooth replaced in its socket within a short time may be successfully reimplanted.

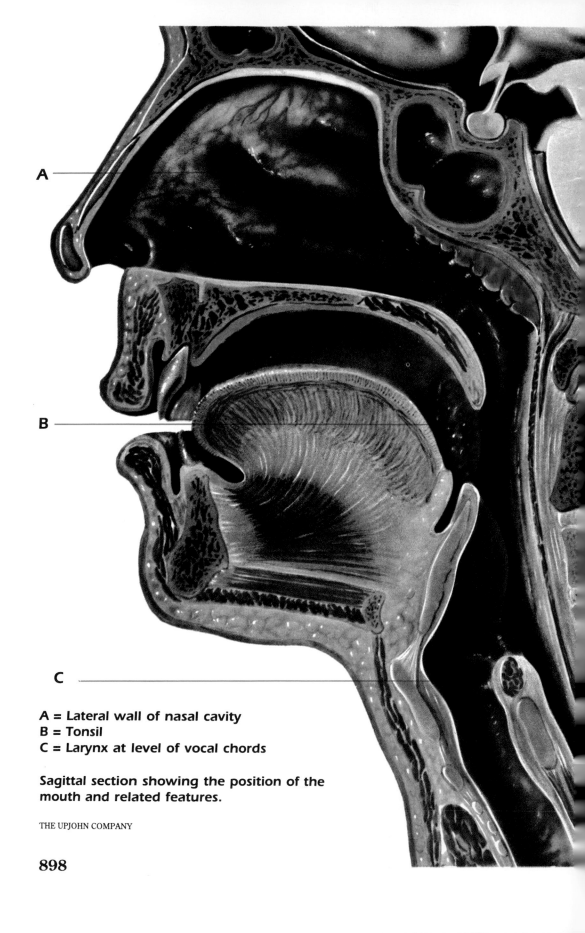

A = Lateral wall of nasal cavity
B = Tonsil
C = Larynx at level of vocal chords

Sagittal section showing the position of the
mouth and related features.

CHAPTER 10

The respiratory system

The respiratory system is designed to convey oxygen-carrying air to the blood, and to carry carbon dioxide waste from the blood out of the body. It consists of the nose, the pharynx (throat), the larynx (voice box), the trachea (windpipe), the bronchi (branches of the trachea), and the lungs. These organs are housed in the head, neck, and chest.

Oxygen is doubtless the most critical environmental need which we have. We can survive weeks without food, days without water, but only minutes without air. Twenty-four hours a day, from birth to death some seventy-five years later, breathing sixteen times each minute, we literally live by the breath of life. At any one time, under ordinary conditions, the body contains 1,200 milliliters (approximately 1.25 quarts) of oxygen—enough to last about four minutes. Actually the body does not store oxygen, so the brain cells, which are so oxygen dependent, receive permanent damage once deprived of their oxygen supply.

Ordinarily, in quiet breathing, about one pint (450 milliliters) of air is taken into the lungs with each breath. This air is drawn through the nose or mouth into the pharynx (throat), passing through the larynx (voice box), down the trachea (windpipe) into the right and left bronchi and on through their terminal branches (bronchioles) to the depths of the lungs. Oxygen from the air is transferred to the hemoglobin of the red blood cells, from where it is transported by the blood to the cells of the body. On the return journey, the red cells bring back the waste carbon dioxide to the lungs, from where it is exhaled.

The passageways through which the air passes from the nostrils to the depths of the lungs are an exquisitely designed air-conditioning system. The air is filtered, cleaned, warmed, or cooled to body temperature, and moistened when needed. The description of the respective parts of the respiratory tract will explain the way this is accomplished.

899

The nose

The nose consists of two chambers side by side, that are separated by a thin plate of cartilage and bone called the **septum.** The hard and soft palates form its base. The two nostrils open on the face, while at the back the nose opens into the throat. On the outside wall of each nasal cavity three shelves of bone increase the surface area. A membrane containing mucus-secreting glands and a rich supply of blood vessels covers the entire cavity.

Inside the nostrils are many hairs moistened by fluid from the eyes (tears), which reach the nose through the right and left tear ducts. This is why your nose "runs" when you cry. These moistened hairs filter out dust particles and other impurities. The lining membrane is provided with cilia (hairlike processes) which beat rhythmically, moving entrapped impurities backward toward the throat. Dry, hot, or cold air is humidified and warmed or cooled as it passes over the blood-rich nasal membrane.

The nose also contains the organs of smell, located high up in the nasal cavity, one on each side. The incoming air is directed into the upper parts of the nasal cavities, where it comes in contact with the smell sensors. A cold or allergy causes the mucous membranes to swell and more mucus to be secreted. The resulting congestion makes it more difficult to smell and breathe.

The nasal sinuses

The nasal sinuses are empty spaces within the bones of the face and head, with openings into the nasal cavities. One of the four pairs is found within the cheek bones; another pair in the bones above the eyes. The two remaining pairs are located above and behind the nasal cavities. The same mucous membrane lines the nasal sinuses as lines the inside of the nose. Sinusitis occurs when these lining membranes become inflamed. Just as the space within the body of a violin improves its tone, so these spaces add quality and resonance to the voice.

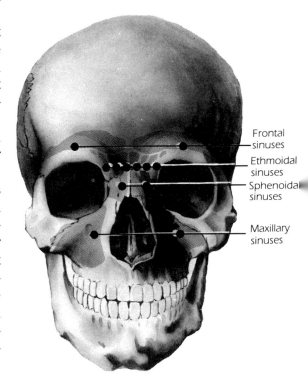

Frontal sinuses
Ethmoidal sinuses
Sphenoidal sinuses
Maxillary sinuses

Blue areas show four pairs of nasal sinuses.

900

The pharynx

The pharynx or throat is a multipurpose space located behind the nose and mouth. Into its upper part open the nasal cavities and the two auditory canals (eustachian tubes). In front is the mouth and back of the tongue, and below are the upper openings of the larynx and esophagus (gullet). Thus the pharynx forms the passageway for both air and food. Somewhat discrete collections of lymphoid tissue virtually encircle the pharynx. Above are the right and left adenoids surrounding the auditory canals. A little below the adenoids are the right and left palatine tonsils (the common tonsils). Between the tonsils are small, somewhat scattered masses of lymph tissue. And finally, on the back of the tongue is the lingual tonsil. As the air we breathe passes these lymph structures, they filter out infectious agents.

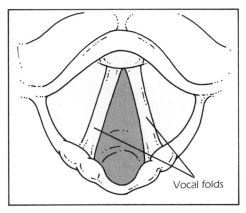

Vocal folds of larynx, viewed from above.

The larynx

The larynx or voice box is located just below the pharynx and directly in front of the upper part of the esophagus. At its lower end, the larynx is directly continuous with the trachea (windpipe). A number of cartilages, attached together with membranes, form the walls of the voice box, making it firm but flexible. Lined on the inside with a mucous membrane, it moves up or down as you swallow or speak. You may feel this movement by placing your finger on your "Adam's apple." As you swallow, the larynx moves up, and a hinged cartilage, the epiglottis, swings down, closing the opening to the larynx and thus preventing food or drink from entering the voice box and trachea.

On either side within the larynx are a pair of shelflike folds of tissue known as the vocal cords. Within the membranes covering these folds lie tiny muscles. Movements of the cartilages to which the folds are attached vary the size of the opening between them. Contracting the muscles allows the cords to tense or relax. When you speak, air coming from the lungs causes the cords to vibrate, producing sound. The level of the pitch depends on whether the cords are tense or relaxed. The volume of air, whether large or small, passing the cords determines how loud or soft the sounds will be. When not in use, the vocal cords fold back against the walls, allowing the air to pass in and out in silence.

The tongue, lips, teeth, and cheeks cooperate in forming words from the sounds produced in the larynx.

A man's voice is deep pitched because of his large larynx and his long cords. As a boy enters manhood

901

his larynx grows rapidly, and his voice changes and becomes deeper pitched. A girl's larynx does not enlarge as much as she becomes a woman; hence a woman's voice remains higher pitched throughout life.

The trachea (windpipe) and bronchi

The trachea is a straight tube that passes from the larynx to the middle of the chest, where it divides into the right and left bronchi. Each bronchus keeps rebranching, penetrating into the depths of its lung. The trachea and bronchi consist of a series of incomplete rings of cartilage secured together by intervening membranes, permitting flexibility but preventing collapse.

As in the nasal cavities, the lining membrane of the trachea and bronchi consists of millions of tall columnlike cells intermingled with goblet-shaped mucus-secreting cells. On the tip of each column cell is a cluster of hairlike cilia. These minute brushes sweep back and forth at up to sixty beats each second. The slow and gentle downward movement toward the lung contrasts with the fast and forceful upward beat toward the throat. A layer of sticky mucus floats on top of the cilia, capturing dust and other impurities in the air. Like an escalator propelled by the beating cilia, the mucous is carried to the throat, where it is swallowed or spat out. In this way each breath of air is cleaned, moistened, and warmed or cooled. When ciliary function is impaired and mucus accumulates, a

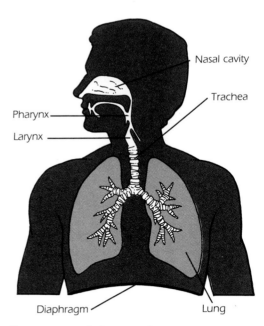

Structures of the respiratory tract.

forceful cough clears the passageways.

The lungs

The lungs, air-filled passages intimately associated with blood vessels, fill the right and left sides of the chest cavity, with the heart in between. Since the heart lies a little more to the left than to the right, the left lung is the smaller of the two. Each lung is divided into lobes; the left has two, while the right has three. Each major bronchus provides a branch to each lobe of the lung. Thereafter, these bronchi redivide about twenty times, continually becoming smaller, the smallest being called bronchioles.

These one million bronchioles further divide until each terminates in a cluster of air sacs (alveoli), num-

902

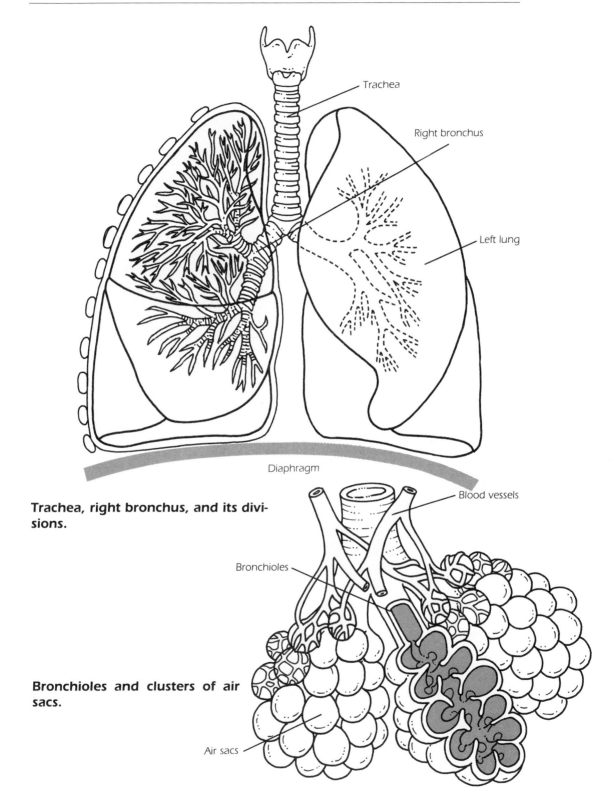

Trachea

Right bronchus

Left lung

Diaphragm

Trachea, right bronchus, and its divisions.

Blood vessels

Bronchioles

Bronchioles and clusters of air sacs.

Air sacs

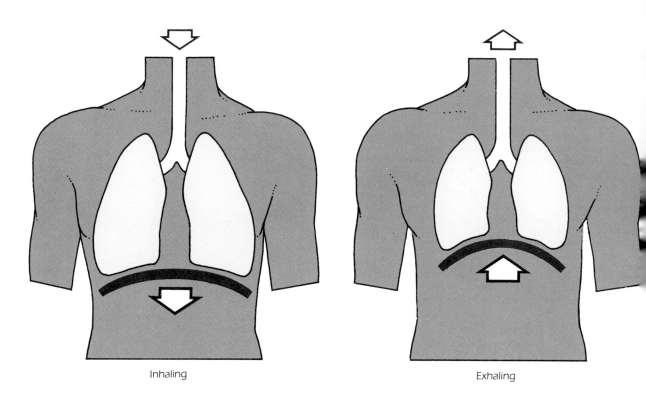

Inhaling

Exhaling

On inhaling, the diaphragm contracts, the chest cavity expands, and the lungs enlarge as they fill with air.

On exhaling, the diaphragm relaxes, the chest cavity retracts, and the lungs shrink as they empty their air.

bering in all approximately a billion. The walls of these sacs are the thickness of a bubble, just a single layer of cells, allowing oxygen and carbon dioxide to pass freely to and from the adjoining capillaries.

The lungs have two sources of blood: the pulmonary arteries, carrying veinous or oxygen-depleted blood, to be reoxygenated in the lungs; and the bronchial arteries, conveying oxygen-rich blood to provide oxygen to the cells of the lung itself. These vessels, also branching,

generally follow the dividing bronchi until their capillaries lie against the air sac walls.

Respiration

The chest cavity, which houses the lungs, is made up of the vertebrae at the back; the sides are formed by the ribs, with their intervening muscles, as they curve forward to join the breastbone in front; the base of the neck is above, and the diaphragm below. The diaphragm, a flat, umbrellalike muscle that attaches to

904

the lower margin of the lowest ribs, divides the chest from the abdominal cavity.

As you inhale, your chest cavity expands; as you exhale, your chest cavity contracts. This is accomplished by the contraction of the muscles of respiration—the diaphragm, the muscles between the ribs (intercostals), and certain muscles in the neck. When the diaphragm contracts, it increases the length of the chest by drawing the floor downward. Since the ribs slope downward and forward, when the intercostals and the muscles in the neck contract, the ribs are drawn upward and forward, increasing the depth of the chest.

The respiratory muscles work together. As the chest enlarges, the lungs expand. Air rushes in to fill the extra space made available. When the muscles relax, the chest returns to its previous size, and the air is forced out the way it came in. When the muscles of the abdomen contract, the contents of the abdomen are pushed upward against the diaphragm, forcing air out of the lungs. Holding your breath and contracting your abdominal muscles increases the pressure within the chest. Controlled, it permits you to modulate the level of your voice as you talk or shout or sing.

Ordinarily, a nerve center in the brain controls the process of breathing automatically. This center sends out nerve impulses to the breathing muscles so that they can contract and relax alternately. It even controls how fast and deeply you breathe, as, for example, when you

exercise. The center may make you stop breathing temporarily. When you swallow, your breathing stops until the food or water passes the opening into your larynx. You can voluntarily override the center by holding your breath. However, it is not possible to commit suicide in this way, because as soon as you lose consciousness, the center takes over again.

The breathing center also controls such actions as **coughing** and **sneezing.** When the lining of the air passages is irritated, the breathing center signals the abdominal muscles to contract quickly. This abruptly forces the air upward through the air passageways. In coughing, the air is forced out through the mouth; in sneezing, through the nose and mouth. The sudden action of coughing and sneezing helps to expel whatever substance caused the irritation.

Snoring is caused by the vibration of the soft tissues in the walls of the air passages as air moves in and out of the lungs. When one is asleep, the muscles that control the soft palate, the pharynx, and the larynx may relax sufficiently to allow the moving air to cause these tissues to vibrate noisily. Changing position may sometimes help. Recently, the surgical removal of redundant tissue in the pharynx has helped some snorers.

The coverings of the lungs (pleura)

The lungs are covered with a smooth, moist membrane. At the roots of the lungs, where the blood vessels enter and leave, and where the bronchi enter the lungs, this smooth covering doubles back on itself and forms a complete lining for that part of the chest in which each lung resides. These two layers of smooth membrane—one that covers the lungs and the other that lines the inside of the chest cavity—are together called the **pleura.** Normally no space separates these two layers; they rest in contact with each other. Because their surfaces are smooth and moist, they glide past each other without friction as the lungs expand and contract.

CHAPTER 11

Diseases of the respiratory system

Disorders of the nose

The nose conditions the air on its way to the lungs. It also contains the receptor organ for the sense of smell. The nasal sinuses which communicate with the nasal cavities give resonance to the voice.

Nosebleed (epistaxis)

Nosebleed is a common occurrence that is usually not a serious problem, and may happen without apparent reason. The blood comes from the rupture of tiny blood vessels in the mucous membrane lining the nasal cavities, usually on one side and in the front part of the nose. Besides injuries, nosebleeds result from picking the nose (removing crusts), breathing very dry air causing cracking of the membrane, inflammation arising from the common cold, high blood pressure, and from any one of the bleeding disorders.

What you can do. It is best to sit up and lean forward, rather than to lie down. This tends to lower your blood pressure, and allows the blood to flow out of your nose rather than into your throat. Frequently the bleeding will stop by itself when you simply hold a handkerchief to the nose. Tightening your lip against a small wad of paper placed between your upper lip and gum may help. Pinching the soft tissues of your nose or pushing your thumb against the side from which the blood is flowing for five minutes will generally stop the nosebleed. Remember not to blow your nose for several hours after it has stopped bleeding lest you dislodge the clot. If bleeding persists, especially if it has occurred repeatedly, see your physician.

What your physician can do. When the bleeding is further back in your nose, simple measures may not work. Your physician may pack your nose with moistened gauze. Occasionally the bleeding vessels must be cauterized or surgically tied. A blood test will reveal if you have an anemia or bleeding disorder, and appropriate treatment can then be instituted.

Anosmia

Anosmia consists of a loss of the sense of smell. The sense organs for smell are hairlike receptors of the olfactory nerves present in the mucous membranes located in the extreme upper part of the nose. Anosmia occurs when the passage of air through the upper nasal cavities is obstructed, as with a nasal polyp. Loss of smell may also result from atrophic rhinitis, in which the lining of the nose deteriorates, or from a skull fracture, in which the olfactory nerve is damaged.

What you can do. See your physician, who can determine the precise cause and institute appropriate treatment.

Boil

A boil is a swelling resulting from a pus-producing infection. It should not be squeezed or lanced.

What you can do. Apply hot salt compresses of gauze outside the nose and cotton inside, allowing the swelling to soften and burst. Do not squeeze the boil, as this may spread the infection. A boil in the nose can be quite serious. If it does not respond promptly, see your physician.

Injury

Your nose is constructed of cartilage and bone, with overlying skin and a mucous membrane lining within. A cartilage and bone septum divides the right and left cavities. Minor injuries will heal by themselves. Serious injuries usually result in displaced cartilages and broken bones. If allowed to be untreated, deformities will result. See your physician.

What your physician can do. He may advise you to see a specialist. Manually or surgically your nose must be reshaped so that when the swelling has subsided and healing has occurred, your appearance is preserved. The septum may have to be straightened. A splint on the outside and packing on the inside may be required.

Obstruction

Obstruction to the flow of air through the nose may result from a number of causes. The most frequent is the common cold (see below). Other causes include a nasal polyp, a benign growth usually resulting from a chronic infection; deformed or swollen turbinates; a malformed or crooked septum; or enlarged **adenoids** (lymphoid tissue) in the back part of the nose. Children sometimes push objects like beans or marbles into their noses, where they become lodged. See your physician.

What your physician can do. Most of these problems will require surgery, except for the foreign object, which can be extracted following anesthesia.

Sinusitis

The sinuses are hollow spaces in the bones surrounding the nose. The mucous membrane which lines the nose is continuous with the mucous membrane lining the sinuses through openings between the two. Inflammation of the mucous mem-

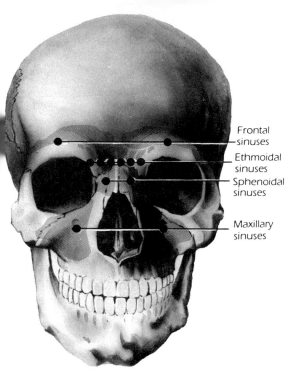

Frontal sinuses
Ethmoidal sinuses
Sphenoidal sinuses
Maxillary sinuses

The nasal sinuses (blue areas) open into the nasal cavity. Infections may travel from the nose into the sinuses. The maxillary sinuses are most commonly infected.

brane of the sinuses, caused by a bacterial or viral infection, results in sinusitis. The organisms usually enter from the nose, frequently following a common cold, although occasionally they may gain access from an infected tooth. A deviated septum or other obstructions make sinusitis more likely.

The frontal sinuses (just above the eyes) and those in the cheek (maxillary) are most frequently involved, exhibiting the symptoms of pain, tenderness of the skin overlying the sinuses, and fever. Headache and a heavy feeling in your eyes or cheeks, especially when leaning forward, are common. Your upper teeth my become tender and painful when the maxillary sinuses are inflamed. The secretions and pus may drain into the nose, or the opening may become blocked.

What you can do. The cautious breathing of steam, from a pan or kettle or vaporizer, often brings relief. You may repeat this treatment three or four times during the day, for ten minutes at a time. A humidifier in a warm room will help. If the condition does not improve rapidly, see your physician.

What your physician can do. He may prescribe a nasal decongestant. This will decrease the congestion in the nose and allow the sinus to drain more freely. An antibiotic to combat the infection may be used. It is generally taken for six days, except in chronic sinusitis when it may be administered for several weeks. If drainage does not occur or if the problem is chronic, the sinus may be drained through a large needle, or an opening into the nose may be made surgically. X-rays are sometimes helpful to precisely define the extent of the infection.

The common cold (acute rhinitis)

The common cold is an infection of the upper air passages (nose, sinuses, pharynx) by any one of possibly two hundred viruses, which attack the lining cells, causing them to pour out mucus. The infection spreads easily from person to person by infected droplets of moisture or dust floating in the air and, 50 percent of the time, by hand contact. Children, who are most susceptible, may spread the virus by touching other children after they have rubbed their noses. You can transmit the virus a few hours

909

before your cold has developed and for as long as five days thereafter. Following exposure, the cold may appear in two or three days, and last from four to seven days, and sometimes even two weeks.

Since any one of many viruses may cause a cold, a specific vaccine is not feasible. Even having a cold makes you immune only to the virus or viruses which caused it. The same virus may infect you repeatedly, as the immunity is relatively short-lived.

The symptoms usually begin with a roughness or irritation in the throat, followed by sneezing and a runny nose. The discharge soon becomes thick and greenish-yellow. You may experience general aching, chilliness, and a low fever. Secondary infection by common bacteria is responsible for the complications that may develop, such as infection of the middle ear (otitis media), sinusitis, bronchitis, and even pneumonia.

Exposure to cold or wind, excessive fatigue, loss of sleep, and other causes of reduced resistance make you more susceptible. This is especially true if you are in crowds or closely associated with someone with a cold.

What you can do. There is no specific treatment for a cold. Staying at home will prevent you from spreading the infection to others. You will be more comfortable if the room air is warm and moistened with a humidifier. Placing the humidifier two to three feet from the patient will protect him against any possibility of a steam burn. Nose drops give relief from congestion, but if used too frequently or for more than a few days, cause irritation and congestion themselves. Cautious inhalation of steam will open the air passages.

Gargling is often recommended, but is essentially ineffective as it keeps the water in front of the pharynx. To stimulate circulation in the throat, drink hot water (do not scald) about once an hour during the day. At night use a heating compress to the neck (see page 593 for details).

Maintain a high fluid intake. Many recommend high doses of vitamin C. No conclusive evidence supports the practice; however, the issue remains controversial. Cough syrup may relieve a troublesome cough. As mentioned earlier, prevention by a healthful lifestyle is the best "treatment."

What your physician can do. Your physician may recommend other symptomatic measures. He can help if you develop complications such as, sinusitis, middle ear infection, or a serious bronchitis or pneumonia. Antibiotics are effective against most organisms.

Hay fever (allergic rhinitis)

Hay fever, an inflammation of the membranes lining the nasal cavities, results from contact with some allergen to which one is sensitive. The allergen releases a substance called histamine, which dilates the vessels and produces congestion. The reaction occurs in the nose, throat, and eyes. The susceptibility appears to be inherited.

The causes include plant pollens from certain grasses, weeds, or trees; house dust containing mites, animal

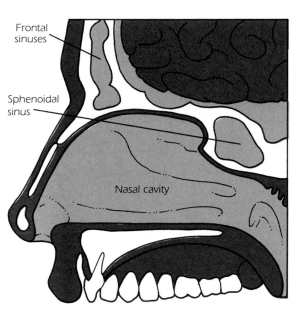

Frontal sinuses

Sphenoidal sinus

Nasal cavity

Section showing area of nasal cavity with adjoining frontal and sphenoid sinuses.

hair and dander, feathers, and plant dust. Some may have seasonal episodes of hay fever when pollens are plentiful. Other may have problems the year round (perennial), depending on the allergen.

The membrane reaction causes itching, runny nose, sneezing, and red watery eyes. A dry cough and fever may be present. Sometimes wheezing occurs, but generally only if one has asthma, a condition similar to hay fever but affecting the lungs and chest.

What you can do. By careful observation attempt to determine the allergen and then avoid contact with it. Staying indoors in a room that is air-conditioned during the height of the pollen season will help. Since allergic reactions release histamine in the body, antihistamine medications, available without prescription, may rellieve the symptoms. Unfortunately these cause dryness of the nose and throat, drowsiness, and slow down your reflexes, which is a serious problem should you have to drive an automobile or operate certain types of equipment.

What your physician can do. Along with antihistamine medication, he may prescribe steroid (cortisone) sprays. These will help the symptoms but will not cure the basic problem. Skin tests may help to identify the allergen to which you are sensitive, and then a series of injections may be given in an attempt to desensitize you against this particular substance. These procedures are not without their risks.

Chronic rhinitis

Chronic rhinitis is an inflammatory swelling of the lining membranes of the nose in which the turbinates are swollen, red, and enlarged. Mucus production is excessive. A chronic infection may be present, causing pus and a postnasal drip. It is seen more frequently in those exposed to chemicals such as house and car painters, photo-lab developers, and those who swim in chlorinated pools. The cause is not due to an allergy.

Avoidance of the offending substance, if known, is obvious, even if it means a change of work. Decongestants, sprays, and steroids may alleviate symptoms.

Atrophic rhinitis (ozena)

Atrophic rhinitis is a condition in which the membrane lining the nasal cavities deteriorates and develops

911

thick crusts, a foul odor, and a tendency to bleed. Loss of the sense of smell (anosmia) usually develops. The exact cause is vague, but repeated infections may be responsible. No cure exists, and the condition can cause extreme discomfort.

Antibiotic or steroid ointments are applied directly to the nasal membranes. Placing a small pledget of lamb's wool in each nostril reduces crusting and drying. Saline irrigations to flush out the nasal cavities may help.

Vasomotor rhinitis

Vasomotor rhinitis is a chronic non-inflammatory swelling of the nasal membranes and turbinates, with a watery discharge from the nose. It affects persons of all ages and both sexes, and is not due to an infection or an allergy. Suffers seem to be sensitive to such things as cold weather, spicy foods, strong odors, cigarette smoke, oral contraceptives, and even emotional disturbances. The presumed cause is some imbalance in the autonomic nerve supply.

As there is no known cure, one must avoid all factors which precipitate an attack. Nasal sprays and nose drops may give temporary relief, but not infrequently aggravate the symptoms by irritating the membranes. Smoking should be avoided, as should the smoke of others.

Diseases of the throat (pharynx)

The throat or pharynx is the back part of the nose and mouth that gives passage for both food and drink for the digestive system and air for the lungs.

Sore throat (pharyngitis)

Sore throat is due to an inflammation of the tonsils (tonsillitis, discussed later), and of the mucous membrane that lines the pharynx. Both are associated with discomfort in swallowing and talking. Your throat will look red and feel raw, and you will frequently feel feverish.

The sore throat may be caused by a virus or any one of a number of bacteria, usually streptococcus or staphylococcus. Sore throat is part of the initial illness in measles, scarlet fever, and whooping cough. It is a symptom in leukemia and infectious mononucleosis, and may accompany such diseases as tuberculosis, syphilis, and cancer. When not accompanied by infection, sore throat may be the result of smoking tobacco, drinking hard liquor, drinking excessively hot fluids, or from using concentrated mouthwashes and antiseptic gargles.

What you can do. For the use of hot water and heating compresses for relief, see page 593 under "common cold." Throat lozenges may provide some relief. Apply hot fomentations to the neck for twenty minutes two or three times a day. If you have a fever, stay in bed, and, despite the discomfort, drink plenty of water and go on a liquid diet (fluid intake should be two to three quarts daily). If the soreness gets worse or persists for more than two or three days, consult your physician. If your sore throat is not due to an infection, remove the cause; for example, stop the use of tobacco or alcohol.

What your physician can do. For an infection your physician will probably prescribe an antibiotic, especially for a streptococcal infection. If it persists, tests can determine if the problem is more serious.

Strep throat (streptococcal sore throat)

This severe sore throat is caused by a strain of the hemolytic streptococcus similar to that which causes scarlet fever. In both, the sore throat is present, but in scarlet fever a rash due to the effect of the toxin on the capillaries of the skin accompanies the sore throat. You may feel very weak. Possible complications of this serious infection include arthritis, infection of the lymph nodes of the neck, middle ear infection, occasionally infection of the lining of the heart (endocarditis), and damage to the kidneys.

Strep throat occurs both in isolated cases and in epidemics. Epidemics usually result from streptococcal contamination of milk or milk products, or other foods handled by someone who carries the organism in the throat.

What you can do. Make every effort to prevent spread of the infection by carefully handling the discharges from the nose and throat and by practicing good hand hygiene. The therapies you can use are similar to those described under "Sore throat." In addition, for tender and swollen lymph glands in the neck, use hot or cold ap-

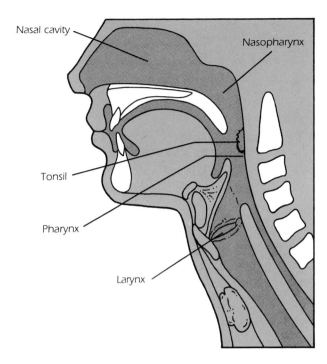

Sore throat results from inflammation of the membrane lining the pharynx and infections of the tonsils.

plications, depending on which provides more comfort. An ice collar can be applied for ten minutes each half hour.

What your physician can do. Streptococcal infections are quite amenable to treatment by antibiotics. They generally reduce the severity of the illness, shorten the duration, and prevent complications.

Tonsillitis and quinsy

Tonsillitis—an inflammation of the tonsils (lymphoid tissue), located on the left and right sides of the throat—commonly prostrates children and young people. It may be caused by a number of organisms, but usually by streptococcus, staphy-

913

The palatine tonsils, on either side of the pharynx, are commonly infected.

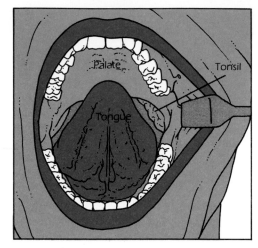

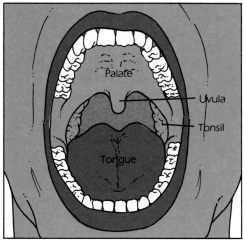

lococcus, or a virus.

Symptoms include intense soreness of the throat, with great difficulty in swallowing; chills, fever (to 104°F (40°C), and aching back and limbs; swollen and red tonsils, with yellow and white patches on the surface; a coated tongue and foul breath; and swollen and tender lymph glands in the neck.

Quinsy is an abscess in the tonsil or in the adjacent tissues, such as the pharynx or soft palate. The symptoms are similar to those of tonsillitis, except that there tends to be more swelling in the throat, the pain of swallowing is more intense, and the sufferer can hardly open his mouth. Complications occur when the abscess bursts, as this may spread the infection into the deep tissues of the neck and down into the chest.

What you can do. The same procedures discussed under "sore throat" will be helpful. However, if prompt improvement does not occur, see your physician.

What your physician can do. Immediate treatment for tonsillitis aims to combat the infection. Here an antibiotic generally proves successful.

Following recovery, and especially if the problem is a recurrent one, it should be determined whether removal of the tonsils is advisable. Should the problem recur three or more times in a year, removal of the tonsils is indicated. In the case of quinsy, the abscess should be drained by a surgical incision and appropriate anti-infective therapy given to prevent complications.

Diseases of the larynx

The larynx or voice box is at the upper end of the trachea and just below the back of the tongue. It contains the vocal cords, which are essential to the mechanism of speech. The two most common problems of the larynx are hoarseness and obstructed breathing.

Hoarseness

Any condition which causes irritation, inflammation, or malfunction of the vocal cords will distort the sounds produced by the cords and will induce hoarseness. Hoarseness, then, can be the result of a number of conditions which include infections of the larynx; prolonged screaming or shouting; improper use of the voice in speaking or singing; inhalation of irritant fumes from tobacco smoke, organic chemicals such as solvents and paint removers; heavy use of beverage alcohol; and benign or malignant tumors of the larynx.

Vocal cord damage. Hoarseness is a warning that the vocal cords are in trouble. Smoking, the heavy use of alcohol, breathing irritating fumes, screaming, shouting, and speaking and singing incorrectly may, if repeated frequently or continued over a prolonged period of time, result in damage to the cords.

Such irritations may cause the appearance of polyps on the cords, or small, firm nodules on the free edge of the vocal cords, or thickening and roughening of the cords. Sometimes ulcers develop in the lining membrane of the larynx.

What you can do. Discontinue any known practice which may have contributed to your hoarseness. Breathing warm steam from a vaporizer may give relief. It is very important that you rest your voice. If you must speak for periods of time in your profession, take lessons in using your voice correctly. Should your hoarseness continue, see your physician.

What your physician can do. A careful examination will reveal the true cause of your hoarseness. Polyps and nodules should be surgically removed. A cancer detected early can be satisfactorily eradicated. Ulcers heal with difficulty and tend to return.

Laryngitis

Laryngitis is an infection, due to a bacteria or a virus, causing swelling and inflammation of the membranes of the larynx, including the vocal cords. Most often a complication of the common cold, it may also occur as part of such illnesses as influenza, pneumonia, whooping cough, and measles. Hoarseness, its most common symptom, is often accompanied by a sensation of rawness and an urge to clear the throat. Speaking

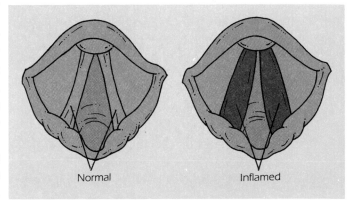

Normal

Inflamed

Looking at the larynx from above. In laryngitis the membranes lining the larynx and vocal chords become inflamed.

915

may be painful, and you may lose your voice. Recovery in a few days is usual. Chronic infection, left untreated, may precede a cancer.

What you can do. Resting the voice and swallowing warm fluids relieve the discomfort. The cautious breathing of steam or warm, moist air hastens symptomatic improvement. Should the problem persist, see your physician.

What your physician can do. Any underlying illness should be treated. As a bacterial infection may damage the vocal cords, antibiotics are frequently prescribed.

Cancers of the mouth, throat, and larynx

At the present writing, more than 40,000 cancers of the mouth, throat, and larynx are reported each year, with an annual death rate of one in three. In India, 40 percent of all cancer deaths are due to cancers in these areas, chiefly as a result of the habit of chewing pan—a combination of pepper leaf, betel nut, and tobacco. In the United States, cancers of the mouth, throat, and larynx are seen most frequently in those who chew or smoke tobacco.

Heavy exposure to alcohol also increases the risk of mouth, throat (pharyngeal), and esophageal cancers. Poor dentures and broken teeth irritate the mucosa and thus are another factor predisposing to cancer development. Persons who are chronically exposed to dust from wood or metal particles, and those who eat generously of smoked or salted fish, also have a higher risk of developing a malignancy in the mouth and adjacent areas.

Symptoms. Any lesion that does not heal within a few days, whether on the lip, tongue, gums, inner cheeks, or throat should be reported to your physician. Cancer of the lip is not uncommon among pipe smokers. A long-continued irritation may result in one or more irregular, hard, milk-white dry patches on the membranes lining the mouth, on the tongue, or on the inner aspects of the lips or cheeks. Such a "white plaque" or **"smoker's patch"** is known as **leukoplakia.** Should the patch appear red, soft, and smooth, it is called **erythroplasia.** Such lesions are considered precancerous.

A sore throat, hoarseness in the larynx, and a persistent dry cough that is not associated with a cold or infection and does not go away in a week or two, should arouse suspicion of a possible cancer and be examined by your physician. Cancer of the vocal cords commonly causes hoarseness but rarely pain. By the time pain is felt, the cancer may have already spread.

What you can do. If you have a poorly fitting denture or a broken tooth, see your dentist. Any hoarseness or cough that you cannot attribute to a cause (such as the flu), or a sore anywhere in your mouth that does not heal within a couple of weeks, should alert you to a possible problem. See your physician. If you smoke, chew tobacco, or use hard liquors, remember that these all increase your likelihood of developing a cancer in this region.

What your physician can do. The diagnosis of cancer is readily confirmed by examining a biopsy (small piece of tissue) obtained from the lesion, either directly or by use of a laryngoscope. Surgical removal is usually the treatment of choice in cancers of the lip, tongue, and mouth. When cancer of the vocal cords is diagnosed early enough, it may be removed by laser surgery. More advanced cancers may require the removal of the voice box (larynx). Once the cancer has spread to the lymph nodes of the neck, these are generally removed and radiation and chemotherapy are employed in the hope of limiting the malignancy.

Loss of the voice box does not mean one cannot speak. Speech therapists can teach you how to trap air in your throat and esophagus and use it to produce recognizable sounds. Mechanical speech devices are also available.

Diseases of the trachea and bronchi

The trachea and bronchi are passageways which carry the air you breathe into the depths of the lungs.

Acute bronchitis

Acute bronchitis is an inflammation of the mucous membranes lining the large bronchi and usually the trachea, and is often associated with a severe cold, pharyngitis, or laryngitis. Generally not a serious problem, it lasts but a few days. Should it persist or there be frequent attacks, the membranes may be damaged, leading to chronic bronchitis.

A deep, productive cough, with yellowish sputum, forms the major symptom. Pain, deep to the breastbone, is aggravated by coughing. A fever may be present. Should the mucus and pus be difficult to cough up, breathing may be difficult.

What you can do. Use many of the procedures discussed under

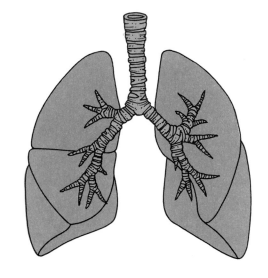

The right and left bronchi are seen entering the lungs. Infections of the lining of the bronchi result in bronchitis.

917

caring for the common cold (see page 910). A warm, humid atmosphere will soothe the inflamed membranes. If a cough medicine is used, it should not completely suppress the cough, but liquify the secretions to make it easier to cough them up and clear the air passages. Should the pain, fever, and cough not improve in two or three days, see your physician.

What your physician can do. To relieve difficulty in breathing, he may order an inhalant to dilate your air passages. He may also prescribe a stronger cough medicine, if he thinks wise, and possibly an antibiotic if it appears you have a secondary bacterial infection.

Chronic bronchitis and emphysema (chronic obstructive lung disease—COLD)

As the bronchi divide and redivide they become smaller and smaller, finally becoming bronchioles. These further divide, terminating in a cluster of minute sacs (alveoli). In chronic bronchitis the principal problem is in the bronchi, while in emphysema it is in the air sacs. A person rarely has just chronic bronchitis or just emphysema; it is usually a combination of the two. If there is more cough and sputum it is chronic bronchitis; if more shortness of breath it is emphysema.

Beginning in 1970 COLD increased alarmingly. By 1980, from this disease alone, 50,000 deaths occurred each year, in number second only to coronary heart disease; another 200,000 were confined to bed; while half a million more were limited in their regular activities. COLD affects some 15 percent of men between the ages of 45 and 75. While many times more frequent among men, the incidence among women is accelerating, due mainly to their having taken up the smoking habit.

In **chronic bronchitis** a smoldering infection makes the walls of the air passageways swollen and inflamed. The outflow of more mucus from an increased number of mucous glands, along with a breakdown of the clearing mechanism of the cilia which normally propel the mucus upward toward the throat, results in coughing and the raising of much mucus or phlegm. Repeated infections damage the walls of the bronchi and bronchioles, causing them to narrow. Because of the excess mucus plus the narrowing, air has difficulty entering and leaving the air sacs, causing breathlessness and wheezing.

In **emphysema,** large-scale destruction of the walls of the air sacs located at the end of the air passages takes place. Once-separate air sacs unite. As the disease progresses, the gradual joining of these air sacs results in the formation of large blebs. The lungs lose their elasticity and stale, oxygenless air is trapped in these blebs. This further damages the lungs. The gradual reduction of the lungs' elasticity and efficiency causes shortness of breath which steadily becomes worse, until life becomes an effort to get one more breath.

Because the lung cannot repair it-

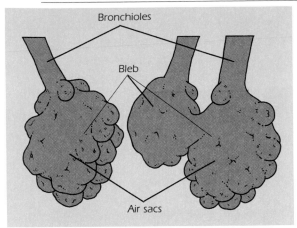

A bronchiole terminates in a cluster of air sacs. In emphysema the walls of the air sacs weaken, break down, and fuse, forming large blebs.

self, emphysema is a serious illness. Its onset is insidious, progressing from mild shortness of breath, to decreasing ability to carry on the ordinary activities of life, to complete incapacitation. Treatment only makes life a little more comfortable, unless detected in a very early stage, when it may be possible to prevent the disease from further development. This will require the removal of the factor or factors which cause or aggravate the disease. The major culprit is tobacco smoke, with minor contributors being cotton fibers, asbestos fibers, coal dust, and a polluted atmosphere at work (certain plastic vapors, welding fumes) or in the environment (nitrous and sulfur dioxides in smog). Some people are born with a genetic defect in the lungs which makes them susceptible.

Both chronic bronchitis and emphysema make one more susceptible to colds and respiratory infections. Each such infection tends to make the condition worse. These diseases also may adversely affect the heart. As they progress it becomes increasingly difficult to pump blood through the lungs, causing right heart failure.

What you can do. To determine whether you have COLD you can perform a simple test. Fill your lungs to the limit with air, and then measure accurately the time it takes to completely expel this air by breathing out (exhaling). With normal lungs and air passages this air can be expelled in three seconds. If the emptying time exceeds five seconds, it is good evidence that COLD exists. To estimate the rate at which the disease is progressing, do a test every few months, recording the results and date of each test.

COLD requires that you stay away from tobacco smoke, and if you are a smoker, to give it up. You may consider finding an occupation where no contaminants are in the air, or move to a warm, dry smogless climate. Avoid contact with people who have colds and other respiratory infections. Exercise regularly within your tolerance.

What your physician can do. To determine precisely your condition, a chest X-ray and pulmonary function tests may be ordered. A bronchodilator may offer relief from difficult breathing. If you frequently get upper respiratory infections, an antibiotic may be prescribed. To relieve obstruction to breathing he may suggest lying in special positions to help clear your lungs of excess mucus (postural drainage). You should regularly receive flu vaccine each

919

fall, and antipneumococcal vaccine should be considered.

Asthma

Asthma is a chronic disease identified by periodic attacks of coughing, wheezing, and difficult breathing. Once air is drawn into the lungs it seems almost impossible to expel it. Attacks last from a few minutes to several hours, and vary greatly in severity, occurring most frequently at night. If not treated, they often end spontaneously.

About one out of every thirty-five people in the population suffer from asthma. Of these, two-thirds develop the problem before the age of five. Boys and men are afflicted more

deaths occur each year, most of which could be prevented with appropriate treatment programs.

An attack of asthma is a hyperactive response of the bronchi and bronchioles to some agent which causes the muscles in the bronchial walls to contract, thus narrowing the passageways; swells the lining of the air passages, further narrowing the openings; and increases the secretion of mucus, clogging the smaller tubes.

An asthmatic episode may begin gradually or suddenly. A feeling of tightness in the chest accompanies wheezing and coughing. In severe attacks the sufferer struggles to force the air out of his lungs, often

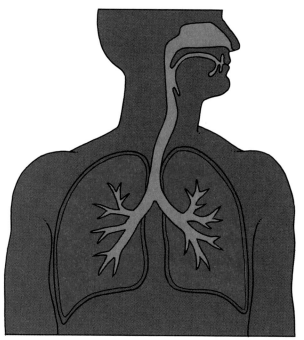

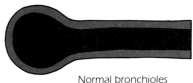

Normal bronchioles

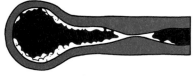

Constricted bronchioles

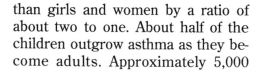

Asthma affects the bronchioles, making the exhaling of air difficult.

than girls and women by a ratio of about two to one. About half of the children outgrow asthma as they become adults. Approximately 5,000

becoming anxious, agitated, and even panicked. The lips and skin turn bluish because of oxygen shortage, accompanied with sweating and rapid heart rate. Coughing expels thick, tenacious mucus. As the attack subsides breathing becomes normal, while the chest may be sore.

Generally the asthmatic has an inherited sensitivity or allergy to factors which trigger an attack. These may include house dust (which contains tiny mites), grain dust, pollens, grasses, molds, dander or hair (from cats and dogs), feathers (in pillows or from pet birds), tobacco smoke, and polluted air. Other agents may be perfumes, hair sprays, furniture polish, detergents, and any of a number of chemical vapors. Some people are allergic to foods, such as sesame seeds, certain nuts and peanut butter, chocolate, orange juice, eggs, and milk. Sudden changes in the weather, physical exertion, fatigue, infections (flu, common cold, sore throat), and even excitement and emotional upsets may provoke an attack.

What you can do. Try to be your own detective and discover what triggers an attack. Keep a detailed record. Observe carefully the circumstances around which attacks occur: the time of day, the season of the year, the activity you were engaged in, whether you were at home or work, what particular foods you have eaten—in fact anything you were doing at the time. You may ask your physician to do some sensitivity tests for foods, pollens, etc.

Once you have identified the cause, try to avoid it if at all possible. Remove from your environment offending materials such as hair sprays, furniture polish, laundry de-

tergents, and even pets. Keep your house free from dust. Should your problem be severe, cooperate with your physician in working out a suitable treatment program. For mild attacks you may find that a warm drink or inhalations from a vaporizer or pan of boiling water may be helpful. Do not allow the steam to burn you. Certain medications available over the counter are effective in controlling an attack, though some may cause drowsiness. Check with your physician as to which are best. Should you get a severe attack which does not yield to measures at hand, call your physician or go to the nearest hospital.

What your physician can do. Available tests can determine sensitivity toward a number of allergens, such as pollens, foods, molds, house dusts, chemicals, etc. He may recommend desensitization against certain of these.

A number of effective medications lessen or prevent an attack. These may be administered through an inhaler or taken orally. If you have seasonal asthma, your physician may advise a routine requiring medication several times a day. Flu shots may reduce infections of the respiratory tract which might set the stage for an asthmatic episode. Work closely with your physician as to the best procedures for avoiding or treating an attack.

Bronchiectasis

In bronchiectasis the midsized or smaller bronchi permanently dilate or expand, forming pockets of chronic infection, in which large amounts of pussy mucus accumulate. Affected areas are usually localized, but on rare occasions are scattered through the lungs. Since the advent of antibiotics, the disease has become relatively rare.

The damage to the air passages frequently results from infections in childhood which follow measles and whooping cough. Other causes include sinusitis, pneumonia, chronic bronchitis, emphysema, lung abscess, lung cancer, inhaled objects, tuberculosis, or a congenital defect. The disease may develop insidiously.

The characteristic symptoms of bronchiectasis are a chronic cough, the raising of large amounts of greenish-yellow, often foul-smelling sputum, at times tinged with blood (hemoptysis), and foul breath or halitosis.The individual coughs most frequently on arising in the morning and upon lying down at night. As the disease advances, he may experience shortness of breath on slight exertion, and his fingertips may become rounded or clubbed.

What you can do. If you smoke, give it up and avoid smoke-filled rooms. Try to develop a healthful lifestyle so as to minimize the possibility of getting upper respiratory infections, such as colds, flu, bronchitis, etc. Learn the technique of **postural drainage,** that is, to put your body in a position in which the accumulations of pussy mucus will drain out and be coughed up. Lie across the bed with your head and chest hanging downward with your elbows resting on a pillow on the floor. Turn your body so that the most seriously affected side of your chest is uppermost. This will promote drainage. You can do this two or three times a day, ten minutes at a time, but especially in the morning.

What your physician can do. Examination of the sputum will identify the infecting organism. An appropriate antibiotic can then be prescribed to control the infection. A bronchoscopic examination (looking at the interior of the air passages), X-ray studies, and a CT scan will precisely determine the area involved. Should the bronchiectasis be localized, surgical removal may reduce if not entirely eliminate the problem.

Cystic fibrosis

Cystic fibrosis is a lethal hereditary disease affecting the glands which secrete mucus and sweat. Those typically involved are the lungs, the pancreas, and the skin. It begins in infancy and continues through childhood, with an average survival of fifteen to twenty years. The mucous secreting glands which line the bronchial tubes produce a thick, sticky mucus which is difficult to cough up. This mucus putrefies and traps germs resulting in infections, such as chronic bronchitis and pneumonia. Bronchiectasis commonly follows.

Severe respiratory infections, most commonly pneumonia, with cough and fever, frequently occur. Antibiotics prolong life and make it more acceptable. However, because of associated problems in the digestive tract, debility is often severe, and ultimately the disease proves fatal.

What your physician can do. To combat infection, antibiotics are used. Medications are also given to thin and help eliminate the mucus. Postural drainage (see under "Bronchiectasis") will provide relief and can be done at home. (For other aspects of the disease, see page 921.) Be sure to ask your physician for information on support groups.

Pneumonia

Pneumonia describes any of the acute infections of the lungs in which the lining of the air sacs is inflamed and swollen, and cells and fluid fill the air spaces, making it difficult to breath. A number of common terms describe various forms of the disease. "Double pneumonia" refers to involvement in both lungs. Involvement localized to one or more lobes of the lung, is called "lobar pneumonia." A scattered or patchy infection in one or both the lungs is called "bronchopneumonia." Still another is "atypical pneumonia" caused by Mycoplasma organisms.

The inflammation can be caused by any one of a number of germs (bacteria, viruses, fungi) to which one is frequently exposed, and irritant poisonous gases. The pneumonia may be mild to severe, depending on the organism and the measure of health of the person. Predisposing factors include heart disease, cancer, stroke, coma, other infections of the respiratory tract (common cold, influenza), inhaled foreign material, alcoholism, malnutrition, drugs given to suppress immunity, and often any debilitating or terminal illness.

The precise symptoms of pneumonia will vary with the infecting organism, and may have an abrupt or gradual onset. Those most commonly observed are cough, fever (up to 105° F), and shortness of breath. Others include chills, sweating, headache, nausea, vomiting, rapid, shallow breathing, chest pain, bloody sputum, and blueness of the skin (cyanosis).

Viral pneumonias, generally mild, are commonly associated with the common cold. In fact, they not infrequently pass as a severe cold. These common pneumonias account for about 75 percent of lung infections. However, influenza A virus pneumonia can be severe, and even fatal. Usually carried by droplets of moisture expelled by sneezing, this virus does not respond to antibiotic therapy.

Bacterial pneumonias—usually more severe and dangerous—are commonly caused by the pneumococcus. If untreated, the disease runs it course in about two weeks, ending in death in more than 30 percent of the cases and in prompt improvement (by "crisis") in the remaining 70 percent. Treatment with antibiotics (penicillin G) or sulfonamides reduces the mortality to less than 5 percent. A vaccine is now available which protects against this type of pneumonia.

Other bacteria which may cause pneumonia include streptococcus, Klebsiella, Haemophilus, and, worst of all, staphylococcus. They also respond to antibiotics. Complications of bacterial pneumonias include pleurisy, empyema, lung abscess, infection of the heart (pericarditis or endocarditis), and meningitis.

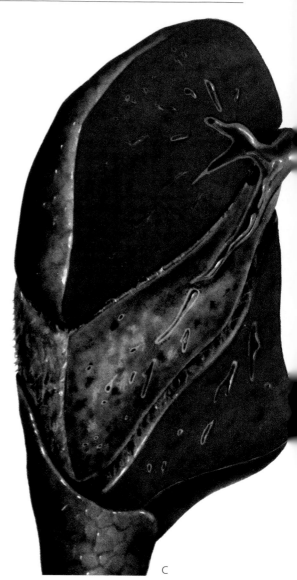

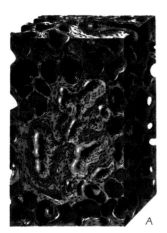
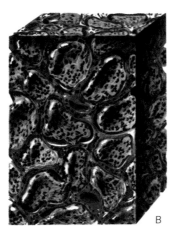

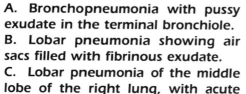

A. **Bronchopneumonia with pussy exudate in the terminal bronchiole.**
B. **Lobar pneumonia showing air sacs filled with fibrinous exudate.**
C. **Lobar pneumonia of the middle lobe of the right lung, with acute fibrinous pleuritis.**

Mycoplasmal pneumonia most commonly appears among adolescents and young adults. It is caused by a tiny bacteriumlike organism, Mycoplasma. The illness starts gradually with a chest cold, dry cough, and fever, and may reach epidemic proportions in the military and in schools. It responds to antibiotics (erythromycins and tetracyclines,

not penicillins). When untreated, spontaneous recovery usually occurs in about ten days. It is spread by droplets produced by the sneezing and coughing of an infected individual.

Legionnaires' pneumonia or **Legionnaires' disease,** first observed in epidemic proportions in 1976 in Philadelphia during an

American Legion convention, is caused by a bacterium named Legionella pneumophilia. Unlike the typical person-to-person transmittal, these bacteria are carried by the air, in some cases by a contaminated air-conditioning system. The symptoms parallel those of a severe pneumonia. The disease progresses rapidly, and the sufferer should be hospitalized and treated with an appropriate antibiotic. A possible complication is kidney failure.

What you can do. Great care should be taken in attempting to treat cases of pneumonia at home. Infants and the elderly (except as a terminal event) are best cared for in a hospital. After a careful evaluation of the condition, your physician will determine what is best. Under his direction, you can carry out certain procedures if you or a family member are treated in your home, or after returning home from the hospital. These are discussed below.

What your physician can do. Your physician will probably hospitalize you and then determine the cause and extent of your problem. Laboratory examination of your sputum, and possibly blood, will reveal the organism involved. X-rays of the lungs will also aid in determining the type of pneumonia. This will direct in the selection of the most effective medication.

Bed rest, the administration of fluids to avoid dehydration, and oxygen, if necessary, will be supportive. The inhaling of steam from a vaporizer or a kettle of water (be careful not to get burned) will open the air passages and help in coughing up mucus. Hydrotherapy treatments in the form of a hot foot bath along with fomentations to the chest and back, repeated twice and given three or four times a day, will be helpful until the infection subsides. For details of the procedure see page 590. Full recovery including regaining strength may take weeks. A program of exercise to tolerance, adequate rest and sleep, and a good nutritious diet will speed recovery.

Cancer of the lung

In 1986, cancer of the lung, or bronchial carcinoma, became the most common cancer of both men and women in the United States, and now causes more deaths in both groups than any other cancer. While a number of other types of cancer can occur in the lungs, bronchial carcinoma is the most frequent and, with rare exception, is due to inhaling tobacco smoke.

That tobacco smoke causes lung cancer goes without question, except in the minds of the tobacco manufacturers. Many factors influence the incidence of smoking-related cancer. These have been discussed in detail under "tobacco" (page 273), and include the years a person has smoked, the number of cigarettes smoked, the length of the cigarette, the depth of inhalation, and the tar and nicotine content of the cigarette.

Cancer types

The majority of lung cancers are either of the squamous cell (flat, scaly) variety or adenocarcinomas (gland cell). Squamous cell cancers go through a precancerous phase, and their cells may be detected in the sputum. They do not spread to distant parts of the body as readily as do the adenocarcinomas.

Symptoms

The most common symptom of lung cancer is cough, but since most smokers have a so-called "smoker's cough" and a chronic bronchitis with sputum, the problem often goes unnoticed until the cough has become quite severe, or the sputum is tinged with blood. Frequently there is shortness of breath, and pain in the chest that increases when inhaling deeply.

Often the first recognition of a lung cancer is the discovery of a cancer at some distant site where it has spread. Common sites to which lung cancers may travel (**metastasize**) are to the other lung, the brain, bones, and liver. A cancer in the brain may cause headaches, mental confusion, convulsions, or a stroke. If the cancer lodges in a bone there is often deep pain, swelling, and often a fracture, or compression of the bone if it is in the vertebral column. Liver involvement is associated with indigestion and jaundice.

General symptoms often include loss of appetite, loss of weight, excessive tiredness, a low-grade continual fever, and progressive weakness.

The prognosis for cancer of the lung is not encouraging since so often the growth has already spread beyond the reach of the surgeon's knife. A light smoker is ten times more likely to develop a lung cancer than one who does not smoke, while a heavy smoker is twenty-five times more liable.

What you can do. You should see your physician at the earliest possible occasion if you notice any of the above signs or symptoms. If you are a smoker, you should stop immediately. If you decide to continue to smoke, and are concerned about getting lung cancer, you should periodically have a Pap smear of your sputum, an X-ray of your chest, and be checked by your physician every six months.

What your physician can do. A number of diagnostic procedures are available. Chest X-rays and the examination of sputum are usually effective. Your doctor may call for a bronchoscopic evaluation, during which washings, brushings, and a biopsy may be obtained. An ultrasonograph or CT scan may be desirable. A needle biopsy or aspiration is helpful if the lesion is located in the outer parts of the lung.

The treatment is usually surgical removal of the involved area of the lung or of the entire lung, together with chemotherapy and radiation therapy. The five-year survival rate is about 10 percent.

Various lung involvements

Pulmonary embolism

A clot that forms within a vessel and is later dislodged and travels in the vessel, is called an **embolus.** Blood flowing through most of the veins of the body passes through the right heart on its way to the lungs. The lungs, as a result, are commonly involved in embolism. Depending on the size or number of the emboli, they will block one or more pulmonary arteries. As a result, less of the lung is oxygenated, and breathlessness occurs. The symptoms can range from mild, to frightening, to fatal. For a detailed discussion, see page 808. Should the embolus arise from the site of an infection, it is called a septic embolus. Drug addicts, who frequently use non-sterile needles, develop infected veins from which infected emboli originate. These infected emboli do all the damage a regular embolus does and more. In the lung they usually result in an abscess. For symptoms and treatment, see "lung abscess," below.

Lung abscess

A lung abscess is a circumscribed area of infection within the lung. The causes may include aspiration or inhaling of infected mucus from nose, mouth, or pharynx (occurring at the time of surgery or by accident); chronic infection from a bacterial pneumonia, bronchitis, or bronchiectasis; an inhaled foreign body (a peanut or piece of popped corn); obstruction of one of the airways by a tumor; a septic embolus; and tuberculosis of the lung.

The symptoms may develop abruptly, rapidly, or slowly, depending on the cause. They include cough, the raising of large amounts of foul mucus containing pus and often blood, fever, and chest pain.

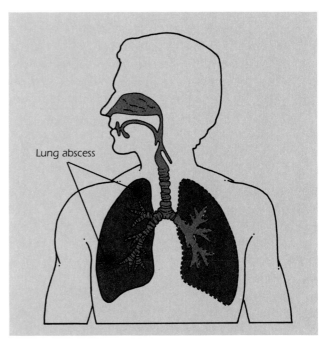

Lung abscess

Lung abscesses in the right lung.

What you can do. Should you have any of the above symptoms, see your physician.

What your physician can do. A chest X-ray and examination of your sputum will help locate the problem and determine the precise germ causing the infection. An appropriate antibiotic, sometimes administered intravenously, will be selected. Lung

927

abscesses heal slowly. Your doctor will seek the source of the infection, such as an infected tooth or vein in the leg. Postural drainage (see page 922) and hydrotherapy (see page 589) may be helpful. In case of severe hemorrage, surgery may be necessary to remove the portion of the lung involved in the abscess.

Pulmonary edema

Pulmonary edema is an acute, life-threatening problem in which the lungs become waterlogged because of an accumulation of fluid in the air sacs. Due usually to failure of the left side of the heart, blood is dammed back in the pulmonary veins, from which fluid seeps into the air sacs. Pulmonary edema appears suddenly, progresses rapidly within a few hours, and, if not treated, can be fatal. It may follow heart failure.

The common symptom is difficult breathing because the air spaces fill with fluid. (See illustration on the next page.) The sufferer grunts as he breathes, is restless, appears anxious, and has a feeling of suffocation. Though unrelated to asthma, the condition is sometimes called cardiac asthma because effort is required to breathe. Other symptoms include a dry cough, which later becomes productive with blood-tinged, frothy sputum; the skin is moist with perspiration and bluish (cyanotic) because of insufficient oxygen in the blood; thready pulse; and pain in the chest.

What you can do. Seek the help of a physician and call for an ambulance. In the meantime, sit up if possible, as this will make breathing a little easier.

What your physician can do. He can order an enriched mixture of oxygen for you to breathe. He may recommend medication to relieve the anxiety, slow and deepen breathing, and reduce the workload of the heart. He may also prescribe a diurectic to eliminate accumulated fluids. A fast-acting form of digitalis may improve the heart's efficiency. Applying tourniquets to three of the extremities for fifteen minutes at a time may decrease temporarily the congestion in the lungs.

Pneumoconiosis (Inorganic dust diseases)

Pneumoconiosis, a chronic lung disease, results from the protracted breathing of irritating industrial dusts, usually occurring in those whose work involves materials that give off fine particles which are carried in the air. Coal, asbestos, graphite, aluminum, talc, cobalt, tungsten, mica, fiberglass, silica, and beryllium are among the offenders. Other people at risk are stone masons, metal grinders, and those working with sugar cane, cotton, and synthetic fibers.

The disease may develop over a period of months, but usually over ten or more years. Areas of irritation occur where the particles accumulate, resulting in scarring and stiffening of the lung. As the lungs become less flexible, breathing becomes progressively more difficult. Additional symptoms consist of a dry cough, and, frequently, clubbing of the fingers.

Eventually serious infections of the respiratory tract, respiratory failure, and heart failure develop.

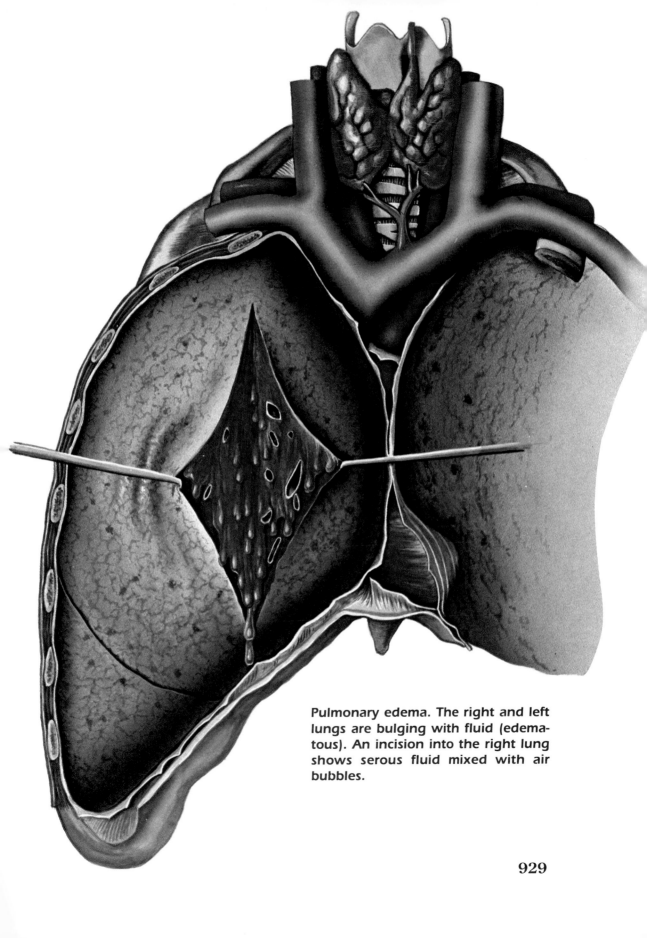

Pulmonary edema. The right and left lungs are bulging with fluid (edematous). An incision into the right lung shows serous fluid mixed with air bubbles.

Black lung or coal miner's disease generally afflicts those who work with hard or anthracite coal, affecting some 250,000 miners each year in the United States. The large majority of those affected show no symptoms and detection is only by lung X-ray. However, in a few, the fibrous areas enlarge and merge with others until little functional lung remains. Death results from respiratory failure, heart failure, or some lung infection.

Silicosis forms a potential problem to hundreds of thousands of workers in industries such as pottery manufacture, glass, tile, and brick making, and in certain foundries that use silica in certain paints, polishes, and abrasive cleaners. Any work which exposes one to fine sand dust, such as sandblasting, tunneling, pneumatic drilling, or breaking up of concrete, poses a possible hazard.

Like other forms of pneumoconiosis, the silica particles irritate the air sacs and terminal divisions of the bronchioles, causing the development of fibrous nodules with a whorl-like appearance, that is scattered throughout the lungs. Some of those heavily exposed develop a rapidly worsening disease causing death in three or four years. In others the condition remains dormant, even throughout life. The symptoms consist of increasing shortness of breath, with cough, loss of weight, and intervening lung infections.

Asbestosis, resulting from exposure to asbestos fibers, is much more serious than exposure to coal dust. The fibers (especially crocidolite and amosite) accumulate around the terminal bronchioles, where they are coated with an iron-protein complex, forming what are called asbestos bodies or crystals. These fibrous masses or fibroids fuse together, resulting in breathlessness, cough, and weight loss. Symptoms gradually increase, death occurring ten to twenty years later.

A number of cancers are associated with exposure to asbestos fibers, the most prevalent being cancer of the lung. Others include cancer of the esophagus, stomach, and intestines, most likely from swallowing sputum coughed up from the lungs. Among those heavily exposed to asbestos, deaths from lung cancer occur five times more frequently than death from lung cancer in the general population. The smoker exposed to asbestos fibers becomes ninety times more likely to get lung cancer than the smoker who is not exposed.

What you can do. Since no known cure for these problems exists, prevention is imperative. If your work exposes you to any of the above mentioned dusts, protect yourself by using appropriate masks. If necessary, change your occupation. If you already have the disease, you should place yourself under the care of a physician, who can follow your condition and recommend treatment as needed. If you smoke, you must give it up.

What your physician can do. Your physician will initially have X-rays and pulmonary functions tests done on your lungs to determine the extent of involvement. Thereafter, periodic examinations are essential. Appropriate treatments for lung infections, respiratory failure, and failure of the heart may be necessary.

Organic pneumoconioses (organic dusts)

A large number of organic dusts encountered in the environment may cause allergic hypersensitivity reactions in certain individuals and lead eventually to lung disease. These dusts contain fungal spores or animal or vegetable products, include moldy hay (causing **farmer's lung**), moldy sugarcane, bird feathers (chickens, turkeys, pigeons, parakeets) and their droppings, maple bark, mushroom compost, wood pulp, animal hair, cotton, hemp, and flax fiber **(Monday fever or brown lung)** and moldy wheat, barley, coffee beans, tea, and paprika.

The symptoms vary, depending on the offending dust and the individual's response. The smaller the particles, the further into the lung passageways they will be carried, affecting the bronchi, bronchioles, and even the air sacs (alveoli). The "dust" may cause spasm of the bronchi or bronchioles, or irritation with the outpouring of mucus. The resulting restriction in the flow of air causes breathlessness, tightness in the chest, and a dry cough.

As seen in **farmer's lung,** certain dusts, moldy hay, moldy sugarcane, mushroom compost, and others, may cause chills and fever. In continued exposure the condition may progress to where the lung becomes inelastic, stiff, and scarred, terminating in respiratory or heart failure.

In **brown lung,** due to cotton, flax, and hemp dust, the tightness in the chest is initially present for only short periods of time. If exposure continues, the tightness begins to persist for longer and longer periods, until it becomes continuous. The persisting irritation may result in chronic bronchitis and emphysema. In most individuals avoidance of the offending dust will bring on prompt recovery.

What you can do. Try to determine the precise cause of your problem. For this you might seek professional help. Once determined, if you cannot avoid exposure during your work, you should consider other employment. If you have already developed a problem, seek your physician's help.

What your physician can do. He may help you to discover the offending agent. By using X-ray and pulmonary function tests, he can determine the presence and extent of your problem. Depending on the stage of your disease, steroids may be helpful on a temporary basis. Should your problem be advanced, he can recommend appropriate care for respiratory or cardiac involvement.

Sarcoidosis

Sarcoidosis is a rare and mysterious disease with no known cause that affects young adults. It involves several organ systems, most commonly the lungs, the skin, and the lymph nodes, but also the spleen, liver, bones of the hands and feet, and the eyes. The symptoms are similar to those of tuberculosis. Small, degenerating   granulomatous

931

nodules develop in the affected sites, frequently combined with fever, weight loss, and painful joints. Involvement of the lungs causes difficult breathing and cough, which may occur in severe paroxysms with vomiting. Other symptoms are related to the organs affected.

When the disease comes on abruptly, it may be followed by remissions, and, even if untreated, it may disappear in two to three years. When the onset is gradual, the disease tends to persist, with a generally unfavorable outcome.

What your physician can do. An X-ray of the chest together with a skin test can determine the presence of the disease. Corticosteroid medication relieves the symptoms and reduces the tendency for the nodules to form scars on healing.

Disorders of the pleura

The pleura consists of two smooth, moist membranes which cover the outside of the lungs and the inside of the chest cavity. The two layers lie next to each other, and between them is a minute space (pleural space). The lungs expand and contract as you breathe in and out, moving without the slightest friction. Inflammation of either surface—called **pleurisy**—causes severe pain at each breath. Should the pleural space fill with fluid, the condition is known as **pleural effusion.**

Pleurisy, pleural effusion, and empyema

Pleurisy is an inflammation of the pleura, usually caused by an infection such as pneumonia or tuberculosis. It may also result from an injury, such as a broken rib.

In pleurisy the pleural membranes become swollen and inflamed, breathing is painful, and the roughened surfaces produce a rubbing sound (easily heard by a stethoscope). When fluid accumulates in the pleural space, the pleural effusion separates the two pleural layers, the pain on breathing disappears, and the rubbing sound

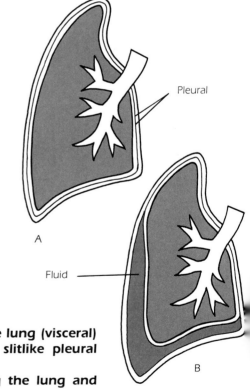

A

Fluid

B

Pleural

A. Normal lung with pleura covering the lung (visceral) and the chest wall (perietal), with a slitlike pleural space.
B. Fluid-filled pleural space constricting the lung and restricting its movement.

932

ceases. However, if the amount of fluid is large, the lung may be compressed and breathing becomes difficult. Should pus-producing germs infect the fluid, the condition is called **empyema.**

These conditions may be limited to a portion of the pleural membrane. When occurring over the diaphragm no pain may occur, or the pain may be felt in the abdomen or pit of the stomach. Pleural pain may be referred to the shoulder or neck.

What you can do. Tightly wrapping the chest wall with elastic bandages restricts chest movement when breathing and may relieve the pain.

Fomentations to the affected side of the chest may relieve the pain and accelerate the healing process (see page 590 for instructions). It would be wise to seek the advice of your physician.

What your physician can do. Your physician will examine your chest and probably order an X-ray, especially if he suspects pleural effusion or empyema. This will also aid in determining the underlying cause, such as pneumonia or chronic bronchitis or some other infection. Sometimes cancer or heart failure may cause an effusion. The precise treatment will depend on the underlying disease. Draining excess fluid or empyema and the giving of an antibiotic may be considered appropriate along with prescribing something for pain relief.

Pneumothorax

In pneumothorax air enters the pleural space, the space surrounding the lungs, and causes areas of the lungs to collapse. Breathing becomes difficult, and one feels a dull, aching pain with a sense of tightness in the chest. Pneumothorax results from penetrating injuries of the chest wall, and from the extension of diseases of the lungs, such as chronic bronchitis, lung abscess, or a growing malignancy, all of which permit air to enter the pleural space.

What you can do. If you have received a penetrating wound through your chest wall, place your finger or a damp cloth over the hole and call for emergency help.

What your physician can do. He will hospitalize you and attempt to determine the source of air entering your pleural space, possibly by using an insrument called a thorascoscope. A physical examination will help, but an X-ray is important. Therapy is directed toward the recovery of the collapsed lung through removing the air by means of a large needle or catheter. Sometimes surgery is required to close the opening through which the air is entering your chest.

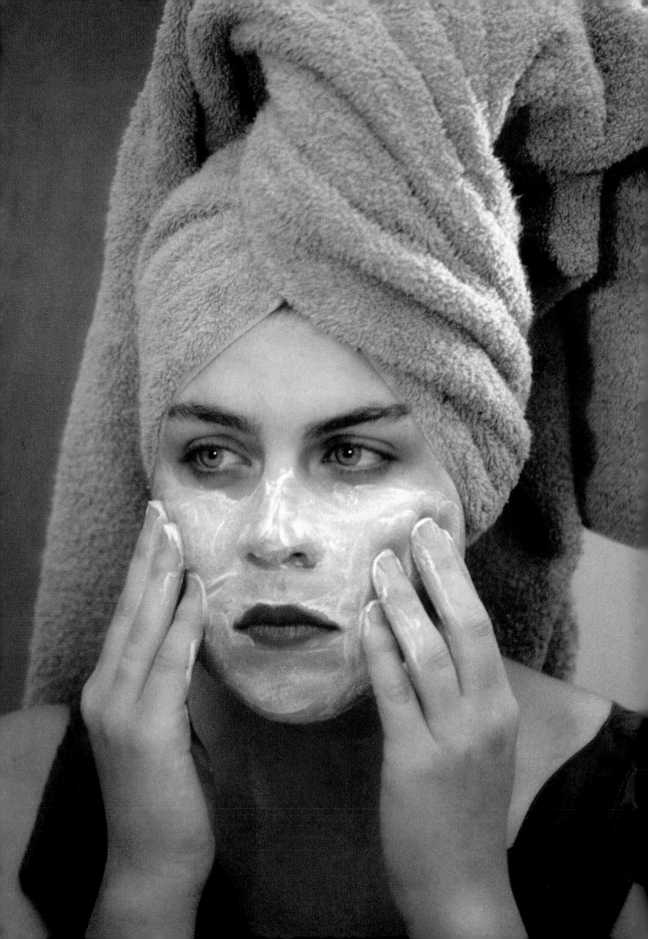

VOL. 3

SECTION 3

**THE SKELETAL
AND CUTANEOUS
SYSTEMS**

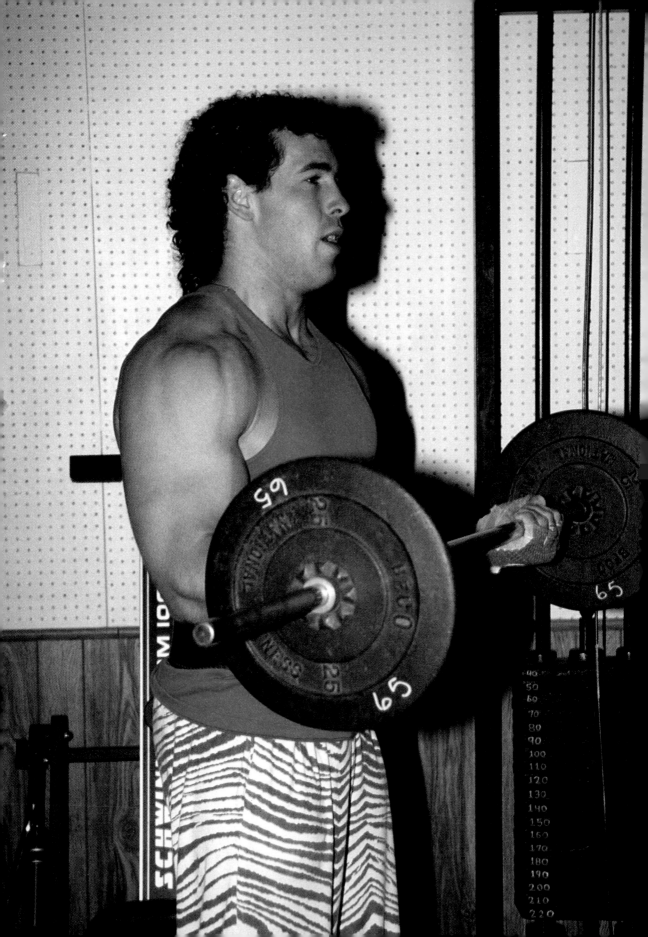

CHAPTER 12

Bones and joints and their disorders

The bones, the major component of the body's framework, join together to form a skeleton, that inner structure which provides support and protection for the body's organs and gives its general shape. The bones are in contact with one another at the joints, which permit flexibility and movement. Along with the bones and joints, the framework of the body includes connective tissue, ligaments and tendons, and cartilage.

The body's skeletal structure

Connective tissue, as its name implies, connects or holds cells together to form tissues, binds tissues together to form organs, and binds organs to one another. It consists of cells and fibers that interlace to form strands and mats. Some fibers are firm and strong; others are pliable and elastic. When tissues are cut or injured in other ways, it is connective tissue that repairs the injury, sometimes leaving a scar (an area of dense connective tissue).

Ligaments and tendons are forms of connective tissue in which most of the fibers run parallel to one another in compact bundles. Though not elastic, they can bend, allowing movement. Ligaments fasten the bones together at the joints. Tendons—fibrous extensions of muscles—like small cables, allow the muscles' pulling force to be exerted on the bones. The tendon that connects the calf muscles to the heel bone is the largest in the body.

In **cartilage,** a flexible, plasticlike substance, called intercellular substance, fills the spaces between the connective tissue fibers. This springy matrix is softer than bone. Cartilage contains no blood vessels and is solid except for the cell spaces within the matrix. When vessels do enter cartilage, they destroy it, except during the growth of bones (at the epiphyses).

Cartilage composes parts of a number of structures, such as the nose, external ears, larynx, trachea, and bronchi, which can bend but do not break. Another type of cartilage covers the joint surfaces of bones, making them smooth and glistening and reducing friction. Still another type forms the disks between the bodies of the vertebrae, cushioning forces of impact and also allowing the spinal column to bend in various directions.

In **bones** the spaces between the connective tissue fibers are filled largely with salts of calcium phosphate and calcium carbonate, along with magnesium and other salts. The elongated, flat crystals are bonded together to prevent "shear." The fibers give great tensile strength, while the calcium salts, as hard as marble, resist compression. The enamel of the teeth is the only substance in the body harder than bone. The ridges and bumps on the bones' surface are for the attachment of muscles, tendons, and ligaments.

Most bones can be classed as either long or flat. The skull and shoulder blades are flat, while the arm and thigh bones are long. Its particular function determines the shape and size of each bone.

A long bone, such as the femur of the thigh, consists of a long, slender shaft, with two large bone masses on either end. The shaft is a hollow tube made of very hard, compact bone with the same strength as a similar-sized piece of cast iron, though much lighter. The rounded ends consist of spongy bone (to further reduce the weight), that is covered by a thin layer of compact bone.

A flat bone, such as one of the skull bones, has an outer and inner plate of compact bone with a layer of spongy bone sandwiched in between. This reduces its weight while keeping it strong. Marrow, which manufactures blood cells, fills both the hollow shafts of long bones and the small spaces of the spongy bone. Thus the Creator wastes no space within our bodies.

Contrary to popular belief, bone is

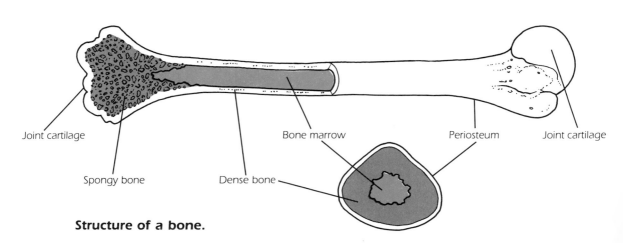

Joint cartilage   Bone marrow   Periosteum   Joint cartilage

Spongy bone   Dense bone

Structure of a bone.

living tissue, containing within its hard, brittle structure millions of living cells provided with oxygen and nutrients by a network of blood vessels. Bone structure is constantly being remodeled by bone-destroying cells (osteoclasts) and bone-building cells (osteoblasts). This dual process of bone destruction and bone production permits bones to enlarge and lengthen, as occurs during periods of growth.

W. Henry Hollinshead and Cornelius Rosse, in their *Textbook of Anatomy,* give some interesting data on bone. "While there are no constant values for the strength of bone, good adult bone is said to have a tensile strength of about 12,000 to more than 17,000 psi [lb. per sq. in.] (that of copper is 28,000 lb, that of white oak along the grain is about 12,500), and a compressive strength of about 18,000 to almost 25,000 (that of copper is about 42,000, that of granite 15,000, and that of white oak along the grain only 7,000)."[1]

Joints are contact points between two or more bones. They may allow little or no motion or free movement, depending on the type of joint. The joint types include ball-and-socket, hinge, pivot, gliding, and saddle. The ball-and-socket joints permit wide movement, as in the shoulders and hips. The knees, elbows, and jaw illustrate hinge joints. And it is the pivot joints which allow you to move your head from side to side, or, with your elbow bent, to make your palm face upward or downward.

Cartilage covers the joint surfaces, permitting free movement. The contact surfaces are further lubricated

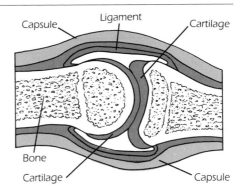

Main structures forming a joint.

with joint fluid, reducing friction to a minimum.

The hand is doubtless the most exquisitely designed instrument in the world. It has the ability, through a variety of joints, for the thumb to touch the tips of any of the fingers or to fold itself across the palm of the hand. That is one of a number of characteristics that distinguishes man from all other animals. These and other movements allow you to thread a needle or ax down a mighty tree. For without our hands, and what they do directly or indirectly, we would have no machines to construct the wonders of modern technology.

The **skeleton** is an arrangement of the bones that gives form and support to the body, while allowing for movement, and provides protection for its vital organs. The infant is born with some 270 bones, many of which fuse to form single bones, reducing the number in adulthood to 206. Five sacral vertebrae, for example, fuse to form the sacrum, a part of the pelvis, while four coccygeal vertebrae fuse to form the tailbone.

Thirty-three vertebrae make up the spine, which extends from the base

939

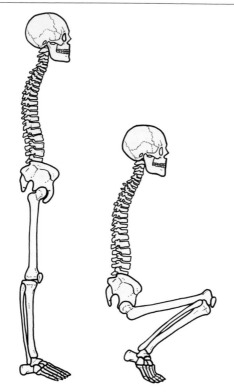

Weight-bearing bony structure of the body.

of the skull to the pelvis. Each vertebra has a flat, rounded, rod-shaped body in front, with a bony arch attached to the back. Three bony spines project from the arch, one extending backward and one on each side directed outward. When the bodies and arches of the vertebrae are placed one on top of another, the bodies form a column (the spinal column or backbone), while the arches form the spinal canal, in which the spinal cord resides.

It is our bones that allow us to carry weight. For example, as one descends the spinal column, the bodies of the vertebrae gradually become larger, allowing each to carry more weight. The spinal canal does just the opposite. It gradually becomes smaller as the nerves which make up the spinal cord pass outward in pairs between the spinal arches, thus wasting no space.

Between the bodies of adjacent vertebrae are disks (intervertebral) composed of dense, fibrous tissue on the outside with a gel-like central core. The disks firmly hold the vertebrae together, act as shock absorbers, and allow the spine to bend and turn.

A pair of ribs attach to each of the twelve thoracic vertebrae. The tips of the first ten pairs join by means of a cartilage to the breastbone, while the last two are short and have no attachment in front (called "floating ribs"). Together the ribs and breastbone form the rib cage or chest.

The skull protects the brain and the organs of sight, hearing, and balance; the vertebral column guards the spinal cord, the chest shelters the heart, lungs, liver, spleen, and kidneys; while the pelvis shields the bladder and certain of the sex organs.

The upper limbs attach by means of the collarbones to the first ribs and breastbone, while the lower limbs articulate with the pelvis. The limbs allow for free movement: the wrist and hands for grasping, the ankles and feet for walking, and the jaw (lower mandible) for talking and chewing. The femur or thigh bone is the largest bone in the body, being one fourth the height of the individual. The three ossicles of the ear are the smallest bones. They transmit sound waves the distance of a few millimeters from the eardrum to the inner ear.

Bone disorders

We will now consider problems and diseases relating to ligaments, tendons, bones, and joints. The collagen vascular diseases are considered here because they involve the connective tissues, which are part of the body's support system.

Fractures

A break in a bone is called a fracture, and is usually caused by a force being applied to a bone that it cannot withstand, as may result from a fall, from a sudden impact (as in a car accident), or from a crushing injury. A **spontaneous** or **pathological** fracture may occur when a bone becomes weakened through disuse, as happens in the elderly; through osteoporosis, commonly seen with advancing age and in those on steroid medications; and through cancer of the bone. A **stress** or **fatigue** fracture is a hairline crack (not seen in early X-rays) that develops from excessive use, observed in new recruits sent on long marches and in athletes and hikers.

A number of other types of fractures exist. In a **simple** fracture the bone is broken, but the skin is not punctured. In an **(open)** compound fracture the broken bone protrudes through the skin, causing tissue

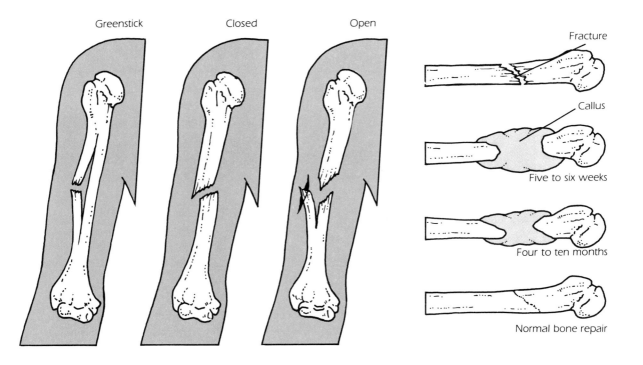

Types of fractures and the process of repair.

941

damage. In a **comminuted** fracture the bone is shattered into many fragments. In a **compression** fracture the bone is compressed or compacted. This occurs when a body of a vertebra collapses under pressure. In a **greenstick** fracture the bone bends and partially breaks. This break is often seen in children, whose bones are less brittle.

The usual indications of a fracture include the following: the injured person felt a sudden "snap" in the involved part of his body; the site of the fracture feels tender and painful and may be swollen and out of shape; the victim is unable or unwilling to move or use the injured part; movement produces a grating of the bones; and the broken limb appears to be shorter than the other limb.

A fracture constitutes a medical emergency. To heal properly, the broken ends must be in contact, with the bones properly aligned. If the bone is not set, healing may not occur, or a deformity may result that requires surgical intervention. Infections from compound fractures must be guarded against. Fractures may damage blood vessels and organs, as sometimes may occur with skull and rib fractures in which the brain or lung is injured.

What you can do. Seek skilled help immediately. Emergency care (see page 548) requires that splints and proper supports be applied to the fractured area so that on moving the injured, no additional damage to vessels or organs will occur. These precautions are especially essential in fractures of the skull, neck, back, and pelvis.

What your physician can do. Examination of the site, along with X-rays, will establish the extent of injury and the type of fracture. If the injured suffers from shock, it must be treated first. The treatment of a fracture requires **reduction**—bringing the fragments into proper alignment. This may require traction if the broken ends have pulled past each other due to muscle spasm. Once aligned, the bones must be immobilized. **Immobilization** may be accomplished with a splint or cast, or by surgically placing screws, a plate, or a rod.

Healing may require weeks to months. Rehabilitation is most important. Follow the instructions of your physician. During this time make every effort to maintain as much activity as possible to preserve good circulation, reduce swelling, and prevent atrophy of the muscles and stiffening of the joints.

Curvatures of the spine

The vertebrae of the neck and low back normally curve forward while the thoracic vertebrae curve backward. Spinal curvature of the upper back, in which the outer curve or hump is directed backward, is called **hunchback** or **kyphosis.** When the curvature in the lower back is directed forward, it is **swayback** or **lordosis.** Sideways curvature is called **scoliosis.**

In kyphosis the person becomes round-shouldered with the chest sunken in. Lordosis in the low back causes the buttocks to protrude backward and the abdomen forward. Increased stress on the muscles re-

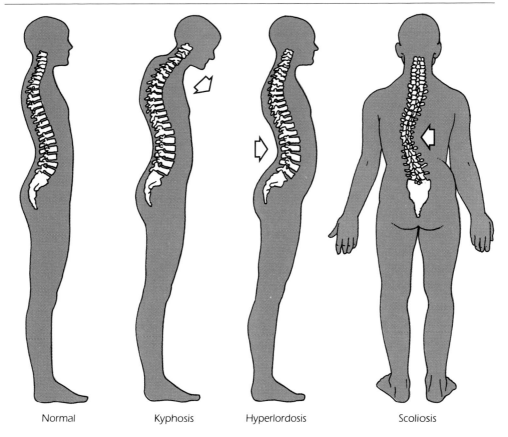

| Normal | Kyphosis | Hyperlordosis | Scoliosis |

Normal and abnormal postures.

sults in lower back pain.

Scoliosis and the other abnormal curvatures may first appear in early childhood, but generally become obvious during adolescence. They occur more often in girls. If scoliosis is not corrected, it progressively becomes worse during growth. The rib cage becomes distorted, and the vertebrae tend to rotate, at times causing difficulty in breathing and frequent chest infections.

The tendency toward scoliosis may be inherited, or it may be aggravated by weakened muscles, by one leg being shorter than the other, causing a pelvic tilt, or by a habit of standing and sitting poorly. However, in most cases the cause is not known.

What you can do. As soon as you observe what appears to be an abnormal curvature, consult with your physician. Postural exercises may improve kyphosis but not scoliosis.

What your physician can do. He can determine whether you need a brace and how long to wear it. In severe and advanced cases he may advise surgery.

Osteoporosis

In osteoporosis, a condition in which the bone substance or matrix is depleted, the bones become thin

943

and weakened. Normally a balance exists between the minerals entering and leaving the bones. When loss is greater than retention, demineralization occurs and osteoporosis develops.

Osteoporosis occurs in certain types of malnutrition, vitamin C deficiency, calcium deficiency, hyperthyroidism, diabetes, and conditions of excess adrenal cortical hormones. Causitive factors include lack of estrogens, especially in women after menopause, cortisone therapy, aging, and **lack of exercise.**

Osteoporosis generally produces no symptoms. Height may gradually decrease as the vertebrae weaken and compress, and the individual becomes increasingly stooped. Backache is also fairly common, and pain becomes severe when a compression fracture occurs in a vertebra as it collapses, or when a hip or arm fractures.

What you can do. Regular exercise and a nutritious diet adequate in calcium and vitamin C and low in protein (high protein intake increases calcium loss) provide both prevention and cure. Sunshine will provide vitamin D (take a supplement if sunlight is not available), which will aid in calcium absorption. Increasing calcium intake alone will not reverse the problem. Many postmenopausal women do not get enough calcium, and so may need a calcium supplement.

What your physician can do. He will try to find and treat any underlying cause, and by means of laboratory tests and X-rays determine the extent of your osteoporosis. If you

are a woman past menopause, he may recommend estrogen therapy.

Osteomalacia and rickets

In both osteomalacia and rickets the bones become weak and soft. Demineralization of the bones, in adults called osteomalacia, in children known as rickets, is due to a lack of calcium and phosphorous, the chief mineral elements in bone structure. These minerals are poorly absorbed from the intestine because of a deficiency of vitamin D.

Vitamin D, often called the "sunshine vitamin," is synthesized in the skin when exposed to sunlight (see page 69) and is essential for the absorption of calcium and phosphorous. Causes of this disorder include shortage of vitamin D, a diet lacking calcium and phosphorous, kidney failure in which phosphorous is lost (called "resistant rickets" in children), and celiac disease.

In **osteomalacia** the outstanding symptoms consist of pain and tenderness in the bones, especially those of the back, chest, thighs, and feet; muscle weakness, which accounts for a shuffling gait and difficulty in rising from a chair; bone deformities (sideways bowing of the thigh bones); and occasional spontaneous fractures.

Rickets frequently occurs in infants six to eighteen months of age. The earliest symptoms consist of restlessness, irritability, and sweating of the head. The junctions of bone and cartilage at the front of the ribs on either side of the breastbone enlarge, forming two rows of hard nodules. Because the skull bones are soft, the head takes on a square shape. Other symptoms include bowlegs or knock-knees, a protruding abdomen, and constipation. X-rays will reveal poor development near the ends of the bones. The pelvis may become deformed, a special problem for girls who, when mature, may have difficulty at childbirth.

What you can do. Both to prevent or cure these problems, eat a nutritious diet with adequate calcium and vitamin D. A wholesome diet (see page 696) will supply the needed minerals, while appropriate exposure to sunlight or a sunlamp will provide needed vitamin D. Otherwise you will need to take a supplement of this vitamin.

What your physician can do. He will order blood tests, which will reveal the levels of calcium and phosphorous. Many postmenopausal women do not get enough calcium, and so may require a supplement. Should the disease be due to an underlying problem, such as kidney failure, he will recommend appropriate amounts of phosphorous.

Bowlegs and knock-knees

Newborn babies normally have bowed legs and flat feet. Changes occur gradually as growth continues through puberty. Arches slowly develop during the preschool years; the child remains bowlegged (ankles touch but knees don't) until he has learned to walk. Although knock-knees are uncommon (more frequent in girls), bowlegs may give way to knock-knees (knees touch but ankles don't). However, usually the feet and legs align correctly by the time growth is complete.

Rarely, bowlegs and knock-knees will occur as secondary disorders of the growing centers of the bones at the knee, or of such diseases as rickets, scurvy, and cerebral palsy. Overweight may also be a causative factor. The habit of sitting on the floor with the knees flexed and the feet and legs to the outside of the thighs ("TV" position) may lead to knock-knees and "pigeon toes."

What you can do. Watch your child to see if growth and development follow normal patterns. A nutritious diet, exposure to sunlight, and plenty of exercise should assure normal development. Should any of these conditions persist beyond the usual time periods or handicap the child, see your physician.

What your physician can do. He may advise braces and/or modification of the shoes to change the direction of the weight-bearing thrust.

Fallen arches and flat foot

The foot has two **arches,** one running side-to-side, the other running the length of the foot, which give the foot resilience and flexibility. The side-to-side arch is not, as is generally believed, at the ball of the foot, but is at about the midpoint of the foot. Some medical authorities consider the long arch to be two arches, side by side. The inner side of the arch is seen on the inside of the foot.

When the muscles supporting the arches fatigue or weaken, the weight is borne by the ligaments which hold the bones of the arch together. As the ligaments stretch, the arch "falls," producing pain that is felt in

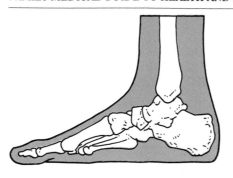

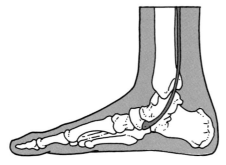

Normal longitudinal arch (top); collapsed arch (bottom) in flat foot.

the foot, calf, knee, hip, and even the back.

In **flat foot,** a common abnormality, the heel twists outward so that the sole of the foot faces away from the body, and the foot is directed outward. It is the result of excess weight being carried on the inside of the foot (medial arch), from overweight, from carrying heavy loads, or from standing for long periods of time. The underlying cause—usually weak muscles and lax ligaments—may be congenital, with faulty alignment of the bones.

The treatment aims to correct, if possible, the factors causing the problem. The doctor may recommend that you lose weight or change occupations if your present occupation requires you to lift heavy weights or stand for considerable periods of time. If you are run down,

build up your general health, walk to strengthen the muscles, and wear well-fitting, comfortable shoes. When walking, do not direct the feet outward (toeing out), but a little inward (toeing in). Should the problem persist, see your physician, who may recommend an appliance.

Club foot

In club foot the ankle twists inward, causing the sole of the foot to face inward, and the person walks on the outer margin of the foot (the opposite of flat foot). The causes of club foot include congenital, nutritional, and positional (intrauterine) factors.

Professional care is essential beginning immediately after birth. Manipulation of a baby's foot with casts to hold it in the correct position for a few weeks or months will bring about normal development. If not corrected by casts in three to four months, surgery is usually required.

Paget's disease

In this disease the normal balance between the breakdown and rebuilding of bone is disturbed so that an excessive amount of new bone develops, which is abnormal in structure. The bones most commonly affected—the skull, vertebrae, pelvis, thigh, and leg bones—become thickened, misshapen, and weakened. The legs may become bowed and the skull enlarged.

Symptoms vary from mild aching to severe pain. The enlarging bones may compress nerves, such as those of the ear, causing loss of hearing. The disease is slowly progressive, of unknown cause, and usually affects about 3 percent of people in the United States above the age of fifty. The treatment consists of pain relief and possibly hormone therapy.

Painful heel ("spurs")

Painful heels are usually due to strain or inflamation of the soft tissues attaching to the heel. This may result from injury or excessive weight on the heel. "Spurs" do not occur on weight bearing surfaces, but where ligaments attach to the bones. They are about as frequent as non-painful heels. The pain can be severe when the soft tissues of the foot press against the spur. A ring-shaped pad around the tender spot and a hot foot bath with massage of the area may provide relief. If pain persists, see your physician, who may recommend an injection of cortisone. Rarely surgical treatment is advisable.

Tumors of the bone

Two classes of tumors affect bones: those that originate in the bone (rather rare), and those which metastasize or spread from other cancers to the bone (quite common). The majority of tumors which arise in the bones are noncancerous or benign. Bone tumors cause swelling of the bones or joints, often with persistent pain. Osteosarcoma is a cancer that originates in the bone, softening the bone, which then tends to fracture.

Many cancers, such as those of the breast, lungs, and prostate, spread to the bones, often before they have been detected in their original sites, Symptoms, together with scans, X-rays, and blood tests determine the precise problem. Treatment will depend on the type and extent of involvement. Chemotherapy, radiation therapy, and surgery are used separately or in combination.

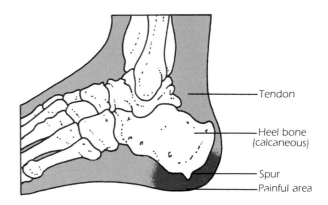

Outgrowth of bone or spur on the heel bone.

Osteomyelitis

Osteomyelitis is an infection of bone and bone marrow. In children (most commonly between the ages of ten and fifteen) the infection spreads through the blood from some distant part of the body, such as a boil, a middle ear infection, or pneumonia. In adults the infection often results from a penetrating injury (gunshot) or an open fracture in which the bone was exposed.

The infection causes severe pain, with extreme tenderness over the infected area, especially when the joint nearby is bent or flexed. Other symptoms include chills and fever, and in children, listlessness, dehydration, and an unwillingness to move the involved limb.

Various germs may cause the infection, but the most common are

947

the staphylococcus bacteria, which erode and destroy the bone. If not treated, the infection will spread into the surrounding tissues and drain through the skin. The bone infection must first be treated. X-rays, CT scan, and laboratory tests of a biopsy will determine the best treatment.

Antibiotics will be directed toward the organism. The infected area may also require proper drainage, with surgical removal of destroyed bone. The infection tends to crop up repeatedly.

Disorders of tendons and ligaments

Tendons, either short or long, attach muscles to bones and may cross joints. Long tendons frequently travel in sheaths, which are lubricated to reduce friction. Sheaths commonly surround the tendons found in the hands and feet.

Tendonitis and teno-synovitis

Inflammation of a tendon is called tendonitis, while that of its sheath is tenosynovitis. **Tendons** become inflamed from injury, stretching, or excessive use. Those most commonly affected are in the shoulder, elbow, hip, back of the knee, and heel. Tennis elbow affects tendons on the outer side of the elbow, resulting from constant grasping (as in playing tennis), from using a screwdriver (rotary movements), or even from shaking hands. The tendon attached to the back of the heel becomes stretched and inflamed when a woman accustomed to wearing high heels transfers to low-heeled shoes. **Tendon sheaths** become inflamed from excessive use or from infections. Those commonly affected are in the palm of the hand or in the sole of the foot. They sometimes becoming scarred and tight.

Symptoms of pain and tenderness occur, especially from infection. Rest and applications of heat and/or cold often give comfort. Sometimes splints or casts give opportunity for healing and antiinflammatory medication and injections of cortisone relieve pain. Healing the infection may require antibiotics and surgical drainage. Surgically splitting a tight sheath will give prompt relief.

Bursitis

Bursitis is an inflammation of the lining of a bursa. Bursas are membranous sacs or pockets situated near a joint, between tendons, or between a tendon and a bone. Their linings secrete a lubricating fluid that reduces friction as the tendons slide by one another or slide over a bone.

Bursitis may develop below the kneecap ("housemaid's knee") and in the shoulder, elbow, and hip. Injury or overuse of the muscles whose tendons are in contact with the bursa cause the bursal lining to become inflamed. The result is swelling due to an increase of fluid, pain on movement, and tenderness on pressure. In chronic bursitis calcium salts may be deposited in the walls of the bursa.

948

What you can do. Bursitis may clear up in a week or two; however, it frequently recurs. Rest, together with hot-and-cold compresses, may provide relief. It is important that you retain full motion in those joints where bursitis occurs. Should your shoulder be affected, lean forward and allow your arm to swing loosely in a rotatory movement. If the bursitis continues, see your physician.

What your physician can do. He may prescribe an anti-inflammatory agent or remove some of the fluid and inject a steroid preparation. If the bursitis persists, or if an X-ray reveals a calcium deposit, surgical removal may be necessary.

Sprain

A sprain is an injury in which one or more of the ligaments which support a joint or the joint capsule stretch or tear. Sprains—most common in the ankle, knee, and wrist joints—result from a sudden twisting of the joint while weight or pressure is placed on it. Because a severe sprain is difficult to distinguish from a fracture, an X-ray is advisable. A sprain causes swelling, tenderness to touch, black-and-white discoloration, and severe pain, especially on use.

What you can do. If the sprain is not severe, use an ice pack for the first twenty-four hours to reduce swelling. Thereafter, use hot-and-cold applications to promote the circulation and speed healing. An elastic bandage will limit motion and relieve the pain. To rest the joint, use a sling for the elbow and crutches for the knee and ankle. When a joint is repeatedly sprained, the ligaments weaken, thus allowing the joint to sprain more readily.

What your physician can do. Severely torn ligaments and capsules may require surgical repair. The physician may recommend a cast to hold the joint in place while healing. He will guide you as to when hot-and-cold applications and exercise of the joint can be undertaken, so as to regain full motion and function.

Ganglion (pl. ganglia)

A ganglion is a cystlike tumor or swelling that develops on a tendon sheath or joint capsule, and occurs most commonly on the back of the wrist and in front of the ankle. Ganglia are about the size of a small bean, are filled with a semisolid substance, and are generally painless. Although the traditional home remedy has been to smash a ganglion with a book, it is wiser to have your physician determine whether the swelling is indeed a ganglion. He will rupture the cyst with pressure. Ganglia may recur or disappear spontaneously, rarely requiring surgical removal.

Dupuytren's contracture

In this condition a tightening of the connective tissue develops beneath the skin of the palm of the hand, and occasionally on the sole of the foot. The shrinkage progresses over years, may involve the tendon sheaths, and eventually causes the ring and little fingers to be permanently bent toward the palm. It does not produce pain. The tendency toward contracture appears to be inherited, occurs in older people, and

949

is seen more frequently in those of European descent. Should the contracture handicap the person, it can be relieved surgically.

Carpal tunnel syndrome

This condition causes pain in the hand and numbness of the fingers, and is usually worse on arising in the morning. It results from pressure on the median nerve as it passes through the wrist. The front of the wrist contains a tunnel formed from wrist bones and ligaments through which pass nine tendons and the median nerve. Swelling of the tissues in this area from injury or arthritis puts pressure on the nerve. The pressure can be relieved surgically by cutting part of the main ligament.

Disorders of the joints

Dislocations

A **traumatic dislocation** has several possible causes: the bones forming a joint are pulled apart, one or more of the ligaments holding the bones together are stretched or torn, or the joint capsule is ruptured or stretched. This causes the loss of the normal range of movement. Dislocations—most commonly involving the shoulder, elbow, wrist, thumb, hip, knee, ankle, or jaw—result from falls, from twisting movements as in athletic activities, and from car accidents. The soft tissues surrounding a dislocated joint (nerves, vessels, muscles) may also be injured.

The dislocated joint becomes swollen, misshapen, hemorrhagic (blood under the skin), and extremely painful. The sufferer is unwilling or unable to move the joint.

Nontraumatic dislocations may be due to a **congenital** abnormality, some disease process, or a previous incompletely healed dislocation. Dislocation of the hip joint, in which the head of the femur has slipped out of its socket, may first be observed soon after birth or when an infant first begins to walk. This condition results from an inherited poor socket or excessively loose ligaments. Early recognition and prompt treatment with appropriate bracing will often avert an otherwise crippling deformity. It should be emphasized that early treatment is of critical importance. Surgery is often necessary if treatment is not started before walking.

Rheumatoid arthritis is an example of a disease affecting a joint (such as the hip), weakening the muscles, tendons, and ligaments so that they no longer hold the bones of the joint together, thus permitting a dislocation to occur. The shoulder joint, once dislocated, may subsequently slip out of place for no apparent reason and may require surgical repair to keep it in place.

What you can do. A dislocation is a medical emergency. Because a dislocation is sometimes difficult to distinguish from a fracture, and sometimes both are present, the patient should be carefully transported to a hospital for professional help (see "first aid procedures," page 548).

What your physician can do.

The physician will carefully examine the joint and prescribe X-rays to provide the detailed knowledge he needs. If the reduction (putting the bones back into place) is not done promptly, an anesthetic may be required. Various joints require different procedures for reduction. Depending on the type of dislocation and the extent of injury to the surrounding tissues, he may have to surgically reduce and repair damaged structures. It is important that he monitor the patient during the period of recovery.

Herniated disk (slipped disk, prolapsed disk)

A disk (see below) is said to be herniated or slipped when the inside gel-like substance (nucleus) either pushes the weakened outer fibrous layer outward or squeezes through it, putting pressure on adjacent nerves. Weakening or degeneration of the disk may occur from unknown causes or may result from physical inactivity, aging, or injury. A sedentary lifestyle, sleeping on soft mattresses, carrying heavy weights, lifting heavy weights incorrectly, and automobile or other accidents may weaken or damage a disk.

The pain resulting from a herniated disk may come on gradually, though usually it comes on abruptly. Depending which part of the spinal column is affected, intense pain may occur in the neck and run down the shoulder and

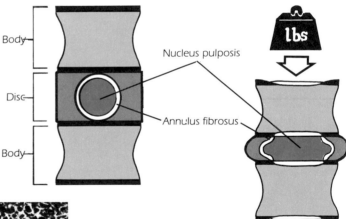

Normal intervertebral disk: when not carrying and when carrying weight.

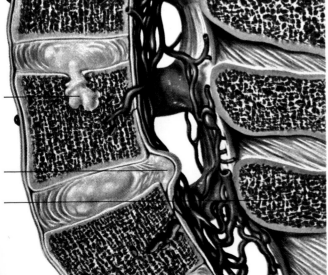

Herniations of the intervertebral disk: (1) herniated into body of vertebra, (2) forced toward spinal canal (which shelters spinal cord), (3) spinous process.

951

arm, or in the low back and travel down the thigh and leg. Not infrequently the hernia puts pressure on the sciatic nerve, in which case the condition is spoken of as **sciatica.** Muscles supplied by the affected nerves may become weak.

What you can do. Depending on the severity of the attack, bed rest may be essential. A physician's guidance may also be necessary. Heat to the neck or back (heating pad, hot-water bottle, or fomentations page 590), and sleeping on an extra-firm mattress should prove helpful. A well-fitting back brace or neck collar often relieves the severe pain and allows you to move about. If you are overweight, you will benefit from losing weight. Keeping your muscles strong, along with standing and sitting correctly, may prevent a recurrence.

What your physician can do. You may have to be hospitalized so that traction can be instituted. At times steroids or medication to relax the muscles may be recommended. X-ray studies and a CAT scan or MRI may be required to specifically determine the problem. Surgical removal of that part of the disk causing the problem should bring relief. He may suggest a specific set of exercises to help you minimize recurrences.

Rheumatoid arthritis

In rheumatoid arthritis the synovial membrane of one or more joints remains chronically inflamed. The membrane becomes swollen, enlarged, soft and spongy, with fluid filling the joint space. The joint becomes stiff as the muscles around the inflamed joint go into spasm, thus limiting the movement of the joint in order to prevent pain. The cartilage covering the ends of the bones gradually deteriorates. Eventually the bones of the joint fuse, losing all movement. The joints most commonly affected are those of the hands and feet, although the knees, shoulders, wrists, ankles, elbows, and neck frequently become involved. In severe cases, every joint can be attacked.

Rheumatoid arthritis usually develops after childhood and before the age of forty, although it may appear as late as sixty or seventy. It occurs three times more frequently in women than men. The disease can be mild to extremely severe, but usually progresses slowly over many years with one or more remissions. Predisposing factors are an infectious agent (virus or bacteria), an endocrine disorder, emotional trauma, and heredity. Rheumatoid arthritis is an autoiumune response in which the body's defenses destroy its own joint tissues.

Eighty percent or more of sufferers carry in their blood a gamma globulin (rheumatoid factor) that combines with its own normal gamma globulin. This new chemical complex, while itself causing inflammation of the synovial lining, also causes the synovia to produce this same inflammatory complex. The synovial lining then attacks and destroys the cartilage and joint.

The inflammation of the joints causes pain, swelling, and stiffness, especially in the morning. The joints appear red and are tender and warm. General symptoms include loss of appetite, loss of weight, with weakness and debility. Anemia may be present.

What you can do. While your general care should be under the direction of a physician, you can do several things. Getting a nutritious diet, adequate rest, and moderate but regular exercise will enhance your resistance. For many, swimming in a pool is well tolerated. Emotional adjustment to the disease and the handicaps it imposes, along with an attitude of peace and tranquility (best obtained through trust in God), will further recovery.

What your physician can do. He can treat and monitor the progress of the disease. The sedimentation rate (the rate at which the red blood cells settle in a tube) indicates the level of inflammation, which must be reduced before any exercise can be in-

stituted. A combination of rest, heat, and gentle massage tends to reduce the inflammation, as do a number of antiinflammatory medications, such as high doses of aspirin, steroids, gold injections, and penicillamine. These agents have serious side effects, and a physician must closely monitor their use.

A physical therapist will direct as to which therapeutic exercises are most appropriate for the particular joint or joints involved. The physician and an occupational therapist should work together to provide the best possible rehabilitation so that the sufferer can function as independently as is feasible. During the early stages of the disease, surgical removal of the inflamed synovial tissues will help to reduce inflammation. In later stages, surgery helps to restore functions by correcting deformities and by replacing destroyed

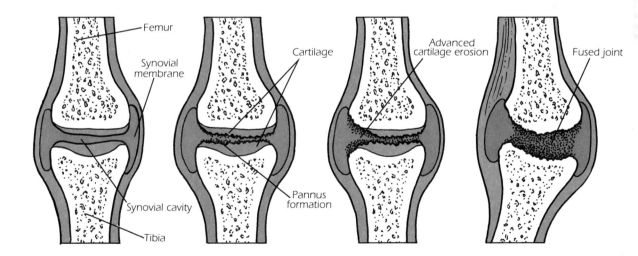

Normal joint with cartilage and synovial membrane. As arthritic process advances, membrane and cartilage are eroded. Joint fusion eventually occurs.

joints, such as the hip, knee, shoulder, and elbow.

Osteoarthritis (degenerative joint disease)

Degenerative joint disease or osteoarthritis (better called osteoarthrosis since there is rarely inflammation) is a degeneration of the articular cartilage (the cartilage covering the ends of bones forming a joint). The cartilage breaks up, and the bone beneath either thins or overgrows irregularly. These bony growths, known as "spurs" or "lipping," grow around the margins of the joint.

Half of those forty years of age and older show signs of osteoarthritis, most commonly in the joints of the spine, hip, knee, and fingers. The precise cause is not known, although it may result from the aging process. Injuries and excessive pressure on a joint from overweight or overuse appear to contribute to the problem.

The process may continue for years without producing any symptoms. Pain usually results from a direct injury to a joint with local inflammation. Range of motion may diminish, and the muscles around the joint tend to weaken due to disuse. Bony overgrowths along the spine may press against nerves, causing pain and muscle spasm. The disease may be handicapping, but is not life-threatening.

What you can do. Since no specific cure for the disease exists, you must adapt to the problem, altering your lifestyle so as to prolong your productive usefulness. You can adopt a number of simple measures which will prove helpful. If you are obese, normalizing your weight will reduce wear and tear on weight-bearing joints (hip, knee, spine). Exercise regularly within toleration, and move each affected joint through its full range of motion each day. Applying dry heat to a painful joint often brings relief. Avoid overfatigue, and sleep on a firm mattress. Refrain from overexerting involved joints.

The market offers an almost limitless number of remedies for the relief and cure of osteoarthritis, but one thing is sure: There is no magic cure. Don't experiment on yourself; seek counsel from your physician.

What your physician can do. He may have blood tests and X-rays done to evaluate your general health and the precise condition of your involved joints. He may prescribe aspirin for severe pain. Steroids are used where aspirin or other non-steroidal anti-inflamatory agents fail to give relief; however, these agents also have undesirable side effects. Cortisone may be injected directly into an inflamed joint to avoid a general response, but the number of times this can be done is limited. Your physician may suggest a series of treatments from a physical therapist.

In severe cases, joint replacement may restore function in the hip, knee, or shoulder.

Infectious arthritis (septic arthritis)

Infectious arthritis is an infection of a joint due to an infectious agent—bacteria, viruses, or fungi—invading a joint. The organism may enter the joint directly, as from a war wound or some injury; migrate into the joint from an adjacent infection (osteomyelitis); or, most commonly, travel in the blood from an infection elsewhere, as from a boil, abscess, gonorrhea urethritis, tubercular lung, coccidiomycosis, candidiasis, German measles, or infectious mononucleosis.

The symptoms are those of an infection: chills, fever, and a warm, swollen, tender joint. Typically one joint is affected—usually a large joint such as the hip, knee, or shoulder. In **gonorrheal arthritis** the knee is affected 50 percent of the time.

What you can do. Should you suspect infectious arthritis, see your physician immediately. The longer the infection lasts, the more damage to the joint, and the harder it will be to heal.

What your physician can do. The organism can be identified by examination of the joint fluid removed by a syringe. Then he will institute appropriate antibiotic therapy. A cold compress or padded ice bag (see page 593) will minimize swelling and relieve pain. He may insist on hospitalization, where the purulent fluid is withdrawn from the knee by a syringe or by surgical drainage. A splint may be applied temporarily to relieve the pain, but he will have you resume movement of the joint, with massage and exercise, as soon as possible to prevent loss of function.

Gouty arthritis

This form of arthritis is caused by crystals of uric acid that are deposited in a joint, usually the knee,

elbow, hand, or foot. The most famous and frequent site is the base of the big toe. It occurs more often among men than women.

Uric acid, one of the waste products found in the blood, is normally eliminated by the kidneys. However, 5 to 10 percent of American males experience excessive levels of uric acid in the blood (hyperuricemia) due to overproduction or inadequate elimination or both. In a few of these (possibly due to an inherited trait), uric acid crystals precipitate in the joint fluid. These needle-sharp crystals cause intense irritation, the joint becoming swollen, warm to touch, and extremely tender. The skin over the joint is tense, shiny, and red.

The first attack usually affects a single joint and, if untreated, runs a course of one to two weeks. The pain is excruciating. Subsequent attacks become more frequent, affect more joints, and become more severe.

What you can do. During an attack, shield the joint from the pressure of bedcovers by the use of a frame. If you are overweight, begin a weight reduction program. Reduce calorie intake slowly but consistently so as not to precipitate an attack. Modify your diet to reduce or eliminate the intake of foods which raise uric acid levels, such as meat, especially organ meats, sardines, anchovies, and legumes. You should abstain from alcoholic beverages because alcohol impairs the ability of the kidneys to excrete uric acid. Begin a regular program of exercise with adequate rest and sleep. Drink an abundance of water (up to 3 quarts a day) to aid the kidneys in eliminating uric acid. It is important to be under the care of a physician.

What your physician can do. He will order blood and urine tests to determine the level of uric acid and the functional capacity of your kidneys. Because it is important to lower the level of uric acid in the blood and tissues, he may order from two types of medication: those which aid in the elimination of uric acid (by blocking its reabsorption by the kidneys) and those which block its production. During an acute attack, colchicine or one of the anti-inflammatory agents will provide relief.

Ankylosing spondylitis

In this disease the joints between the vertebrae of the spinal column first become inflamed, and then adjacent bones fuse, causing the spine to become bent and rigid. The first joint affected is usually the sacroiliac, between the sacrum and pelvic bones. Occasionally other joints are involved (hip, shoulder, hands, feet, and jaw).

The disease develops mainly in young men. The main symptoms consist of stiffness and pain in the morning, especially in the low back. Fatigue, weakness, fever, and general lassitude may also occur. Should the disease affect the rib-bearing vertebrae, breathing may be difficult and painful.

Seek the help of your physician. He can prescribe medications to relieve pain. However, with the help of a physical therapist, a program of exercise and training will help retain the best possible posture to maintain

adequate breathing. Surgery is sometimes performed to correct a badly deformed back.

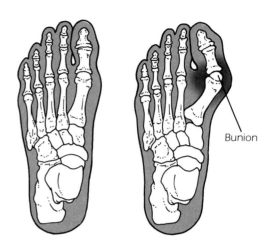

Bunion

Bunion. Note how the bones of the big toe are directed toward the little toe instead of forward, as shown in the normal foot at left.

Bunions

A bunion is a tender, painful enlargement caused by inflammation of the soft tissues (bursal sac) and bone at the outer edge of the base of the big toe. The great toe bends toward the little toe and may overlap the second toe. The skin over the protrusion rubs against the shoe and forms a callus.

Bunions usually develop at the same time on both feet. Hereditary factors include a wide foot, muscle imbalance, and relaxed ligaments. Tight-fitting, pointed, high-heeled shoes, seem to force the toes into this abnormal position. The longer the irritation continues, the greater the deformity.

Rest, foot baths, and cutting away

the shoe at the site of the bunion will relieve the pain in most cases. You should wear shoes of such size and shape as to allow the great toe to assume its normal straightforward position. Placing padding between the first and second toes will help push the big toe toward its more normal position. Night splints are available commercially. In severe cases surgical repair may be the only satisfactory solution.

Collagen vascular diseases

In collagen vascular diseases, collagen, a major protein component of connective tissue, is affected, resulting in widespread inflammatory changes in the body's connective tissues and blood vessels. An abnormality in the body's immune system apparently causes it to attack its own collagen; hence these disorders are autoimmune diseases.

Systemic sclerosis (scleroderma)

Scleroderma means thickening of the skin, and in this disease the skin becomes thick and inelastic. The disorder also affects the small blood vessels, causing them to become narrowed. When the hands are affected, the skin becomes tight and glistening, and the joints of the fingers become prominent. Ulcers often develop as the skin is injured. In some sufferers, exposure to cold causes blanching of the hands and feet (Raynaud's disease). Internal organs may also be affected: the air sacs of the lungs may thicken, causing difficulty in breathing; the pericardial sac around the heart may become stiff and constricted, resulting in heart failure; the esophagus may stiffen, making it difficult to swallow; and the kidney may be damaged, causing hypertension.

The sufferer should be under the care of a physician. No known cure for this slowly progressive disease exists. There may be remissions and relapses. Physical therapy with active and passive exercises help the hands. Local infections should be treated promptly. Steroid medications have proved ineffective.

Systemic lupus erythematosus

This disease, often referred to as SLE, is the most prevalent of the collagen diseases. It occurs in two forms: the cutaneous (discoid) form, which primarily affects the skin; and the systemic (disseminated) form, which may affect the kidneys, heart, lungs, digestive organs, or nervous system. However, the majority of those with the skin type develop the systemic disease, while only a few of those with the systemic disease develop the skin disorder.

This autoimmune disease may develop at any age, but occurs most frequently between the ages of twenty to forty, and is five to ten times more frequent in women than men. While the symptoms vary with the type of disease and the organs affected, the sufferer typically experiences fatigue, loss of appetite and weight, pain in certain joints, skin rash (especially in areas exposed to the sun), fever, and general debility.

The progress of the disease is generally chronic, but varies from person to person, usually with a series of remissions and relapses. The skin lesions are red, rounded, slightly raised scaly patches typically appearing on the bridge of the nose and cheeks in a "butterfly" pattern, giving a wolflike appearance (from the Latin word *lupus*). The skin lesions may sometimes be widely disseminated and are aggravated by exposure to the sun.

The systemic symptoms depend on the organ or organs affected. Kidney failure, problems of digestion, difficulty in breathing, and inflammation of the joints resembling rheumatoid arthritis may be present.

What you can do. Avoid exposure to the sun, and use sunscreen ointments when going outdoors. Avoid stress and get adequate rest, appropriate exercise, and a nutritious diet. Certain medications may precipitate an attack, so indicate to your physician that you have lupus.

What your physician can do. Therapy is directed toward hastening a remission or delaying or preventing a relapse. He may prescribe steroid medication, topically (for skin lesions) and systemically; antimalarial drugs for cutaneous lupus; or antirheumatic and autoimmune suppressants.

Polyarteritis nodosa

Polyarteritis nodosa is a form of **vasculitis** characterized by an acute inflammation and destruction of small and medium-sized arteries. When healing occurs in patches along the artery, lumps or nodules develop (hence the name nodosa) which can be felt in superficial areas. The cause of this disease, which is seen three times more frequently in men than women, is unknown.

The usual symptoms include fever, weakness, loss of appetite and weight, muscle and joint pain, and general illness. Other symptoms relate to the organs affected when the blood supply of an area is cut off due to closure of an artery. The kidneys are most frequently affected, resulting in nephritis and hypertension. Blockage of the coronary arteries causes chest pain and heart failure. The digestive organs, the nervous system, the lungs, and the skin may also be involved.

If untreated, the disease is usually fatal within a year. The use of steroids proves generally helpful and may prolong periods of remission. Supportive treatment depends on the particular organ affected.

Polymyositis and dermatomyositis

Polymyositis is an inflammation of the muscles with destruction of muscle tissue. When the disease also attacks the skin it is called dermatomyositis. The muscles of the shoulders, arms, pelvis, and thighs are the most frequently affected, resulting in weakness in these areas. The disease may involve other muscles, such as those of the pharynx (causing difficulty in swallowing), diaphragm and chest wall (causing difficulty in breathing), and heart (causing irregularities in rhythm). Skin involvement produces a purplish rash, usually over the face and upper chest, especially over the bony prominences. Arthritis is often present.

The cause of the disease is not known, but researchers suspect an autoimmune problem. The disease, occurring twice as often among women as men, can be diagnosed by means of a myogram (testing how the muscles contract) or by a biopsy (microscopic examination of a small sample of muscle tissue). Steroids, sometimes given in combination with cytotoxic drugs, generally slow muscle destruction. Immunosuppressives are also used. Plasmapheresis, a process in which your own blood is withdrawn and the red blood cells removed and then returned to your bloodstream, may help when medications fail, perhaps by reducing the substances affecting the muscles.

1. W. Henry Hollinshead and Cornelius Rosse, *Textbook of Anatomy*, 3rd ed. (New York: Harper and Row, 1984), p. 21.

CHAPTER 13

Muscles and muscle disorders

By weight your body is more than 50 percent muscle, comprising more than all the other organs and tissues combined. There are three kinds of muscles. **Voluntary** or **skeletal muscles,** which make up 80 to 90 percent of the muscle mass, attach to your bones and give your body both form and movement, beauty and grace. The remaining 10 to 20 per-cent—**involuntary muscles**—are of two types: **heart muscle,** which forms the walls of that organ, and **smooth muscle** or **visceral muscle,** found in the walls of the blood ves-sels, in the walls of the digestive, uri-nary, and genital organs, and even in the hair follicles of the skin.

Your voluntary muscles, at your will, allow you to make all the move-ments you take for granted: to walk or run, stoop or stand, scratch your nose or wash your hands, chew your food, or open and close your eyes. Your heart muscle performs its work throughout your lifetime, beating about 100,000 times a day, pumping blood to the farthest cell in your body.

Smooth muscle in the walls of your stomach and intestine churns your food and propels it downward through your digestive tract. Smooth muscle adjusts the size of your pupils to allow just the right amount of light to enter your eyes. Smooth muscle changes the shape of your lenses to focus for either near or far vision.

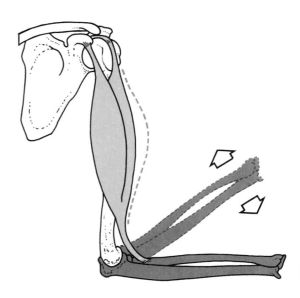

Muscles contract or shorten, thus making movements.

Muscles are designed to contract or shorten, and thus all body movement results from pulling rather than pushing. The specific shape and size of each type of muscle differs to meet its functional needs. Each voluntary muscle fiber contains several hundred to several thousand myofibrils. Each myofibril, in turn, has 1,500 myosin and 3,000 actin filaments lying beside it. These minute filaments, when stimulated by a nerve impulse, shorten or contract.

The length of a skeletal muscle fiber varies, depending on the size and location of the muscle. Some may be several inches long while others are shorter. Heart muscle is very similar to voluntary muscle but has shorter, differently shaped fibers. Smooth muscle fibers are short, except for those in the wall of the uterus, which during pregnancy enlarge and lengthen.

As mentioned earlier, muscles are stimulated to contract by means of nerve impulses. The voluntary nervous system controls the skeletal muscles, while the involuntary or automatic **(autonomic)** nervous system activates heart and smooth muscles. The heart muscle is unique in that, while controlled by autonomic nerves, it has its own pacemaker and a special type of tissue to conduct the contraction impulse throughout the heart.

After a muscle fiber has contracted, it must rest and recuperate. A muscle can be used continuously because each muscle possesses hundreds and thousands of muscle fibers, and not all work at the same time. While some work, others rest. They go on and off work shifts automatically. As more and more fibers are inadequately rested, the muscle tires or fatigues.

Obviously, for muscles to move bones, they must be attached to them. This attachment may be through a tendon—a fibrous extension of the muscle—or directly to the bone itself. The large muscles which give movement to your fingers are located on the front and back of your forearms. Their long tendons cross the wrist before attaching to the bones of the fingers. By locating the sites of the attachments on opposite sides of a bone, the bone can be moved in opposite directions. This way your fingers can bend toward the palm or extend straight out.

The power or strength of a muscle depends on its size and the use to which it is put. A muscle that is exercised or used consistently and judiciously will be strong, function efficiently, and have endurance. If used infrequently it will weaken, function inefficiently, and tire rapidly. If not used at all, it will atrophy. In the machine-age culture of today, our sedentary lifestyle does not demand that we exercise. For this reason we suffer from many diseases resulting from inactivity.

Fortunately, you do not have to give conscious attention to the various muscles that are required to make a certain movement. Some movements are programmed, while others are learned. Your brain and the related parts of your nervous system are organized in such a marvelous manner that the right combination of muscles activate automatically at your slightest thought. Thus you can move your arm back and forth, and the appropriate muscles will pull your arm in one direction and then the other.

Posture

More than 200 bones and 600 muscles make up your body framework. While the bones move at their joints, this movement is accomplished by the pull of the muscles. If it were not for muscle pull or a certain degree of muscle tension, you would fall in a heap, a crumpled mass. The alignment of your bones while standing and sitting (and to some extent while lying) determines your posture.

Good posture, whether standing or sitting, is determined by your bony framework, the muscles attached to them, and the organs within being related one to another in their proper positions with a minimum of effort, tension, or strain. Standing and sitting correctly requires little effort. For example, when standing upright—head up, back straight, shoulders back, chest out, abdomen in, and pelvis flattened—you are so balanced that the large muscles of your back (calf, thigh, buttocks, back, shoulders, and neck) pull you slightly backward with neglegible effort. With good posture you are tipped slightly forward, so should you suddenly faint when standing correctly, you would always fall face down.

Why should you strive for good posture? For both physiological and psychological reasons. The organs in your chest and abdominal cavity are suspended from your spine or vertebral column. Standing or sitting incorrectly disturbs their normal alignment, not only putting extra stresses and strains on your bones, joints, and muscles, but also impairing their function.

Your diaphragm, which lies between your chest and abdominal cavities and is the major muscle of respiration, cannot contract as efficiently when your standing posture is poor. The same holds true when you sit incorrectly, especially with your thighs crossed. This posture cramps your diaphragm and pushes your spine into abnormal curvatures, affecting adversely your respiration, circulation, and digestion.

Developing proper posture is not difficult, but it takes constant thought and effort until the habit is fixed. First you must become posture conscious. This means that you should

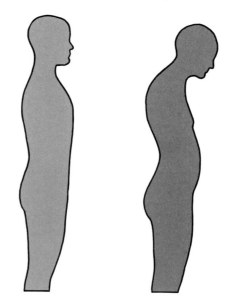

Good and poor posture.

constantly think about how you are standing and sitting.

The secret to good posture is to learn to flatten your pelvis, because this determines the forward and backward curvatures of your spine. To accomplish this, contract your large gluteal muscles (those of your buttocks) while standing. This throws your pubis upward. You cannot do this while walking, but practice it whenever you are standing. Then stand and sit tall, holding your head erect with your chin out. Allow your arms to hang naturally by your sides. If you have developed rounded shoulders, you may have to pull them backwards for a period of time.

Good posture is a real asset. It will improve your health and appearance. It will give you poise and grace. It will provide you with a positive influence and make you more readily accepted by others. You will look and feel better.

Disorders of muscles

Muscle cramps

Muscle cramps occur when muscles in certain localized areas go into violent spasm, most commonly seen in the muscles of the calf, back of the thigh, and feet. While the precise cause has not, as yet, been determined, certain factors appear to precipitate their occurrence. These include severe cold, poor circulation to the affected area, overexercise of the muscle, stretching the muscle too much, pointing the toes forward (extending the foot), and dehydration (lack of sufficient water intake).

Night cramps frequently wake some people up with extreme pain. However, the condition is harmless. Something in the muscle (lack of oxygen, excess lactic acid, faulty relaxation) triggers a reflex response from the spinal cord. This contraction, in turn, further stimulates the sensory nerves, causing another response from the cord, which increases the spasm.

Swimmer's cramp is similar to the cramp discussed above. It occurs more frequently among swimmers who kick with their feet stretched out (extended). Avoid overextending your feet while swimming. Some of the procedures described below may be helpful.

What you can do. Once the cramp has occurred it will relax of its own accord. However, to hasten its relaxation, try contracting the muscles that produce a movement in a direction opposite to that which the cramping muscles are pulling. For instance, if your calf muscles are in spasm and drawing your foot downward, hold the foot in that position while trying to draw the foot upwards (towards your shin). This may provide immediate relief. Do not stretch the cramped muscle too far. Another suggestion: stand on the balls of your feet while raising and lowering your heels.

Some people obtain relief by gently massaging the affected muscles.

963

Raising the foot of the bed helps others. A warm footbath, which increases the circulation in the legs and feet, will also give relief, and if taken before going to bed will frequently prevent their occurrence. Heavy bed clothes which force the foot forward (toward the sole) may precipitate an attack. Try using a cradle or pillow under the covers to remove the weight of the covers from the feet. Drink plenty of water, especially during hard physical exercise and especially in hot weather.

A simple exercise done during the day may also help. Stand erect in stocking feet. Lean forward, keeping your heels on the floor until you feel a pulling sensation in the calf muscles. Hold for ten seconds, then repeat after a five-second interval of rest. Do this five times, two or three times a day, until the night cramps disappear.

What your physician can do. Should the above measures fail to bring relief, have your physician determine if there is some underlying cause for the problem. Quinine (a toxic drug used to treat malaria) for some unknown reason gives relief. However, it should only be used on your physician's advice.

Claudication is pain and spasm that occurs most commonly in the muscles of the calf, and is brought on by walking. It results from an inadequate blood supply to the cramping muscles. The cramps may be triggered by vigorous exercise beyond that for which your muscles are conditioned or from advancing atherosclerosis, which is gradually reducing the flow of blood through your arteries.

What you can do. Rest will promptly relieve the spasm and pain. If your problem is one of inactivity, go on a regular exercise program. Should you suspect atherosclerosis, consult with your physician. He will evaluate the underlying cause and advise an exercise program, hot-and-cold contrast baths, or a medication which will increase circulation in the area.

Wryneck (torticollis)

Wryneck, a spasm of the muscles on one side of the neck, twists the neck and draws the head over in an unnatural position to that side.

The causes may include a temporary contraction of the muscles due to exposure to cold, to an injury, to enlargement of the lymph glands of the neck (from infection in the neck or pharynx), to local irritation of the muscles, or to emotional problems. It may result from a congenital disorder in which the muscles of one side of the neck shorten and become fibrous or the skin of one side of the neck contracts.

What you can do. In mild cases, apply heat (moist or dry), massage the area gently, and stretch it five times a day. This may relieve the situation. If the problem does not respond to this treatment in two or three days, see your physician.

What your physician can do. He can determine and treat the underlying cause. Wryneck, observed early in infancy, may require surgical intervention to release the contracted muscles, and then a splint or cast to hold the head in proper position for a period of time.

Myofascitis (myofascial pain, fibrositis)

In **myofascitis,** stiffness, aching, and deep pain occur in certain parts of the body. The neck, the shoulders, the lower back, and the thighs are the areas most often affected. The sufferer complains of stiff neck, pain in the thigh, or arthritis, all worse in the morning, and often with tender swellings or "knots" in the muscles. The cause of this discomfort, which generally occurs in those forty to sixty years of age and is sometimes associated with inability to sleep, is unknown.

What you can do. The condition is not serious and lasts from a few hours to a week or two. Rest, together with heat applications (hot baths, heating pad, heat lamp, or fomentations) and gentle massage will bring relief. If the discomfort persists, see your physician.

What your physician can do. He may prescribe a muscle relaxant and something to relieve pain. Injections of a steroid into the tender, painful areas are often helpful.

Muscular dystrophy

Muscular dystrophy comprises a group of congenital disorders showing progressive weakness and wasting of the muscles. The most common form, **Duchenne dystrophy,** appears only in male infants or very young boys. The weakness starts in the muscles of the hips, thighs, and calves, and may progress to the shoulders and elsewhere in the body. The child walks with a waddling gait, falls frequently, and has difficulty in standing up again. There is no known treatment, and the illness is progressively unfavorable.

Juvenile dystrophy usually begins during adolescence and affects both sexes equally. The weakness often starts in the shoulders and then affects the face and upper arms. Eventually the muscles in the hands, feet, and back become involved. The back becomes swayed, and the arms and legs are held in abnormal positions. The disease may become arrested spontaneously.

What your physician can do. Laboratory tests, including a biopsy of a muscle, will determine the precise diagnosis. Genetic counseling should be sought as to the risks involved in marriage and having additional children. The physician will direct treatment toward maintaining as much functional activity as long as possible. Physical therapy and surgery to correct deformities may prove helpful.

Polymyositis and dermatomyositis. See under "collagen diseases," page 957.

Skin and hair

The skin covers the entire surface of your body, an area of more than 18 square feet, and weighs twice as much as your heart or liver—approximately 10 pounds (4.5 kilograms). An area of skin the size of a postage stamp (2.2 x 3.6 centimeters) is made up of more than 25 million cells, containing approximately 560 sweat glands, 90 oil (sebaceous) glands, and 60 hairs, with thousands of sensory nerve receptors for touch, pain, cold, heat, and pressure. Besides these, there are numerous muscles and yards (meters) of nerves and blood vessels.

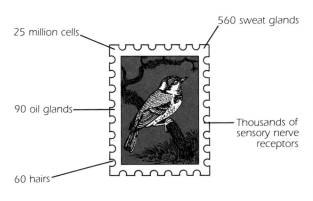

Note the many structures in a piece of skin the size of this stamp.

25 million cells

560 sweat glands

90 oil glands

Thousands of sensory nerve receptors

60 hairs

The skin is what you first see of others, and what they first see of you. Soft, smooth, and elastic, it adds beauty and color to the form and contours of your body. But it differs in thickness and design in various areas of the body, depending on its functional needs. It is paper thin on the eyelids, but strong and thick on the palms of the hands and soles of the feet. It is an organ of many purposes.

The skin consists of three parts: the epidermis on the outside, the dermis beneath the epidermis, with the subcutaneous tissue deep to both.

The **epidermis** contains no blood vessels—but layer upon layer of cells. Nourished by tissue fluid, its deepest cells are alive and constantly produce more cells like themselves. The new cells are pushed toward the surface, and thus are gradually removed from their source of nourishment. As they die, they undergo a chemical change to form keratin, a horny material that is tough, insensitive, and impermeable to water. Eventually, as they reach the surface, they are rubbed off. As fast as surface cells are lost, new cells form so that the skin is virtually indestructible.

This epidermal layer of skin protects the body from outside assault: from physical injury, for the skin is tough even though it is soft, resilient, and pliable; from chemical attack, for while the skin can absorb many chemicals, it blocks the penetration of most and retards the entry of others; and from germs, both bacteria and fungi, for the human skin is covered with an acid coat that hampers the growth of these microorganisms. The skin also protects the body's inner environment, for without it, vital body fluids, containing life-preserving substances, would soon be lost.

The **dermis** is a mat of strong interlacing fibers containing blood vessels, lymph channels, nerves, muscles, sweat and sebaceous glands, hair follicles, and a vast array of sense organs, which give us the sensations of hot and cold and the feeling of touch, pain, and pressure. Furthermore, the skin can repair itself following injury.

Just beneath the dermis is a layer of **subcutaneous tissue,** a loose network of fibers (connective tissue) with an abundance of fat cells. This layer of subcutaneous fat is thicker in women than in men, deeper in some places than others, and fills in the hollows between the deeper structures, giving the skin a smooth and beautiful appearance. This layer of fat provides protection from injury, insulation from the entry of cold or the escape of body heat, and serves as a depository of fuel, a store of energy for time of need. These fat stores increase when you put on weight.

The amount of melanin, a pigment

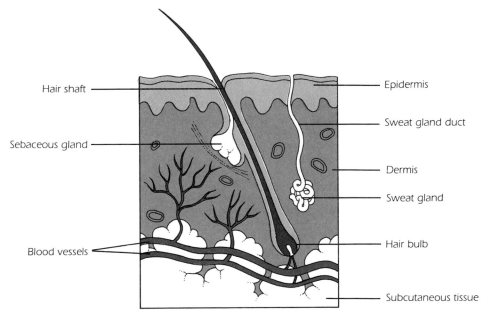

The layers of the skin and its many structures.

Hair shaft

Sebaceous gland

Blood vessels

Epidermis

Sweat gland duct

Dermis

Sweat gland

Hair bulb

Subcutaneous tissue

produced by some 5 percent of the cells in the epidermis, and the amount of blood momentarily present in the dermis determine the color of the skin. The more melanin present, the darker the complexion. The rosy complexion seen in fair-skinned people is due to a greater flow of blood in the dermal layer. And interestingly, the skin can reveal the state of your emotions: pale and bumpy (goose pimples) when afraid, red when angry, flushed or blushed when ashamed, and wet with sweat when stressed.

The skin's **sweat glands,** shaped like tiny coiled tubes, extract water and salt from the blood capillaries and secrete them on the skin's surface. A large and different type of sweat gland found in the armpit and groin secretes a sweat which develops a distinctive odor. The majority of the **sebaceous** or **oil glands** are located adjacent to the hair follicles and produce an oily substance (sebum) that keeps the skin pliable and the hairs from becoming dry. Drying sweat mixed with sebum collects dust and dirt, and becomes offensive. This is an excellent reason for washing and bathing.

The skin of a child is soft and smooth, but gradually changes with age. During adolescence the oil glands become more active, especially on the face. The skin may appear greasy, and blackheads and pimples tend to develop (see page 983). With maturity the secretion of oil slows down, and with advancing age, oil production further decreases. The skin becomes less elastic, which largely accounts for the appearance

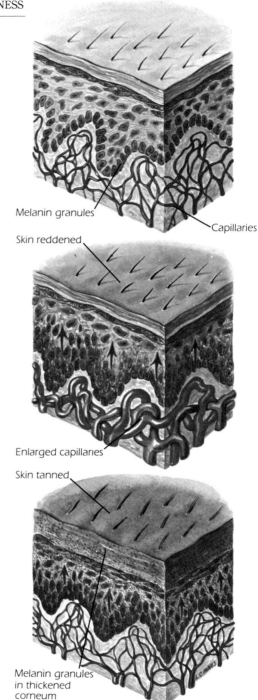

Melanin granules

Capillaries

Skin reddened

Enlarged capillaries

Skin tanned

Melanin granules in thickened corneum

Effects of exposure of skin to sunlight: upper, normal skin; middle, twenty-four hours after exposure (redness from blood-filled capillaries); lower, one week after exposure (tan coloration due to increase in granules of melanin).

of wrinkles. Drying, wrinkling, and aging of the skin can be delayed by avoiding too much exposure to sunlight and wind, and from smoking cigarettes.

The surface of the dermis is not a straight plane but undulates with ridges and valleys. These, in turn, fit into corresponding valleys and ridges on the undersurface of the epidermis and are reflected on the surface of the skin. These ridges and valleys seen on the tips of your fingers and toes, when pressed on a smooth surface, leave behind **fingerprints** (and toeprints), each with a particular pattern, unique for each individual. This unevenness of the skin on the hands and feet allows a person to grip objects more surely and walk more securely.

The skin contains millions of **sense organs** located on the undersurface of the epidermis. These include the receptors for pain, touch, heat, cold, and pressure. There is approximately one pain receptor for every square millimeter of skin, or the size of this *o*. The number varies, however, depending on the area of the skin, being less numerous on the back than on the fingertips. This is also true of touch. Almost twenty-five times as many tactile bodies occur on the tips of the fingers and toes as on the back.

Our skin sensors not only tell us that something is cold or warn us when something is hot, but also help us to maintain a remarkably constant **temperature,** regardless of our environment. When the body tends to overheat, blood is rushed to the skin, where heat is dissipated, aided by the evaporation of sweat. To reduce the radiation of heat from the body when exposed to cold, the blood vessels in the skin constrict, sweat production ceases, and the oil glands pour out more oil, which spreads on the skin and further reduces evaporation.

Tattooing involves injecting an insoluble dye (black or colored) into the dermis. Once the dye is placed, it is extremely difficult to remove without leaving a scar. Another serious problem is the danger of contracting an infection, such as AIDS or hepatitis, from a needle that was not properly sterilized.

When a large area of skin has been destroyed by a burn or injury, to hasten healing and to prevent scarring, a surgeon may make a **skin graft.** Generally a split-thickness graft is used, in which a thin layer of skin is shaved off some other area, such as the abdomen, back, or thigh and bandaged in place on the denuded area until attached. Sometimes a pedicle graft is necessary, in which a piece of skin close at hand is partially removed and stretched over the destroyed area. More recently, grafts taken from neonatal (newborn) foreskin and autographs (a person's own skin) grown in culture are being used to replace the dstroyed skin.

Fingernails and **hairs,** produced by cells of the epidermis **(keratinocytes),** are keratin structures similar to the cells on the skin's surface. Nails are produced by cells that proliferate at the base or matrix of the nail, while hairs are made by similar cells reproducing in hair follicles.

The process parallels that which takes place in the epidermis. As new cells form in the nail matrix or hair follicle, they are pushed toward the surface, become removed from their source of nourishment, die, and become hardened keratin.

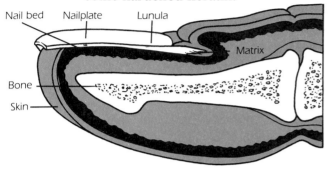

A section showing the major structures of the nail.

Within the hair follicle are pigment-producing cells which intermingle with the hair cells. As the pigment cells die, they leave their pigment granules behind, giving color to the hair. The loss of this pigment is responsible for the graying of hair. This pigment is also responsible for the repigmentation of a person with vitiligo. Because the nail matrix has no pigment-producing cells, nails are clear colored.

It is estimated that a person has from one-third to half a million hairs on the skin. Fair-haired people have more and finer hairs. Hairs on the beards of men, scalp, eyebrow, and pubis grow longer than do those elsewhere on the body.

CHAPTER 15

Diseases of the skin, nails, and hair

Skin diseases affect all age groups. While many similarities exist among the various skin disorders, important differences often point to the specific cause and indicate the best treatment.

Dermatitis

Dermatitis, frequently referred to as eczema, is an inflammation of the skin. Such disorders may result from an inborn sensitivity (inherited), acquired sensitivity, exposure to some agent, or to emotional stress. Thus skin diseases have many causes and take many forms. Only the more familiar will be discussed.

The common characteristics of dermatitis are reddening, swelling, blistering, oozing, crusting, and itching. Depending on the condition, there may also be scaling and changes in the color or pigments of the skin.

Atopic dermatitis

This condition is an inflammation of the skin resulting from an inherited hypersensitivity. Seventy-five percent of sufferers have relatives who are troubled with asthma, hay fever, and hives. While it may occur at any age, it is most likely to occur during infancy and childhood.

The disorder varies in intensity from time to time. In infants it affects the face and outer surfaces of the arms and legs. In children it usually affects the skin on the inner surface of the arms and legs. From adolescence onward the lesions tend to be more dry with the formation of plaques, especially in the skinfolds of the arms and legs, on the neck, face, hands, and in the crotch. At all ages scratching further aggravates the situation. The problem tends to become less severe as one gets older.

A number of factors may provoke or intensify atopic dermatitis. These include marked changes in tempera-

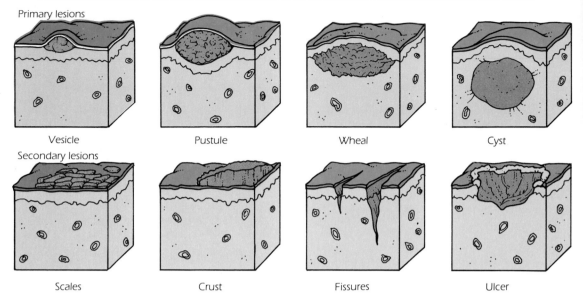

Primary lesions

| Vesicle | Pustule | Wheal | Cyst |

Secondary lesions

| Scales | Crust | Fissures | Ulcer |

Common lesions of the skin.

ture (cold weather, heat and humidity), profuse sweating (from vigorous physical activity), exposure to certain chemicals (grease, solvents, detergents), excessive clothing (especially woolen and coarse-textured garments), psychological stress, and allergens. In general, food allergies and pollens carried in the air are not related to the disorder.

What you can do. Since there is no cure, you must try to avoid anything which will trigger an episode, while treatment is directed toward relieving the symptoms. Itching causes scratching, and scratching intensifies the itching, aggravates the lesions, and encourages infections. Wet dressings help to clean the lesions and reduce itching while the eczema is wet and oozing. Bathing and soap may intensify the problem. Cleansing creams may be used instead. Constant lubrication with a soothing cream or ointment is a necessity. When washing clothes and bed sheets, avoid detergents, use a mild soap, and thoroughly rinse the wash.

What your physician can do. He will instruct you how to cleanse and care for your lesions. Cortisone ointments as well as purified tar preparations with cautious ultraviolet light exposure will reduce both the itching and the inflammation. In severe cases oral antihistamines and steroids may sometimes be recommended. An appropriate antibiotic will control a secondary infection.

Contact dermatitis

Contact dermatitis, as the name suggests, is an acute inflammatory eruption resulting from direct contact with an irritant material or to some substance to which an acquired sensitivity (allergy) has developed.

Irritant dermatitis can occur from a number of commonly used agents which include detergents, bleaches, toilet bowl cleaners, strong alkalis and acids, furniture polishes, aerosols, swimming pool disinfectants, adhesive bandages, rubber gloves, elastic components in stretch garments, and industrial solvents and oils.

Allergic dermatitis results from a sensitivity to a substance developed from a previous exposure to it. Almost 75 percent of the population react to contact with **poison ivy** and **poison oak.** One can acquire sensitivity to almost any substance: the dyes in leather, the elastic in garments, fingernail polishes, and to metals in jewelry, such as nickel.

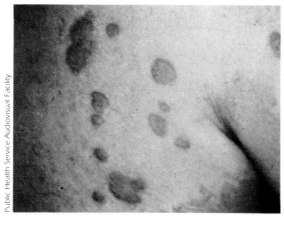

Public Health Service Audiovisual Facility

Rash caused from administration of penicillin.

Dermatitis from irritants causes reddening, blistering, drying, and cracking. Painful fissures and ulcers may develop. Itching, if present, is mild. In response to a substance to which you have become sensitive, the skin becomes red, and small to large blisters form. These break to ooze and weep. The eyes and face may be puffy. Itching may be intense. As healing occurs, the lesions will dry and crust. Allergies to metals develop slowly and cause itching, scaling, and redness.

What you can do. Try to avoid contact with any substance to which you respond adversely. To determine whether you will react to a substance, try a patch test. Put a drop or a tiny amount of the material on a very small piece of gauze, place it in contact with the skin of your abdomen or inner thigh, cover the gauze with wax paper, and attach it with a piece of adhesive tape. Leave it in place for forty-eight hours unless itching and irritation occur earlier, at which point it should be removed. If you have no reaction, the substance is likely safe for you to use.

Your physician may be able to do sensitivity tests for things to which you have become allergic. Careful observation on your part as to the circumstances under which you develop dermatitis will greatly aid him in recognizing the offending materials.

For irritant dermatitis, protect yourself from exposure. Wear cotton gloves inside rubber gloves when doing dishes or other chores in which your hands might come in contact with an irritant. Should you become exposed, wash the material off as quickly as possible. For exposure to poison oak or ivy, use soap to remove the waxy or resinous toxic material, and thoroughly wash all clothes involved.

Many of the procedures for treating contact dermititis are similar to those discussed under atopic dermatitis. Wet dressings, mild ointments, and calamine lotion should reduce itching and bring relief.

973

What your physician can do. He can test for agents to which you might have become sensitive. Depending on the severity of the inflammation, steroid ointments and antihistamines may be recommended. An appropriate antibiotic will care for a secondary infection.

Other inflammatory skin disorders

A number of inflammatory skin disorders similar to atopic and contact dermatitis, but which do have certain differences, are briefly presented.

Seborrheic dermatitis is a common condition in which thick, yellowish, greasy (sometimes dry) scales affect the scalp **(dandruff),** the sides of the nose, corners of the mouth, and the crease behind the ears. Often the eyelids and lid margins become red and scaly **(blepharitis).** More severe cases involve the face and neck, and the armpits, groin, and genital regions **(intertrigo).** It may come and go, or persist for years. While the cause is unknown, there appears to be a hereditary tendency.

Certain shampoos are quite effective in controlling scalp problems. Low-dosage cortisone-containing lotions, creams, and ointments give effective relief. See your physician before using cortisone-containing preparations for prolonged periods or around the eyes, as damage to the skin and eyes may occur. Should intertriginous seborrhea become infected, wet dressings, and antibiotic or antifungal agents used topically or systemically, are helpful.

Chronic dermatitis, similar to atopic dermatitis but more localized, may appear in any age group. Itching is intense, and the skin thickens through constant scratching. Chronic dermatitis commonly affects the shins, ankles, inner thighs, and the cleft between the legs, neck, and forearms. Frequently the cause of the itching is not known. Protecting the affected areas from scratching, together with a steroid ointment and antihistamines, often brings relief.

Xerotic eczema is a dry, scaling irritation of the skin, seen especially on the lower legs in the elderly. Severity increases in dry weather and improves as the humidity rises. Moistening of the skin with soothing lotions and bath oils, and bathing less frequently and without detergent soaps, provide relief. When the air is dry, a humidifier may be beneficial.

Dyshidrosis is an inflammatory eruption occurring along the sides of the fingers, on the palms of the hands, and on the soles of the feet. It produces mild itching and burning. Small blisters form which break and ooze, or dry up and turn brown. The skin may peel later. The cause is not known; however, it may be related to atopic dermatitis in adulthood. The disorder goes in cycles, may be induced by stress, and is worsened with increased exposure to water. A subtype, "housewife's eczema" ("dishpan hands"), occurs in those whose hands are frequently exposed to the chemicals listed under contact dermatitis. The skin becomes red, chapped, dry, cracked, and fissured. Small to large blisters may develop, which break and weep. For treatment, see under "contact dermititis," page 972.

Stasis dermatitis

This disorder shows red, scaly patches of skin on the front and inner side of the lower leg and ankle. It may or may not itch and results from failure of the circulation in the veins. The skin may break down and an ulcer form. Stasis dermatitis is often associated with varicose veins or thrombophlebitis.

What you can do. Avoid standing for long periods of time. Do not cross one thigh over the other. When seated, try to elevate your feet to the level of your hips. In stubborn cases, elevating the foot of your bed about four inches may help improve veinous circulation. If you have prominent leg veins, wear support hose or an elastic bandage to decrease stagnation of blood in the veins.

Walking will improve the circulation in your legs. Be careful not to injure the lower leg. Should your problem persist and these simple treatments prove ineffective, see your physician.

Nummular dermatitis

This eczema appears as round, coin-shaped lesions (*nummulus* means "coin"), mostly seen on the extremities of older men and young adult women. It may develop as a single lesion or several lesions that may recur in episodes. The cause is unknown but may be related to a bacterial infection and dry weather. The condition may worsen with contact with wool, soaps, medications applied to the skin, and frequent bathing.

What you can do. When bathing, hydrate the skin by using oil additives. Keep the skin from drying by the generous use of body creams.

What your physician can do. He can prescribe an appropriate coal tar preparation or a topical steroid.

Bacterial infections of the skin

Bacterial infections may be caused by a variety of organisms, but the most common are staphylococcus and streptococcus. The infections are usually contagious. The lesions become red, blister, create pus, and form a crust. The neighboring lymph glands may be tender and swollen. Some people develop fever and general illness. Treatment is appropriate antibiotics.

Impetigo

Impetigo, a common, acute, contagious, superficial skin infection oc-curring in adults but most often in children, is usually caused by staphylococci or by streptococci. The lesions ordinarily appear around the mouth and nose. If caused by streptococci, small red blisters break and fuse, forming pustules that ooze. As they dry, loosely attached golden-yellow or honey-colored crusts form in one to two days. The infection spreads along the margins, is itchy but not painful, and generally disappears by itself in two to three weeks. If caused by staphylococci, small blisters form that easily break, leaving a denuded base.

The disease is seldom dangerous, except in infants, where it can become widespread, and if streptococci are involved, may cause a serious kidney disease (glomerulonephritis).

What you can do. Keep your fingers away from the crusts and do not scratch them, as this tends to spread the infection. Your face cloths, towels, and linens should not be shared by other family members. Children with this disorder should be kept out of school. Gently wash the lesions with soap and water. However, because of possible complications, you should see your physician.

What your physician can do. He will probably recommend an anti-infective ointment to rub on the lesions after washing. An antibiotic by mouth or injection is effective, and the condition should clear up in about a week.

Folliculitis

Folliculitis is a superficial infection of one or more hair follicles, usually caused by staphylococcus bacteria. The follicle becomes red, fills with pus, forms crusts, spreads to adjacent follicles, and most commonly affects the bearded area of men or any hair-bearing skin. Young bearded adults can suffer from chronic recurrent folliculitis.

What you can do. The treatment is similar to that for impetigo: gentle cleaning of the infected area with an antibacterial soap, the nonsharing of towels and linens, the use of an antibacterial ointment following shaving, and, when necessary, an antibiotic by mouth provided by your physician.

Boils (furuncles)

A boil is a hard, red, very painful infection affecting a localized group of hair follicles (a complication of folliculitis), that is caused by staphylococcus bacteria. It commonly develops under the arms, on the face, on the scalp, on the inner sides of the thighs, and on the buttocks. As the boil enlarges, a core forms, the surface skin softens and then ruptures, allowing the pus within to escape. A boil that develops on the eyelid is called a sty.

Avoid the dangerous practice of

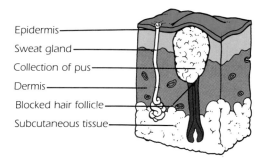

Epidermis
Sweat gland
Collection of pus
Dermis
Blocked hair follicle
Subcutaneous tissue

Boil resulting from an infected hair follicle.

picking or squeezing a boil (or pimple), as this may force the germs into surrounding tissues or into the bloodstream (septicemia). This is especially true of boils forming in the area between the nose, upper lip, cheek, and eyebrow, and inside the nostril, as the infection may travel to the brain.

When a number of boils develop in the deep layers of the skin adjacent to one another, the lesion is called a **carbuncle.** Often accompanied with fever, carbuncles have multiple heads and are commonly seen on the back of the neck, back, and thighs.

976

What you can do. The same principles of treatment apply to boils as to folliculitis. Warm, moist compresses (several layers of gauze wrung out of hot water) applied several times a day will hasten the boil's coming to a "head" and discharging its contents.

What your physician can do. Your physician may choose to open (lance) the boil rather than allowing it to rupture by itself. Should the boil persist, he may prescribe a suitable antibiotic. He will also determine if some underlying problem, such as diabetes, obesity, or anemia may be a contributing factor.

Cellulitis

Cellulitis, a serious infection affecting the tissues beneath the skin as well as the skin itself, is usually caused by staphylococcal or streptococcal bacteria which gain entrance through a break in the skin. The infection spreads along the lymph channels, causing red streaks in the direction of the lymph nodes that service the area. The nodes become enlarged and tender, while the affected skin is hot, red, and painful. The sufferer feels ill and has chills, fever, and headache.

Erysipelas, sometimes considered a form of cellulitis, is also a serious infection caused by streptococcus bacteria occurring in the more superficial skin layers. The affected area, frequently the face, reddens and swells, spreads in all directions, and itches and burns. The firm margins of the infection are easily felt (in contrast to cellulitis), and, if on the face, stop abruptly at the hairline. The general symptoms are the same as for cellulitis.

What your physician can do. If untreated, cellulitis, and especially erysipelas, can be fatal, as the organisms may enter the bloodstream, causing septicemia (blood poisoning). Effective antibiotics are available to treat these infections. Hot compresses may give local relief.

Fungal infections of the skin

Fungal infections tend to be persistent, but seldom form true pus or cause fever. Fungi are more complex than bacteria and multiply by means of spores. In general these infections do not respond to antibiotics. Some are extremely common, and most people have at least one fungal infection. The most common conditions are ringworm infections (dermatophytosis), yeast infections (candidiasis), and tinea versicolor (changing color).

Ringworm infections (dermatophytosis)

Ringworm infections (tinea) are not caused by a worm as the name would suggest, but by fungi. The term *ringworm* stems from the observation that the lesions tend to heal at their centers and continue to spread in a widening, ringlike fashion. Although these infections are spread by contact with people and pet animals, or by contact with infected objects used by others (towels, combs, etc.)

977

the affected person probably has an inherited inability to combat a particular fungus. This is the reason why, in a camp or family, only certain people develop the disease.

Athlete's foot (tinea pedis)

This infection is a form of ringworm occurring between the toes in which the skin softens, turns white, and tends to peel and flake. Blisters and cracks appear. Secondary infection is common, resulting in the formation of ulcers and pus with itching and burning. Probably the most common infection of the skin, it is quite contagious and is spread from contaminated shoes, showers (especially public), and areas surrounding swimming pools. The hands may be affected in two ways: (1) Painless "blisters" develop on both hands as an allergic response to toxins produced by the infection in the feet (carried in the blood to the hands—dermatophytid reaction). (2) Scaling of one hand (2 feet, 1 hand disease), which is also affected by the fungus.

What you can do. Wash your feet daily (or more often), dry thoroughly between the toes, use an antifungal powder (antifungal creams tend to keep the skin moist), use absorbent socks, and, whenever possible, wear sandals and air your feet. Should the problem continue, see your physician for systemic medicine.

Ringworm of the scalp, body, and groin (tinea capitis, t. corporis, t. cruris)

Ringworm of the scalp—most common in children—presents small, round, reddish, scaly spots with blisters. The spots enlarge rapidly, become grayish in color, and show definite boundaries. The affected hair shafts break off, and patchy hair loss results. If this persistent inflammation is left untreated, permanent hair loss may result.

Ringworm of the body may affect all areas of the skin except the scalp and groin. It first appears as pea-sized reddened patches, which, while growing rapidly, heal in the center, thus forming rings. The outer edges show tiny papules and small blisters. There is mild itching.

Ringworm of the groin (jock or crotch itch) presents brownish-red scaly patches with tiny blisters at the spreading edges. There is mild itching and smarting. It affects the inner surfaces of the upper thighs and the genital and anal areas. Heat, moisture, profuse sweating, and chafing by clothing aggravate the infection. This disorder is seen more frequently in men.

Ringworm of the beard (barber's itch) is an inflammation in and around the hair follicles. Superficial nodules appear in groups, become deep-seated, discharge a thin pus, itch, and are mildly painful.

Ringworm of the nails affects either fingernails or toenails, which become thickened, brittle, broken, white, and often ridged. Frequently only one nail is affected.

What your physician can do. After an appropriate diagnosis, your physician will prescribe an ointment containing a fungicide, or an oral antibiotic (griseofulvin is commonly used, as it is secreted through the skin). Some fungal infections tend to be persistent (of the beard and nails); hence their treatment will be prolonged. In ringworm of the beard the hairs should be clipped, not shaved.

Yeast infections

Yeast organisms (species of Candida) cause infections **(candidiasis)** in the mouth (thrush), fingernail folds, body folds, and areas around the vagina and anus. Whitish curd-like deposits develop or red, raw lesions. There may be mild burning and itching. Warmth and moisture aggravate the condition.

This benign organism—found in the mouth, vagina, and intestine—does not normally inhabit the skin. For reasons not known, the organism may cause serious infections in debilitated people, in those taking antibiotics by mouth for a long period, in women taking birth-control pills, in the obese, in diabetics, and in those who sweat profusely,

Skin folds should be kept dry. Ask your physician to advise as to the best anti-infective ointment or oral antibiotic.

Tinea versicolor ("sun fungus") is a curious, but harmless, skin infection that affects some young adults. The lesions are small, rounded, velvety, flat spots, which scale and itch slightly. The yeast organism attacks the pigment-producing cells of the skin on the chest, shoulders, armpits, and abdomen. The spots may lose their pigment and may not tan, or they may become pigmented (hence the name "tinea versicolor"). Treatment consists of an antifungal medication by mouth, antifungal creams, or a sulfur/salicylic acid soap or shampoo.

Viral infections of the skin

A number of common skin disorders are due to viruses. These include cold sores or fever blisters, shingles, and warts.

Cold sores or fever blisters (herpes simplex, facial herpes)

Cold sores are caused by the Herpes Simplex Type I virus, and most often, though not always, occur along the margins of the lips. The virus is highly contagious. (Herpes virus Type II is usually found in the genital parts of the body.)

The initial **(primary herpes)** attack is generally severe and, besides the lips and mouth, may involve other areas of the skin and even the eyes. The tiny blisters that appear on the lips, lining of the mouth, tongue, and gums often fuse, forming painful ulcers that make eating difficult. A fever accompanies swollen, tender lymph nodes in the neck. The symptoms appear six days, more or less, after exposure, and the illness lasts about two weeks. The body produces antibodies against the virus, which, however, remains present in the tissues throughout life. In the genital region it may be severe enough to cause painful urination and retention.

Recurrent attacks **(recurrent**

979

herpes) occur from time to time on the lips. A crust forms, which disappears in about ten days. Attacks are triggered by exposure to sunlight, dry winds, injury to the lips (dental work), menstrual periods, fever, general illness, and emotional upsets.

What you can do. Use a lipstick or cream to *prevent* sunburn or drying. Once the problem has developed, a drying lotion or camphor-containing compound may provide relief. Usually no treatment is needed. In initial herpes, or if the involvement is severe, your physician may use an antiviral capsule or ointment early on in therapy, which may be effective in shortening the course. For chronic, frequently recurring herpes, a continuous plan of medication under close supervision may be needed. (See page 846.)

Shingles (herpes zoster)

Shingles is characterized by lesions similar to those of herpes simplex, or cold sores, but is caused by the chickenpox virus, which has remained inactive since the sufferer was exposed to the disease. Shingles appears on one side of the face or body, due to an irritation of one or two sensory nerves. A tingling sensation is followed by the eruption of blister clusters along the nerve path. Crusts form that heal in two to four weeks. Shingles causes extreme pain in the affected area, sometimes even before the eruption occurs. In a few individuals the pain may last for a few weeks to many months after the lesions have healed (postherpetic neuralgia).

What your physician can do. If the infection is severe and painful,

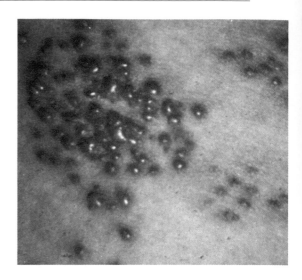

Shingles, with typical blisters.

your physician may prescribe a high dose of an antiviral capsule, as well as systemic corticosteroids to prevent long-lasting pain. After the skin lesions have cleared, moist compresses applied for thirty minutes three to four times a day, with the lesions gently dried in between, may relieve the discomfort. A drying agent (calamine, etc.) may also help. For severe pain your physician can recommend an ointment containing an analgesic to apply to the skin, or he may suggest a medication to take by mouth. Secondary infections can be controlled with appropriate antibiotics. For severe post-herpes pain, the treatments available in a pain-control center may be needed.

Warts (verrucae)

Warts are small benign tumors on the skin, most commonly on the hands and soles of the feet, in persons who have temporarily lost their immunity to the virus that invades the cells. They are spread by contact.

Common warts are firm, raised, have sharp margins, and may or may not be darker than the surrounding skin. **Plantar warts,** on the soles of the feet, are firm, produce pain on pressure, may appear in groups, and are compressed by the body's weight. (See also "calluses and corns," page 985.) **Genital** or **venereal warts** (condyloma) occur on the moist surfaces of the genital areas of males and females. They are skin-colored or gray, occur separately or in groups, and may be flat or cauliflowerlike. They are transmitted by sexual contact.

What you can do. Most warts, given time, will disappear on their own. For common and plantar warts, medications (containing trichloro-acetic acid or salicylic acid), applied as paints or plasters, can destroy the warts. For persistent warts and venereal warts, see your physician.

What your physician can do. Satisfactory treatments for common warts include electrocautery, chemical cautery, freezing (with liquid nitrogen), and intra-lesional injection with interferon or an anticancer agent. Laser surgery may sometimes be necessary. Your physician will determine the procedure most suitable for venereal warts. Women with recurrent flat condyloma are more at risk to develop cancer of the cervix. Therefore partners of women with condyloma and the women themselves should be vigorously treated.

Parasitic infestations of the skin

Temperate-zone parasites that attack the skin from the outside are the itch mite and blood-sucking lice. Their attacks produce severe itching. With appropriate treatment they can be cured and spreading can be prevented.

Scabies (itch mite)

Scabies is an irritation caused by the itch mite, which burrows into the superficial layers of the skin, where it lays its eggs. The condition causes intense itching, especially at night, and a dermatitis due to scratching. The scratching allows bacteria to produce a secondary infection with blisters, pus, and crusting. The mite prefers the most tender skin areas: the webs between fingers; the inner surfaces of the arms, thighs, and legs; and the armpits, breasts, buttocks, and navel. The face and head are rarely affected. The eggs hatch in six days, grow rapidly, and are spread through intimate contact, clothes, and bed linens.

What you can do. Treatment requires killing the mites on your person, as well as those in your clothing. Secondary infections can be handled with an anti-infective ointment. Your physician can prescribe a pesticide-containing shampoo for the pubic area, and an ointment or lotion for your skin from your neck down. Before applying the medication, thoroughly scrub your body with soap and water. Clothes and linens should be laundered, while bedding and clothes which might be harmed should be left unused for five or six days to allow the mites to die.

Lice (head, body, and pubic)

Lice infestations (pediculosis) cause intense itching, followed by scratching, and are often aggravated by a secondary bacterial infection. **Head lice** live in the hair, lay their eggs (nits) on the hair shafts, and feed by sucking blood from the scalp. **Body lice** live in the seams of clothes, lay their eggs in the seams, and come out on the skin to suck blood. **Pubic lice** or **crab lice** attach themselves to the pubic skin, lay their eggs on the hair, and suck blood. Lice are spread by close contact or by the common use of objects such as combs, brushes, and beds. Crab lice are dispersed by sexual contact or occasionally by heavily infected toilets.

What you can do. Cleanse the hair with a pesticide-containing shampoo; carefully comb with a fine-toothed comb to remove the nits (eggs). Repeat the procedure according to directions. Wash the clothes and bed linens thoroughly. Pressing the seams of clothes with a hot iron kills lice and eggs. Bathe with a medicated soap. Remove pubic lice by shaving or clipping the hair, which should then be burned. Use a pesticide-containing shampoo, and sterilize clothing, bed sheets, and toilet seats. Nits occurring on the eyelashes can be smothered with petroleum jelly for twenty-four hours. Treat secondary infections with appropriate ointments. Itching that continues after the infestations have been cleared may be relieved by an antihistamine or a steroid cream.

Miscellaneous skin disorders

The following section will include disorders affecting any of the several layers of the skin and those of the sebaceous glands.

Acne (pimples, simple acne, acne vulgaris)

Acne or pimples are small, localized swellings on the skin which frequently become infected. Pimples generally appear during adolescence and clear up after maturity is complete. However, in some they appear at various times and may continue into adulthood. Most commonly occurring on the face, they may also appear on the neck, chest, back, buttocks, arms, and thighs. About 80 percent of teenagers experience some degree of acne, while 20 percent suffer from the more severe form.

The oil or sebaceous glands of the skin secrete a material (sebum) which lubricates the skin. During adolescence the male hormone (testosterone) is secreted in larger amounts by both the testes and ovaries. This stimulates increased production of sebum. The hair follicle into which the sebum is secreted bulges, and if the outlet is plugged, a

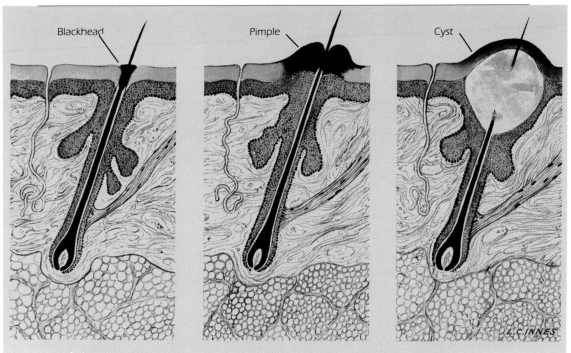

Blackhead **Pimple** **Cyst**

L.C.INNES

Skin sections showing how a blackhead forms in relation to a hair follicle and how it can develop into an infected cyst.

"whitehead" forms. Sometimes melanin is present and appears as a **"blackhead"** (comedo). If the material becomes infected, inflammation around the hair follicle occurs, pus may form, and a full-blown pimple develops.

Pimples appear at a time when the adolescents are most conscious of their appearance, and the blemishes make them sensitive and embarrassed. The precise cause is not known. Since a genetic tendency to develop acne exists, blaming the teen-ager for his condition may result in serious emotional problems.

What you can do. To keep your skin as free from oil as possible, cleanse your skin two to three times each day with warm water and a soft, nonirritating soap. It is best not to use cosmetics, but if used, they should not be oil-based products. Do not pick or squeeze pimples, as this tends to aggravate the problem. Blackheads, if removed, should be removed with a blackhead remover (available in the drugstore), and preferably by a professional. Try to keep your resistance up by maintaining good health habits (see page 124).

What your physician can do. Depending on the severity of the condition, he may prescribe a vitamin A–like product topically or systemically, an antibiotic in a cream or systemically, or topical benzoyl peroxides of sulfur on the skin. When scarring has occurred, a dermabrasion (planing the skin), face peel, punch graft removal of pits, or collagen may be used to correct the defects.

983

Rosacea (acne rosacea)

Rosacea is a chronic permanent enlargement of the tiny blood vessels of the skin involving the nose, cheeks, brow, and chin. The affected areas appear flushed, varying in color from pink to a deep red to a purplish-red. The skin may thicken and pustules form, resembling pimples (hence the name). The nose may become greatly distorted. The cause of rosacea is unknown. This harmless ailment occurs between the ages of thirty and fifty and is three times more common in women than men.

What you can do. Avoid anything which tends to make you flush, such as emotional stress, hot drinks (tea, coffee, soups), spicy foods, alcoholic beverages, and environmental factors of excessive heat, cold, wind, and sunlight, as they aggravate the condition.

What your physician can do. Medications can be taken by mouth or applied topically in the form of cream. Enlarged blood vessels can be electrically desiccated. Overgrown tissue on the nose may be surgically removed.

Psoriasis

Psoriasis is a thickening of the skin with the formation of red patches covered with shiny silvery scales that shed continuously. The lesions— mildly sore and itchy—usually affect the elbows, knees, buttocks, back, and scalp, although the plaques may develop elsewhere (finger- and toenails, genitals, anal area, and skinfolds). One to two percent of Americans have some degree of psoriasis,

while 10 percent of these have a severe, incapacitating form. About one in twenty have an associated arthritis, commonly of the fingers and toes, but sometimes of the spine.

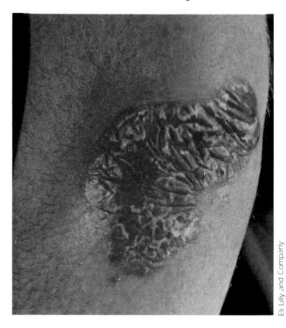

Eli Lilly and Company

Psoriasis with characteristic reddish patches.

The fundamental cause of psoriasis is not known. One in three appear to have some hereditary factor. The essential problem is an overproduction of epidermal cells. These cells are normally replaced every twenty-eight days. In psoriasis, because of rapid production, replacement occurs in three to four days. The severity of the illness varies widely. An acute attack usually ends spontaneously, but the condition usually recurs. Hot weather, humidity, and sunlight aid, while cold weather hinders, recovery. Emotional stress, an infection such as a sore throat, an injury of the skin, alcohol, and general debility tend to precipitate an attack.

In psoriasis the nails characteristically become pitted, contain spots of yellowish discoloration, and toward the tips may separate from their beds. (See the illustration on page 991).

What you can do. Keep in good health by adopting a healthful lifestyle (see page 124). Sunbathing (without getting sunburned) or exposure to a sunlamp (ultraviolet) will aid recovery. Avoid emotional upsets. After gently washing the lesions with mild soap and water, apply an ointment suggested by your physician.

What your physician can do. The usual treatment includes the use of creams, coal tar preparations, and ultraviolet light treatments. A new regime, called PUVA (used in the resorts at the Dead Sea), uses psoralens, either topically or by mouth, to enhance the healing quality of the long wave ultraviolet light (UVA). (Your physician should check recent reports of an increase in skin cancers in those who have undergone this therapy.) Steroids can be used in ointments or be injected into the lesions, but systemic steroids are rarely appropriate. Anticancer drugs, vitamin A–derived preparations, and recently vitamin D and immunosuppressant agents have been used, but should be monitored closely under a specialist's guidance.

Pemphigus

In pemphigus blisters develop on the skin and, in 60 percent of the cases, on the lining of the mouth and other mucous membranes (esophagus, vagina, cervix). The blisters break open and superficial crusted ulcerations form. Body fluids are depleted, and secondary infections occur frequently. It is believed to be an autoimmune disease in which the body attacks its own skin. Occurring more commonly in persons of Mediterranean origin, pemphigus usually proves fatal if left untreated.

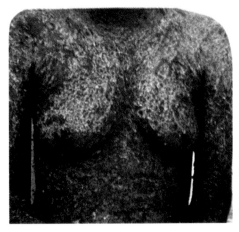

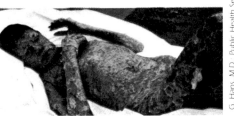

Skin lesions of pemphigus.

What your physician can do. He will prescribe immune suppressant medications, especially steroids, to be taken by mouth. Body fluids lost through open skin lesions must be replenished. Infections developing in the ulcers can be treated by appropriate antibiotics.

Calluses and corns

A **callus** is a patch of thickened surface skin (epidermis) commonly occurring on the soles of the feet or palms of the hands, caused by pro-

985

longed friction and pressure. A **corn** is a small, pointed, localized thickening of the skin (one quarter inch or less in diameter), with the point directed inward, usually seen on the feet or toes. With corns, pain occurs on pressure. Ill-fitting shoes or a bone defect cause most calluses and corns. Some people are more prone to these problems than others.

What you can do. Choose shoes that fit properly. Calluses, if they bother you, can be thinned or removed by soaking them in warm water and then by rubbing them with a rough cloth, pumice stone, or callus file. Placing a felt ring around a painful corn will give relief, and may provide time for it to disappear. You can destroy both corns and calluses chemically. These plasters and paints should be used as directed, repeatedly removing destroyed skin, until you obtain relief. If pain increases or infection develops, see your physician or podiatrist, who occasionally may need to remove the corn or callus surgically.

Bedsores

Bedsores are ulcers of the skin, usually seen on the buttocks, spine, sides of the knee, and elbows. The prolonged pressure from the weight of the body destroys the skin, which first becomes tender, then inflamed, turning from red to bluish-gray, before breaking down to form an ulcer. These ulcers heal slowly.

What you can do. You can prevent bedsores by keeping the sheets free from food crumbs and creases, by frequently turning the patient to new positions in the bed, by keeping the skin clean, and by toughening the skin with regular alcohol rubs. Frequent ultraviolet exposure (without sunburning) will strengthen and thicken the skin. Soothing ointments will help to relieve the pain. Healing will not occur unless the pressure is relieved. This can be accomplished by the use of pillows, air mattresses, or a sheepskin. Should the ulcer fail to heal or a secondary infection start to develop, see your physician. Antibiotic therapy and sometimes surgery with grafts may be needed.

Pigment disorders

Skin and hair normally contain a certain amount of pigment, called melanin, manufactured by special cells in the skin called melanocytes. Normal exposure to sunlight causes an increase in the melanin in the skin, recognized as tanning. Certain disorders of the skin may result in an abnormal decrease or increase in this pigment.

In **albinism**—an inherited disorder occurring in about one in 20,000 individuals—the skin, hair, and eyes lack melanin, because the melanocytes cannot manufacture the pigment. Albinos' lack of sufficient pigment in their eyes makes them intolerant of bright light. They are also more prone to sunburn and skin cancer. They should use sunglasses and sunscreen lotions to protect exposed areas.

Vitiligo is present when patches of skin lose their pigment. The cause of this condition is unknown, although there may be an inherited propensity to develop the disorder. Often symmetrically distributed, the non-pigmented areas may increase or decrease in size. Should the skin of the scalp be involved, the hairs in the patch may lose their pigment, and nonpigmented areas sunburn readily. While vitiligo is a harmless condition, it may rarely be associated with more serious conditions (thyroid disease, pernicious anemia, diabetes, Addison's, halo nevi, alopecia areata). Skin dyes, self-action tanning creams, and makeup are available for cosmetic purposes. The only medical treatment available is PUVA (see under "psoriasis," page 984) which can be combined with small grafts of normal skin to the affected area.

In **chloasma** (melasma) pigmented blotches, brownish in color, appear in women during pregnancy or while taking birth control pills. The blotches appear on the skin over the cheekbones, forehead, and upper lip. Seemingly related to changes in hormone levels, they may disappear a few months after delivery or when oral contraceptives are discontinued. Avoiding direct exposure to sunlight and using sunscreen ointment and a bleaching cream on exposed areas of skin may be helpful.

Freckles are spots of skin with more than the usual amount of pigment (melanin). They are not harmful, occur more often in blonds and redheads, and are more prominent after exposure to excessive sunlight. Should the freckles adversely affect the appearance, they can be made less conspicuous by the use of creams and lotions which make the skin peel, but these should be used only on the advice of your physician.

Liver spots are small darkened (hyperpigmented) areas of skin due to chronic exposure to sunlight, which appear most commonly on the backs of the hands in the elderly. They tend to persist despite protection from sunshine (by use of sunscreens or gloves). Freezing with liquid nitrogen may be helpful.

Sweating disorders

Lack of sweat (anhidrosis) is present even when the body becomes overheated. A disorder of the nerves controlling the sweat glands or a complication of psoriasis or scleroderma causes the condition. While there is no cure, applying a moisturizing cream and avoiding overheating relieves discomfort.

Excessive sweating (hyperhidrosis) results from overactive sweat glands. Two main types are seen: thermogenic and emotional.

A disturbance in the temperature-regulating mechanism in the brain causes **thermogenic hyperhidrosis.** The body responds as when in excessively warm surroundings. It is seen in certain diseases, such as tuberculosis, hyperthyroidism, gout, diabetes, and certain cancers. The underlying cause should be treated by your physician.

Undue stress triggers **emotional hyperhidrosis,** with the sweat occurring mainly in the face, under the arms, and in the skin of the hands and feet. Frequent bathing and the use of antiperspirants and dusting powders on the feet are helpful.

Bromhidrosis (foul-smelling sweat) is caused by bacteria acting on the sweat after secretion and occurs most often in the armpits and on the feet. Frequent bathing, the use of clean garments, and the application of an appropriate lotion should cure the complaint. Your pharmacist can make up this lotion: copper nitrate 2 grams; benzoic acid 4 grams; acetone 20 milliliters; and ethyl alcohol (90 percent) up to 120 milliliters. Apply three or four times a day to the affected areas with a moistened cotton ball (held with tweezers to avoid staining the fingers).

What your physician can do. Medications that decrease sweating, aluminum salts locally applied, tap water electrophoresis, and glutaraldehyde and tannic acids soaks (made up with a concentrated solution using tea bags) may be helpful.

Ichthyosis (fishskin)

Generally, four main types of ichthyosis are recognized. In this condition, aggravated by dry air and cold weather, the outer layer of skin thickens and becomes dry, rough, and scaly. Cracks form and the surface tends to peel, giving the skin a fishlike appearance. The face, hands, and feet are rarely affected. Treatment consists of lubricants containing lactic acid. Some of the types may improve with an oral vitamin A–derived preparation (retinoids).

Prickly heat (miliaria)

Prickly heat—a skin eruption in which the sweat glands have become obstructed—occurs in very warm climates or when one is overclothed. Prickly heat affects areas in which two skin surfaces come together,

such as at the bend of the elbow and knee, under the breasts, and in the groin. Wearing lighter clothing, moving to a cool climate, avoiding overheating, and applying a soothing ointment or lotion (calamine) to the eruptions will relieve the discomfort.

Sunburn

Sunburns are usually first-degree burns, causing redness, swelling, and tenderness. Sometimes blistering, oozing, and severe pain develop, suggesting a second-degree burn. If large areas of the body are involved, chills, fever, weakness, and even shock may ensue.

Sunburn is an acute overexposure to the ultraviolet rays of the sun. These rays—most intense between nine in the morning and three in the afternoon—can penetrate haze and overcast skies, 70 to 80 percent reaching the skin. Ultraviolet is more intense at high mountain altitudes and is reflected off snow (100 percent) and sand (25 percent).

Long-term harm to the skin can occur from exposures that do not cause a burn but are repeated over and over, because the damage is cumulative and cannot be reversed. The skin becomes prematurely aged, wrinkled, and tough. People with fair skin, blue eyes, and red or blond hair are much more susceptible to burning than those who have dark eyes and dark skin, and they face a greater risk of skin cancer from long-term exposure.

What you can do. Wear protective clothing (light clothes will permit some ultraviolet to pass through). Consistently used, sun-

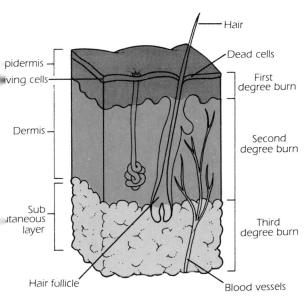

Epidermis —
living cells —

Dermis —

Sub
cutaneous
layer

Hair follicle

Hair

Dead cells

First
degree burn

Second
degree burn

Third
degree burn

Blood vessels

Depths of tissue affected by first, second, and third degree burns.

screen lotions either block or absorb the ultraviolet rays. These lotions are graded by a Sun Protection Factor (SPF) number—the higher the number the greater the protection. A mild sunburn will heal rapidly. Wet dressings and a soothing lotion (calamine) will bring relief to more severe burns. A mild cortisone cream can be used in a first degree burn. Drink plenty of water. If a large area is involved, especially with blistering, see your physician.

What your physician can do. Besides wet dressings, he will guard against shock and replace lost body fluids. Sometimes hospitalization is necessary. He will prevent or treat secondary infections with antibiotics.

Chilblains

Chilblains are swollen, bluish-red spots on the skin of the fingers, toes, and ears that burn and itch. The condition is caused by off-and-on exposure to low temperatures. Healing occurs in about two weeks, with the skin turning brown and scaling. In severe cases, the lesions may blister and ulcerate or become infected. Keep the affected areas warm and dry. Improve circulation by hot-and-cold hand or foot baths (see page 589). Apply a soothing ointment or oil. Protect against infection.

Hives (urticaria)

Hives are red, itchy areas of the skin that develop firm, elevated wheals (0.5 to 2.5 cm), often with a white spot in the center. Hives may fuse together to form giant hives. They usually fade away within minutes or hours. A severe response involves tissues deep under the skin with marked swelling of the eyes, lips, face, and larynx, known as **angioneurotic edema.** Breathing becomes difficult and life may be threatened. Nausea, dizziness, headache, and a drop in blood pressure may occur **(anaphylactic shock).**

A single hive is usually due to an outside cause, such as a bee sting or an insect bite. An allergic response to certain foods, pollens, house dust, feathers, molds, or drugs can cause multiple hives. They can also result from an underlying infection (parasitic, sinusitis, yeast infection, tooth abscess), as well as an underlying disease (hepatitis, connective tissue disease, cancer). Hives can be trig-

989

gered by physical factors such as exposure to cold, heat, sunlight, pressure, or even water. Urticaria can also develop as a result of stress. In fact, in more than 60 percent of cases no definite cause is found.

What you can do. For immediate relief of itching use cool compresses, a warm soaking bath, or a soothing lotion. A paste of baking soda and water will provide comfort. Then try, by careful observation, to identify and then avoid the cause which triggers an attack, whether it be a food, a pollen, or a drug. Hives should break out soon after exposure.

If you have become sensitized to insect stings (ants, bees, wasps) or react violently to any allergen, you should have available an emergency first-aid kit (with adrenaline and antihistamines). A violent reaction is a medical emergency. Go to a hospital or see your physician.

What your physician can do. He can help you determine what is causing your problem, but this is sometimes difficult. In an emergency, an injection of adrenaline or steroids is life-saving. In resistant cases antihistamines may be advisable.

Other skin disorders

Cutaneous lupus erythematosus. See page 957.

Scleroderma. See page 957.

Burns. See page 537.

Frostbite. See page 555.

Nail disorders

Both local injury or infection and a number of illnesses affect the nails, causing them to become discolored, deformed, or both. Nails may be injured by shoes that are too tight and short, by being squeezed as in a car door, or by being struck with a heavy object such as a hammer. Systemic nail disorders include bronchiectasis, endocarditis, iron deficiency, psoriasis, and AIDS.

Injury to the nail may cause blood to accumulate beneath the nail. If the amount of blood is small, it will grow out with the nail. However, if the amount is large, the nail may be lifted from its bed and later it will fall off as the new nail forms.

Infection of the nail by ringworm (tinea unguium) causes the nail to thicken, crack, and crumble. A yeast-like organism (Candida) may invade the nail, resulting in its becoming yellow, hard, and thick, and sometimes separating it from the nail bed **(onychomycosis).** (See the illustration on page 991.)

Illnesses (general medical disorders) may produce distinct patterns in the nails, affecting their shape, color, and strength. A decrease in protein (Terry's nail) in patients with cirrhosis can produce a white nail at the base with a small pink area at the top. Yellow nails can be seen in those with chronic edema (bronchiectasis, lymphatic disorders). Separation of the nail bed from the nail plate may develop in thyroid disease, allergy, psoriasis, and contact dermatitis. Longitudinal ridging can be a change due to age (senile nail). Spoon nails

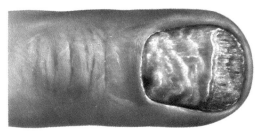

Onychomycosis. From fungi invasion.

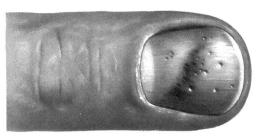

Psoriasis. Note typical depressions.

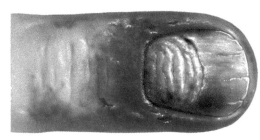

Eczema. Longitudinal splitting distinctive.

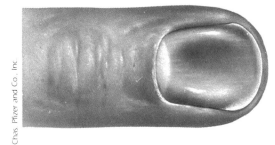

Koilonychia. Gives "spoon nail" effect.

Chas. Pfizer and Co. Inc

(see illustration below) can occur following chronic trauma, iron deficiency anemia, and as a normal variant. Endocarditis may produce small linear splinter hemorrhages; and pitting may result from psoriasis, hair loss (alopecia areata), eczema, and trauma.

What you can do. Time will generally cause injuries to disappear. Infection, especially with fungi, tend to be resistant. If local application of a fungicidal ointment does not relieve the problem, see your physician.

What your physician can do. For persistent infection your physician may prescribe an antibiotic (griseofulvin) to be taken by mouth. Steroids may sometimes be helpful. When the particular systemic disease is passed, the nail should grow normally.

Paronychia

In **paronychia** the tissues surrounding one or more of the fingernails (sometimes the toenails) are swollen, extremely tender, and ooze pus. This causes the loss of the cuticle and a secondary infection. The nail plate becomes thickened and discolored with transverse ridges. Bacteria followed by fungi, particularly Candida, invade the tissues, especially when constantly immersed in water. Diabetics and those in poor nutritional state are highly susceptible.

What you can do. After washing your hands, dry them thoroughly. Keep your hands away from water as much as possible. Use water-resistant gloves, with cotton gloves next to the skin, when you must immerse your hands in water. Apply a

991

medicated cream at night, rubbing it into the tissues around the nail. Should the infection persist, your physician may prescribe an antibiotic or antifungal agent.

Ingrowing toenail

As the toenail grows, one or both of the front corners of the nail of the great toe cut into the flesh, which becomes swollen and painful. The problem is caused by wearing shoes that crowd the toes, making the nail curve under at the sides. Another cause is cutting the toenail too short. Sometimes a secondary infection may develop.

What you can do. Wear well-fitting shoes. Cut the nail straight across so the corners are just beyond the flesh. If the toe has become infected, unless you are a diabetic or suffer from decreased circulation in your feet, use hot and cold foot baths to relieve the inflammation and swelling. Should the pain and infection continue, see your physician. It may be necessary for him to remove a slender lengthwise strip of nail plate in the involved area.

Hangnail

The cuticle that surrounds the base and sides of the nail splits and creates a fissure, which as it tears into the living tissue causes pain. It may become inflamed. However, do not pull the loose tissue off. Gently trim the tissue away with a pair of scissors or with a small cuticle cutter (available at any pharmacy) designed for this purpose. The fissure will heal. Use a mild cream to keep the tissues soft and pliable.

Hair disorders

Hair loss (alopecia, baldness)

Baldness, a lack of hair on the scalp, occurs whenever the rate of loss exceeds the rate of replenishment. Hair loss, with resulting baldness, has many causes. The cause may not be known (alopecia areata), but the following are known causes: hereditary factors (male pattern baldness); severe physical or psychological stress (telogen effluvium); systemic illnesses, such as iron deficiency anemia or hypothyroidism; certain drugs; traction; and certain diseases and chemicals which directly affect the scalp.

Alopecia areata is a spotty loss of hair in oval or round areas of the scalp, and occasionally on other parts of the body. In a minority, the hairless areas enlarge until the entire scalp becomes bald, and in fact may progress to involve hair regions of the entire body. This disease is thought to be autoimmune in nature, and can be associated with thyroid disease, pernicious anemia, vitiligo, Addison's disease, and Down's syndrome.

This disorder requires the attention of a trained physician to prevent total hair loss. Treatment may include topical steroids, local injection of steroids, the introduction of an irritant dermatitis, localized PUVA (see "psoriasis," page 985), or, more recently, immunomodulation.

Male pattern baldness is a progressive loss of hair that begins at the temples, and later on the crown of the head. Hair loss continues until the bald areas fuse. Occasionally the entire scalp becomes bald, but usually hair remains on the sides and back of the head. It also occurs in women some fifteen to twenty years later, but is generally not as severe. Heredity (from the mother's side), the level of androgens (male hormones), the response of the follicle to androgens, and aging, appear to be responsible.

To date no specific cure has been found. The many creams and lotions on the market purporting to grow hair are ineffective. Topical nunoxidil ("Regane") can be helpful in early cases with a variable response in 20 to 25 percent of people. Hair pieces are worn by many. Hair transplants and scalp reductions are helpful in good candidates, and are the only permanent solution. Artificial "hair" should not be used.

Stress-related hair loss (telogen effluvium) is a temporary hair loss that occurs some two months after a stressful event. Stress alters the hair cycle from the growth to the resting phase. Following the hair loss, the growth phase resumes, and the hair is restored. Many possible causes exist: psychological stress, surgery, acute illness, high fever, pregnancy, and drugs.

Other causes of hair loss include exposure to certain drugs, especially from those used to treat cancer (cytotoxic); excessive intake of vitamin A; the habit of pulling the hair, such as too tight ponytails (traction hair loss); chemicals used for curling and straightening hair; thyroid disorders; and diseases of the scalp. The hair growth generally resumes when the causative factor is removed.

Gray hair

Gray hair is caused by the failure of the hair follicles to form pigment. This part of the aging process starts at various ages in different families. Hair dyes and rinses to conceal the grayness are available, but you should check for skin sensitivity.

Benign and malignant tumors

Skin cancers occur more often than all other cancers combined. Most can be cured if detected early and treated promptly. Since most of the skin can be seen, the total deaths from malignancies of the skin are far fewer than from many cancers occurring less frequently, but whose presence is difficult to detect. It is often hard to distinguish normal from abnormal skin, but the axiom should be, when in doubt see your physician.

Vascular tumors (vascular nevi, hemangiomas, birthmarks)

The ordinary birthmark is a cluster of tiny blood vessels in the skin with a reddish or purplish color, the size and shape varying greatly, from a spot to a large area. Because they may occur on any part of the skin, they are primarily a cosmetic problem, but rarely become cancerous, unless they break down and ulcerate. The majority of birthmarks lighten in color or disappear by age seven, even if untreated. Depending on their size, shape, and color they carry different names: spider nevus, salmon patch, strawberry and cherry hemangiomas, and port-wine stain (nevus flammeus).

What your physician can do. Home remedies do no good. Small lesions may be made less conspicuous with a lotion or powder. A dermatologist should determine which available treatment to use: tattooing, surgery, freezing, radiation. However, laser therapy appears to be the most effective.

Moles

Moles are a benign growth of melanin-producing cells (melanocytes) with sharply demarcated edges. Many moles—some dark

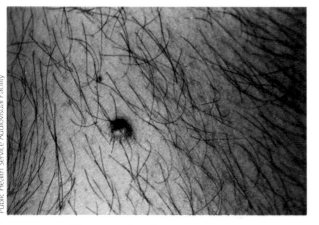

Some moles become cancerous.

colored, others remaining the color of the surface skin—do not become apparent until adulthood. Generally, moles are harmless and one need not try to remove them, unless they are a cosmetic problem or are subject to irritation from clothing. However, occasionally a mole may become cancerous—a condition that is indicated by a sudden change in its shape, color, or size.

Epidermal inclusion cyst (sebaceous cyst, wen)

This type of cyst usually results from a defective hair follicle tumor. It may have a central pore opening, as well as a cheesy malodorous content composed of keratin (sebum).

These harmless cysts range from pea to orange size. They may be white, pink, or purple, and feel either soft, doughy, elastic, or firm to the touch, but rarely tender or painful, unless infected. When infected, they become red, inflamed, and painful, and may burst, expelling thick pus. Enlarged and infected cysts are removed by a simple surgical procedure.

Fatty tumor (lipoma)

A lipoma is a benign, painless, encapsulated mass of normal fat cells developing in or just beneath the skin. They commonly form on the neck, forearms, and trunk, vary widely in size, and are generally round, rubbery, and movable. Various kinds of lipoma—fibrolipomas (with fibrous tissue), angiolipomas (with blood vessels), and myolipomas (with muscle cells)—are satisfactorily treated only by simple surgical removal. Should one suddenly enlarge, see your physician.

Keloid

A keloid is an overgrowth of scar tissue forming nodules or irregular tumor masses. Following an injury such as a burn or laceration of the skin, the scar continues to grow beyond its need, causing mild prickling and burning and becoming tender and painful. Fortunately, keloids are not malignant and tend to run in families, more commonly in blacks than whites. Keloids should be treated by a dermatologist, as after removal they tend to recur. Injecting a steroid into the surgical wound appears to give the best results.

Seborrheic keratosis

Seborrheic keratoses appear as small, slightly raised tumors consisting of masses of skin cells, mainly those of the epidermis. Sharply demarcated, round to oval in shape, and slightly darker than the surrounding skin (sometimes dark brown or black), these lesions are covered with a loosely attached soft, greasy crust, which when removed reveals a raw and pulpy base that bleeds slightly. They do not tend to become malignant.

The tumors develop in the middle aged, and are the most common skin tumor in the elderly. They appear on the face, forehead, neck, chest, and back. The size may vary from a few millimeters to several centimeters across. Itching—sometimes severe— is the only symptom. Your physician should determine that it is not a more serious condition. Application of a freezing agent or curettement easily removes keratoses.

Actinic keratosis (solar or senile keratosis)

Actinic keratosis, the most common pre-cancerous skin lesion, is a reddish or tan spot, round or irregular, slightly elevated, flat, rough, dry, and often scaly. Varying in size from a few millimeters to over a centimeter, they develop most frequently on the areas of skin exposed to the sun, such as the face, back of the hands, forearms, and bald scalp. Approximately one in ten of those with actinic keratosis develop signs of squamous cell carcinoma, characterized by sudden enlargement, elevation, and inflammation or ulceration of the lesion.

What you can do. Prevent actinic keratosis by guarding against undue exposure to sunshine. Cover exposed areas with appropriate clothing, or use a sunscreen lotion or cream. All actinic keratoses should be seen by your physician.

What your physician can do. A keratosis can be frozen (liquid nitrogen), chemically peeled, electrically desiccated, or removed surgically. If the lesions are numerous, a sclerotic chemical can be applied to the area in a lotion or cream.

Basal cell carcinoma

A basal cell cancer appears as a dome-shaped nodule, whitish to pink in color, with a raised pearly border. It may scale, crust, or ulcerate in the center (rodent ulcer). It rarely spreads to distant areas, but can destroy neighboring tissue, whether

995

skin, muscle, or bone. In this most common skin cancer, two of every three occurrences develop in areas exposed to the sun—and most often in people over forty. Your physician will remove all such malignancies, either with surgery, electrodesiccation and curettage, or with X-ray irradiation. Occasionally superficial lesions are frozen.

Squamous cell carcinoma

A squamous cell cancer—a firm, red lesion with a rounded raised border and a shallow ulcerated center—can be invasive and can spread. This cancer most frequently affects the skin of the face, scalp, ears, and the backs of the hands. Excessive exposure to the sun is the predominant cause, although X-ray exposure, irritant chemicals, and chronic infections can predispose to this type of malignancy. Removal by surgery or radiation, if done early, is curative.

Malignant melanoma

Among skin cancers, melanomas cause the most deaths and are one of the most dangerous. They usually occur between the ages of 30 and 60. Persons with fair skin, blue eyes, and blond or red hair, are highly susceptible. While heredity may play a role, the duration of exposure to the sun appears to be the most important predisposing factor.

The superficial spreading mela-
noma is the most common. It begins as an irregular, small brown lesion and grows along the skin for one to five years. Nodules indicate invasion of the deeper layers of the skin. Early recognition before deeper invasion has occurred is extremely important, since such lesions are easily removed by surgery.

Melanomas commonly appear on the head, neck, and body of men, and the arms and especially legs of women. The major features that distinguish a melanoma are its asymmetrical growth, its irregular border, various colors in the lesion, and a diameter of 6 mm or more. As the lesion grows horizontally, the edges may be notched by finger-like growths that reach into adjoining areas. While melanin is light brown to almost black, shades of red, white, or blue may be present. Red indicates inflammation, white scarring, and blue that the pigment is deep in the dermis. Itching, scaling, and tenderness are also significant signs. The thicker and deeper the tumor, the poorer the prognosis.

Report to your physician immediately any lesion that changes size suddenly and is irregular in shape and variegated in color.

Immediate and complete surgical excision, including surrounding tissue, is the best treatment. Immunotherapy and chemotherapy may be used if the disease has spread internally (metastasized).

VOL. 3

SECTION 4

THE ENDOCRINE
AND NERVOUS SYSTEMS
AND THEIR DISORDERS

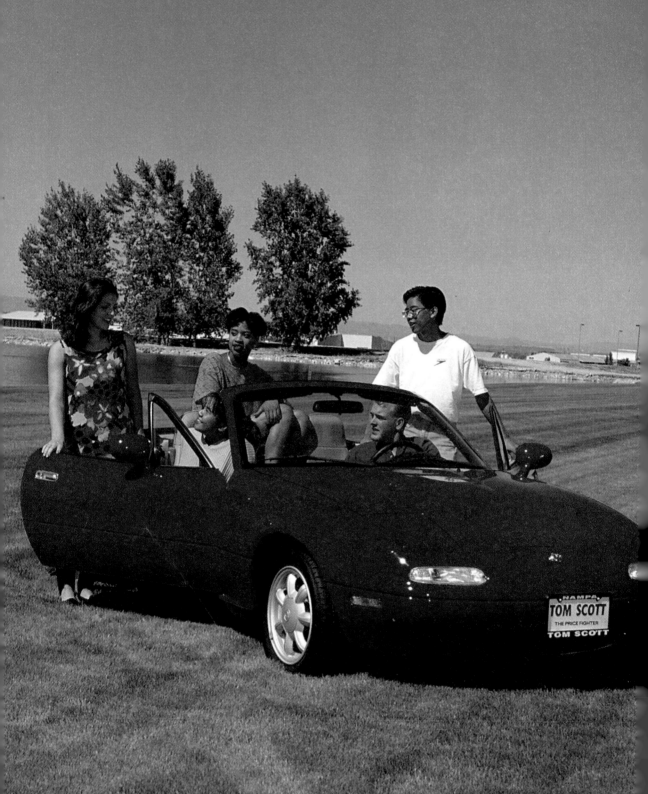

CHAPTER 16

The endocrine glands

The chemicals or hormones excreted by the endocrine glands, together with the nervous system, form a highly complex but beautifully integrated system to control and regulate the physiological functions of your body.

A hormone is a chemical substance manufactured by a cell or by a group of cells that form an endocrine gland. Hormones secreted directly into body fluids have a local effect and are called **local hormones.** Others, carried by the blood to distant parts of the body, are called **general hormones.** Both types control the activities of specific tissues, called target cells or target organs. Usually the greater the amount of a hormone produced, the more active its target organ. While each hormone performs a separate and unique task, certain hormones alter the functions of others, and even control the production level of other hormones.

Local hormones have a variety of functions. Acetylcholine is a local hormone released at the end of certain nerve endings (parasympathetic and motor nerves). Secretin, formed in the wall of the duodenum, is carried by the blood to the pancreas, where it stimulates pancreatic secretion. Cholecystokinin, released by the wall of the small intestine, stimulates the gallbladder to contract and activates enzyme secretion in the pancreas.

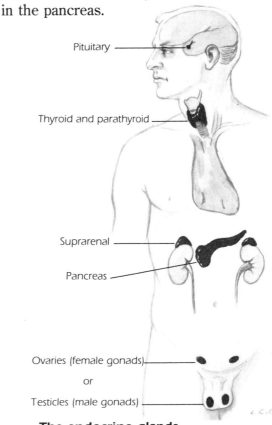

Pituitary

Thyroid and parathyroid

Suprarenal

Pancreas

Ovaries (female gonads)

or

Testicles (male gonads)

The endocrine glands.

The general hormones are produced by the pituitary, pineal, adrenal, thyroid, parathyroid, pancreas, ovary, testicle, and placenta. Singly and together they influence all aspects of life, modifying behavior and causing the distinctions of age and sex.

The pituitary gland

The hormones produced by the pituitary gland, for the most part, regulate the activity of other glands. This "master gland" plays a dominant role, picturesquely described as the conductor of the endocrine orchestra. It is surrounded by a bony chamber, located in the base of the brain. Connected to the hypothalamus by a tiny stalk, the gland is divided into two lobes, anterior and posterior.

Hormones of the anterior lobe. These include six important and several less important hormones. The **growth hormone** regulates general physical growth, especially by influencing protein formation. **Prolactin** stimulates the breasts to develop and produce milk. **Corticotropin (ACTH)** acts on the cells of the adrenal cortex to produce its hormones, as does **thyrotropin** on the thyroid, and **gonadotropin** on the sex organs (gonads). The anterior pituitary produces two kinds of gonadotropins: **follicle-stimulating hormone (FSH),** which causes the ovaries to produce and liberate the female sex cells (ova) and the testes to produce male sex cells (sperm) and **luteinizing hormone (LH),** which in women develops the corpus luteum and stimulates the ovary to produce estrogens, and in men stimulates the testes to produce testosterone.

Hormones of the posterior lobe. Two important hormones—vasopressin and oxytocin—are stored and released by the posterior lobe. **Vasopressin (ADH)** is an antidiuretic hormone that acts on the tubules of the kidneys to control the amount of water allowed to pass into the urine. When the body fluids become too dilute, the production of vasopressin decreases so that more water is allowed to escape from the body. When the body fluids become too concentrated, production of vasopressin increases so less water passes into the urine, thus conserving body water.

Oxytocin has no effect in men. In women it has two actions: it causes contraction of the uterus during childbirth and acts on the breasts to aid in the release of milk.

Pineal gland

Hormones and maturity. Certain wavelengths of visible light act on the pituitary, which, in turn, influences the sex organs, delaying the onset of maturity. Children born blind mature or adolesce sooner than do children of the same age who have sight. Should a child lose his sight some years before adolescence, the time of adolescence will be advanced.

In response to light, the retina in the back of the eye sends a signal to the pituitary gland located in the center of the brain. The pituitary then, via a chemical messenger or hormone, transmits the signal to the ovaries or testicles. These glands respond by causing the maturing process to proceed at the appropriate pace.

Biologic rhythms appear to be influenced by the light cycles of day and night. Your cortisol levels peak in the morning and gradually fall during the day, being lowest in the evening. Should you decide to work nights, it takes five to ten days to reverse the cycle! Visible light, entering the eye, affects the production of **melatonin,** a hormone produced by the tiny **pineal gland,** located in the back and center portion of your brain. Light blocks the production of this hormone, so the concentration of melatonin is lowest toward sundown. When darkness comes, the amount of this hormone rises—an appropriate cycle because melatonin encourages sleep!

The adrenal glands (suprarenal glands)

The right and left adrenal glands sit atop the right and left kidneys. Each gland consists of the cortex which surrounds the medulla, and which can be roughly compared to the filling of a sandwich lying between two slices of bread—the cortex. Because the cortex is essential to life, its hormones must be replaced artificially if the cortex is destroyed by disease.

Hormones of the adrenal cortex. Some thirty steroids, called corticosteriods or adrenal corticoids, have been found in the adrenal cortex. Only the best understood will be described.

One group, the **mineralocorticoids,** helps maintain the body's water balance by influencing the absorption of certain mineral ions. In this group, **aldosterone,** the best known, acts on the kidneys to favor the elimination of potassium and the retention of sodium.

Another group, the **glucocorticoids,** plays a number of important roles, one of which is the conversion of carbohydrates (starches), protein, and fat to energy. **Hydrocortisone (cortisol)** is the most active in this group; **cortisone** is somewhat less active. These hormones play a part in maintaining blood pressure and promptly respond to a variety of forms of physical stress (injury, infection, extremes of heat and cold, and debilitating disease). They also have an anti-inflammatory action by blocking many of the factors that promote inflammation, and effectively reduce allergic reactions. However, in large doses they reduce the level of the body's immunity.

The third group are the **sex hormones.** The androgens play a very important role in women as well as in men, although they are overshadowed in men by the testes. Androgens and estrogens are produced by both sexes, but the dominant hormones are the androgens in men, and the estrogens in women. The testes and ovaries also produce these hormones.

Hormones of the adrenal medulla. Two hormones, **epinephrine (adrenaline)** and **norepinephrine,** are produced by the adrenal medulla in a ratio of about four to one. Their actions differ only in the degree to which they affect various organ systems.

As these hormones circulate throughout the body, they marshall the resources of the body for fight or flight. They cause virtually all the blood vessels to constrict, the activity of the heart to increase, and the blood pressure to rise. They suppress gastrointestinal action, dilate the pupils of the eye, raise blood sugar levels, and increase the metabolic rate up to 100 percent above resting.

The adrenal medulla composes part of the body's alarm system and functions as an integral part of the sympathetic nervous system (which is part of the autonomic, or automatic nervous system). The release of hormones from the adrenal medulla is the body's way of declaring a state of emergency. It prepares the body to meet a crisis. Medullary hormones have the same effect as stimulation of the nerves of the sympathetic nervous system, except that the effects last for a minute or two instead of a few seconds, as is the case with sympathetic nervous stimulation.

The thyroid gland

The thyroid gland, shaped like a butterfly, is located below the larynx. Its two lobes (wings) lie in front and on either side of the windpipe (trachea) and are connected by a strip of glandular tissue (the body). The gland receives an abundant supply of blood, about five times its weight each minute, an amount possibly exceeded only by the adrenal cortex.

The thyroid is composed of thousands of small "follicles," each consisting of a single layer of cells on the outside with a core of gelatinous substance (colloid) on the inside. The colloid, largely glycoprotein thyroglobulin, provides the storage reservoir for excess thyroid hormones. The cells forming the shell of the follicle can direct the hormones they produce into either the blood (capillaries surround each follicle) or into the central storage area, depending on the body's needs.

The thyroid produces three hormones: **thyroxine (T4), triiodothyronine,** and **calcitonin.** While the actions of thyroxine and triiodothyronine are the same, the thyroid produces nine times as much thyroxine as triiodothyronine. Interestingly, much of thyroxine is converted to triiodothyronine, which is four times more potent. Thyroxine and triiodothyronine contain the element iodine, generally obtained in the diet. The production of thyroid hormones is under the control of thyrotropin (TSH), a hormone made by the anterior pituitary.

These thyroid hormones control virtually all chemical (metabolic) reactions in the body, increasing the oxygen requirement of most of the body's tissues. They play an important role in growth and skeletal development in children, working with the growth hormone (GH) of the anterior pituitary. And they improve a person's ability to think. When these hormones are in short supply, thinking is retarded, sometimes extremely.

Calcitonin plays a role in maintaining the precise level of calcium in the blood, and to do this, works with the parathyroid hormone.

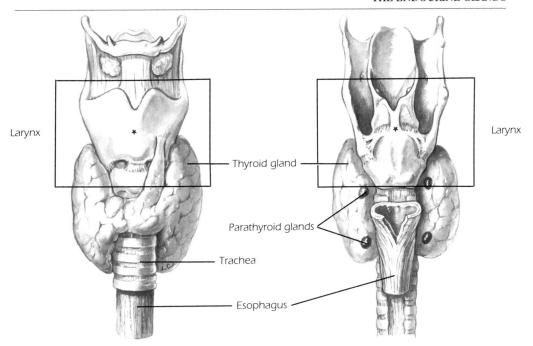

Larynx

Larynx

Thyroid gland

Parathyroid glands

Trachea

Esophagus

The thyroid and parathyroid glands. The thyroid gland straddles the trachea just below the larynx. The **parathyroid glands lie on the back surface of the thyroid, usually two on each lobe.**

Parathyroid glands

These four small glands are located on the back surfaces of the thyroid lobes. They produce the **parathyroid hormone,** which works with calcitonin and vitamin D to maintain the proper concentration of calcium and phosphate in the blood. Vitamin D increases the absorption of calcium and phosphate from the gut. Calcitonin encourages calcium and phosphate storage in the bones, while parathyroid hormone and vitamin D promote the release of calcium and phosphate from the bones. The balance between release and storage maintains a precise blood level.

The pancreas

The pancreas is located crossways in the back part of the abdomen, below and behind the stomach, and extends from the duodenum to the left kidney. It contains two types of glandular tissue: one that produces digestive juices (exocrine), another that produces hormones (endocrine). Clusters of the hormone-producing cells are scattered mainly through the tail of the pancreas. These clusters (called islets of Langerhans) contain cells of three types: alpha-producing **glucagon,** beta-releasing **insulin,** and delta-secreting **somatostatin.**

These three hormones work together to maintain the proper level of glucose in the blood. After it has been absorbed from the intestine, the glucose coming from carbohydrates and protein passes through the liver. More than half of this is

1003

stored in the liver as glycogen, making the liver the body's major storehouse for glucose. The remainder circulates in the blood and is used as fuel by the brain, red blood cells, and muscles. Some is converted to fat and held in fat cells.

When the amount of glucose in the blood increases (after a meal), the production of insulin increases correspondingly. Insulin facilitates the entry of glucose into muscle and other tissues and also facilitates its storage in the liver. Should the level of glucose drop, glucagon is secreted. This influences the liver to convert glycogen back to glucose and release it to the blood. While the functions of the newly discovered pancreatic hormone somatostatin are not fully understood, it appears to limit the secretion of both insulin and glucagon.

The ovaries

Besides being the organs which produce the female sex cells (ova), the ovaries produce two types of hormones, the **estrogens** and **progesterone.** While six or more natural estrogens have been isolated, those in significant amounts are estradiol, estrone, and estriol. Of the three, estradiol, the major estrogen, is twelve times as potent as estrone, and eighty times more powerful than estriol.

In the female, the estrogens regulate the functions of the reproductive organs, the adrenal androgens, and the desire for sexual activity. In the adolescent girl they stimulate the development of the feminine characteristics.

New follicles begin to develop in the ovaries about every twenty-eight days, activated by the gonadotropic hormones of the anterior pituitary. During the growth of the follicles, estrogens are released. After the ovum is freed, the follicle form a corpus luteum (a yellow mass), which secretes estrogens and progesterone in large quantities.

Progesterone is produced not only by the corpus luteum, but also in smaller amounts by the adrenal cortex and by the placenta. This hormone prepares the lining of the uterus to receive and nourish a fertilized ovum, and the breasts to give milk. If no pregnancy occurs, most of this lining tissue is eliminated at the time of menstruation.

The testes

The right and left testicles, found in the scrotal sac, have two functions: to produce the male sex cells (sperm) and the male hormones called **androgens.** The androgens are produced mainly by the interstitial cells, which lie in clumps between the tubules that produce the sperm.

The principal androgen is **testosterone.** In adolescent boys it brings about the development of the secondary male characteristics, while in the adult male it maintains these characteristics and stimulates the desire for sexual activity. It also promotes a feeling of wellness and vigor.

CHAPTER 17

Endocrine gland disorders

Since the endocrine glands through their hormones activate and regulate the functions of cells and organs throughout the body, any dysfunction of these glands will produce widespread disturbances in major physiological functions.

The endocrine glands and their normal functions are described in the preceding chapter.

Pituitary disorders

Diabetes insipidus

In diabetes insipidus, a rare disorder, huge quantities (20 quarts or 19 liters) of dilute urine are produced daily, causing constant urination and severe thirst, day and night. The urine does not contain sugar (glucose) and should not be confused with diabetes mellitus.

The difficulty results from the failure of the posterior pituitary to receive or release normal amounts of the antidiuretic hormone (ADH or vasopressin). Vasopressin activates the cells of the kidney tubules to reabsorb water and thus prevents excessive loss of urine. Head injury, a tumor growth, surgery, or radiation therapy in the area of the pituitary may cause the problem. Often the cause is not known.

What you can do. Drink as much water as needed, and see your physician.

What your physician can do. If possible, he will determine and remove the cause. When this is not possible, you may be able to drink adequate water to care for mild cases. Otherwise, a synthetic ADH (desmopressin) can be taken by nasal spray one to three times per day or by an injection.

Abnormal milk production (galactorrhea)

Production of the hormone **prolactin** sometimes occurs because of a tumor that has developed in the anterior lobe of the pituitary. This condition is rare in women (except after pregnancy) and very rare in men. The excess prolactin activates the breast tissue to produce milk. The amount of milk may be so small that it can be observed only when the nipple is compressed. The condition may cause cessation of menstruation in women and impotency in men.

What your physician can do. Examination may reveal a pituitary tumor. If the underlying problem cannot be resolved, an endocrinologist may recommend hormonal treatment to suppress milk production.

Gigantism and acromegaly

These disorders result from an overproduction of the **growth hormone (GH) somatotropin,** usually resulting from a tumor made up of cells located in the anterior lobe of the pituitary which produce GH. The tumor growth may be slow or rapid. If the overproduction occurs during childhood, **gigantism** results, with an adult height of six and a half feet or more. However, one must not suppose that all tall children are afflicted with this disorder. Most tall children are merely genetically determined to be tall.

When the overproduction of GH begins in an adult, **acromegaly** results. In this disorder no apparent increase in the person's height occurs, but the hands and feet gradually become larger, and the jaw, lips, nose, and ridges above the eyes become more prominent.

What your physician can do. Surgical removal of the tumor, or its destruction by radiation are standard procedures but carry serious risks, even in the hands of a specialist. Your physician may also attempt hormonal treatment.

Dwarfism

Restriction of growth or dwarfism may result from inadequate secretion of the growth hormone, often caused from pressure exerted by a tumor on the anterior pituitary gland. However, other causes for short stature include disorders of the thyroid, the adrenals, and the sex glands; malnutrition; and debilitating diseases. Again, one must not suppose that all short children are afflicted with dwarfism. Most are genetically determined to be short.

In dwarfism due to inadequate secretion of growth hormone, the body's proportions are usually normal, but sexual development is often deficient. Treatment with growth hormone during the growing years may be successful.

Hypopituitarism

In this disorder one or more hormones that are manufactured in the anterior lobe of the pituitary fail to be produced in adequate quantities. Since many of these hormones are responsible for controlling the hormonal output of other endocrine glands, these inadequacies produce widespread effects.

The symptoms of hypopituitarism include atrophy of the sex organs with infertility, absence of menses in women, reduction of axillary and pubic hair, and premature aging, along with weakness, low blood pressure, low body temperature, loss of appetite, and dwarfism in children.

One cause of this disorder is bleeding into the pituitary after delivery of a baby. Another is a tumor which destroys the substance of the gland. Possible treatment includes the removal of the tumor and the administration of multiple hormones. For example, hormones from the thyroid, adrenal, ovaries, or testicles, along with others would be necessary, and should be given under the direction of a specialist.

Tumors of the pituitary gland

These tumors may be benign or malignant and show symptoms as already mentioned under dwarfism, gigantism, acromegaly, galactorrhea, hypopituitarism, and diabetes insipidus, along with Cushing's disease. Should they extend beyond the bounds of the pituitary they may cause headaches and visual problems.

Surgical removal or destruction with radiation may be attempted, but involves high risks.

Adrenal disorders

Addison's disease

This disease develops when the cortexes of the adrenal glands atrophy, usually due to an autoimmune disorder in which the body's own defense cells attack the functioning cells of the adrenal cortex. Other causes include tuberculosis, cancer, or an inflammatory process.

Symptoms develop after about 90 percent of the glands are destroyed and include chronic fatigue, exhaustion, low blood pressure, loss of appetite, nausea, gastrointestinal distress, dizziness and fainting, a dark pigmentation of the skin, and inability to handle stress. Even minor infections, surgery, or injury may precipitate an "addisonian crisis" which, if not promptly treated, leads to shock and death.

Treatment consists of daily replacing hydrocortisone, together with synthetic mineralocorticoid—a hormone formerly provided by your glands. In acute adrenal failure intravenous sodium chloride and cortisol should be administered immediately. An individual suffering from Addison's disease should carry adequate identification to alert medical personnel of his problem in case of accident or illness.

Cushing's syndrome (and Cushing's disease)

In both of these conditions (the symptoms are similar) there is an excess of glucocorticoids (cortisol and cortisone), hormones produced by the adrenal cortexes. In Cushing's disease an excess of these hormones results from overproduction of ACTH (corticotropin) in the anterior pituitary, which stimulates the adrenal cortexes to excess activity. Usually this is the result of a tumor

1007

in the anterior pituitary. Cushing's syndrome, more common in women than men, may result from ACTH production elsewhere in the body by a malignant tumor (lung, thymus, pancreas, kidney); from a glucocorticoid-producing tumor in the adrenal cortex or cortexes; or from excessive intake of glucocorticoids (hydrocortisone, cortisone) as a medication.

The usual symptoms include obesity (involving the face and trunk), muscular wasting and weakness, excessive growth of hair on the face and chest, thinning and reddening of the skin, high blood pressure, suppressed menstruation in women and decreased sex desire in men, thinning of bone structure (osteoporosis), increased liability to infection, and diabetes mellitus.

What your physician can do. He will attempt to determine the cause. A tumor in one adrenal can be readily removed. A tumor in the pituitary may be surgically removed or destroyed by radiation (the risks are high). Sometimes both adrenal glands are removed, which requires hormonal intake for the rest of your life. If excess intake of corticoids (as may occur in the treatment of arthritis or some other disease) causes the condition, your physician will gradually reduce the dosage. (Do not abruptly discontinue steroid intake.)

Hyperaldosteronism

Excess production of aldosterone, usually due to an aldosterone-producing tumor, causes this disorder. This hormone controls the retention of sodium and the elimination of potassium in the kidneys and elsewhere. Excessive sodium retention and potassium depletion results in high blood pressure, muscle weakness with cramps, and passing of large amounts of urine, especially at night. The treatment usually involves removal of the tumor, but sometimes, suppression of aldosterone secretion may be accomplished with medication.

Adrenal virilism

This condition results from an overproduction of the masculinizing androgen hormone, due either to overactive secreting cells in the adrenal cortex or to an androgen-producing tumor. Occurrence in early childhood causes early onset of sexual maturity. Development in adulthood causes accentuation of masculine characteristics in both men and women.

Treatment includes the surgical removal of the tumor or the suppression of pituitary ACTH with cortisol, combined with the essential hormonal replacement therapy.

Pheochromocytoma

A pheochromocytoma is a life-threatening tumor in the medulla of the adrenal gland. Excessive epinephrine and norepinephrine (adrenalin) production results in high blood pressure, severe headache, racing heart, sweating, and faintness. Episodes may be triggered by exercise, exposure to cold, or an emotional upset. A CAT scan or an angiogram can localize the tumor, which, when removed, generally cures the condition.

Thyroid disorders

Goiter

Goiter is a common term for any enlargment of the thyroid gland. In some goiters an excess of thyroxine is produced, and in others a reduced amount.

Nontoxic goiter. In this condition the thyroid gland enlarges in an effort to produce more thyroxine. Because the hormone is in short supply, the pituitary gland stimulates the thyroid to compensate for the deficiency. Factors which provoke

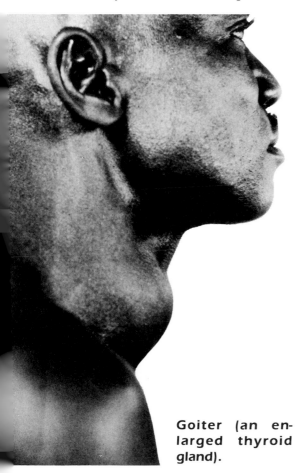

Goiter (an enlarged thyroid gland).

this response include a shortage of iodine (a constituent of thyroxine) in the food or water; an overuse of thyroid-depressing drugs; and Hashimoto's disease, in which the glandular tissue of the thyroid is destroyed.

Treatment is to provide thyroxine.

Other goiters. These may arise from benign or malignant tumors, or more commonly from toxic nodular goiter and from chronic thyroiditis (Hashimoto's disease). These will be discussed in the following pages.

Overactive thyroid (hyperthyroidism)

A number of forms of overactive thyroid exist; however, the most common problem is overproduction of thyroxine, in spite of a suppression of thyroid-stimulating hormone by the pituitary. Excess thyroxine speeds up all the chemical (metabolic) activities of the body, affecting both physical and mental functions.

Graves' disease or thyrotoxicosis occurs eight times more often in women than in men, and is thought to be a disturbance in the body's immune system. Less common causes include tumors of the thyroid, pituitary, and placenta. The usual symptoms consist of nervousness, intolerance to heat, rapid heartbeat, weight loss despite increased appetite, excessive thirst, tiredness, difficult breathing, weakness of the muscles, fine tremor of the hands, frequent urination, and diarrhea.

1009

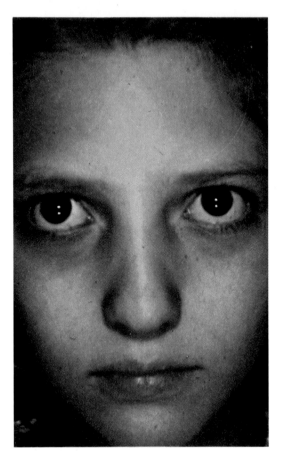

Thyrotoxicosis (Graves' disease). The eyes appear to bulge and are abnormally prominent.

The thyroid usually enlarges (goiter), and in many cases, the eyes have a "staring expression" and appear to bulge (exophthalmic goiter). If the condition remains untreated, the heart may fail through overactivity.

Toxic nodular goiter usually occurs as a late complication of nontoxic goiter and in most cases develops later in life. The symptoms are less extreme, develop more slowly, and do not include bulging of the eyes. Heart damage may occur in neglected cases.

What your physician can do. Depending on the severity of the condition, your physician will recommend the most desirable of several methods. A radioiodine scan may help determine the extent of the problem. Antithyroid drugs are used to suppress overactive hormone production, but often the benefit is temporary. The most successful therapy is a single treatment of radioactive iodine, which concentrates in the gland and destroys overactive secreting cells. Many patients become hypothyroid and require replacement hormonal therapy.

Underactive thyroid (hypothyroidism)

In such conditions the thyroid gland produces inadequate amounts of thyroxine, thus slowing down all body processes. The causes include a congenital defect—the baby being born with an underproducing thyroid or no gland at all; an autoimmune problem in which the body's own immune system gradually destroys the gland (Hashimoto's disease); a deficiency of TSH (thyroid stimulating hormone) of the pituitary; and a complication of treating an overactive thyroid. The effects differ, depending on the age of the person.

Cretinism. Children with this condition do not grow as rapidly or symmetrically as they should, and their minds develop slowly. No abnormality may be seen at birth, but within a few weeks the skin begins to thicken, and the cry becomes hoarse. The tongue becomes large, and the facial expression, piglike. The teeth develop late. If untreated,

---

children become cretins and remain deformed, feebleminded dwarfs. Little improvement is possible once the growth years are past.

The condition can be recognized immediately after birth by testing blood samples to determine whether a deficiency of thyroid hormone exists. If treatment begins before the infant is three months of age, the prospects of normal development are better than if it is delayed.

Myxedema. Myxedema is, typically, a disease of adults, and the symptoms develop slowly. Body functions gradually decelerate. The heart becomes weaker, and the heart rate and breathing become slower. The heart may become dilated. Perspiration is scanty, and susceptibility to infection increases. Body temperature is below normal, and the individual feels chilly, wears more clothing, and uses more bedcovers. Body weight increases despite decreased food intake. The skin becomes puffy, red, and thickened; the hair becomes dry and falls out easily; the nails are brittle and cracked. The body appears fat and soggy. The voice often sounds hoarse and harsh, hearing is impaired, and the sufferer appears depressed and mentally dull.

In **Hashimoto's disease** (sometimes called chronic thyroiditis) the gland is not inflamed, but the glandular tissue is gradually replaced with connective tissue (scar tissue), and sometimes it is infiltrated with white cells (lymphocytes). While thyroxine production is gradually reduced, the gland enlarges **(goiter)** two to three times its normal size. Occurring

twenty times more frequently in women than in men, this condition can be treated simply by administering thyroxine.

Thyroiditis

As the name of this condition implies, the thyroid gland is inflamed. In **acute thyroiditis** the gland becomes inflamed by an invasion of bacteria from an infection in the surrounding tissues of the neck or from an infected thyroid cyst. The symptoms include fever, with localized pain and swelling. Treatment with an appropriate antibiotic will eradicate the infection.

In **subacute thyroiditisa,** apparently caused by a virus, the gland becomes enlarged and painful. In mild cases, the illness subsides spontaneously after days or a few weeks. In severe cases, if untreated, remissions and relapses may occur over a period of months to a year or two. The condition responds favorably to corticosteroids.

Cancer of the thyroid

Cancer of the thyroid has shown a marked increase in recent years. Much of this may be due to having received radiation of the head or neck in childhood. It may occur in individuals who have had a goiter, but also develops independently of any thyroid disease. An enlargement of the gland, difficulty in breathing, or pain in the thyroid area are signals to see a physician, who will prescribe a thyroid scan to outline the swelling (benign tumors do not spread).

Surgical removal of malignant tumors is followed by administration of radioactive iodine to seek out and destroy any remaining islands of malignant cells, whether the cells are local or have migrated (metastasized) to other parts of the body. After removal of part or all of the gland, the individual must take appropriate amounts of thyroxine for the remainder of his life in order to restore the amount of thyroid hormone the body requires, and to suppress TSH in an attempt to prevent the growth of any malignant thyroid tissue which might remain.

Parathyroid disorders

The principal disorders are hyperparathyroidism or hypoparathyroidism, conditions characterized by either an excess or a shortage of the parathyroid hormone.

Hyperparathyroidism

In this disorder, the overabundant secretion of parathyroid hormone causes the bones to release excessive amounts of calcium. Because of the large amounts of calcium being eliminated through the kidneys, kidney stones form. Permanent damage to the kidneys may result from calcium being deposited within their tissues. The bones become demineralized and tend to fracture. Other symptoms include excessive thirst, excessive urination, pains in the back and in various bones and joints, and loss of appetite, sometimes accompanied with nausea and vomiting.

A benign tumor in one or more of the parathyroid glands is usually the cause of hyperparathyrodism. However, excessive secretion of parathyroid hormone can also occur in association with chronic kidney disease and in rickets. Certain malignant tumors elsewhere in the body can produce a hormone similar in function to parathyroid hormone, even to the extent of producing symptoms of hyperparathyroidism.

Treatment consists of surgically eradicating the offending tumors. Should kidney stones be present, they will also require removal.

Hypoparathyroidism

In hypoparathyroidism the inadequate amount of parathyroid hormone secreted causes low calcium and high phosphorus levels in the blood. Failure of the gland itself (possibly from an autoimmune disorder), or an inadequacy of other glands such as the thyroid or adrenals causes this condition, which occurs more commonly in childhood. Numerous symptoms include stunted growth, malformed teeth, and mental deficiency. The acute phase produces painful spasms and cramps (tetany) of the muscles of the abdomen, hands, feet, and throat, along with difficult breathing, sensitivity to light, and convulsions. When chronic, cataracts tend to develop, and permanent brain damage occurs.

In adults, hypoparathyroidism usually develops after thyroid surgery and results from injury to or loss of the parathyroids. The resulting lack of calcium causes muscle spasms and convulsions.

The treatment requires the administration of calcium and vitamin D, and must be continued throughout life.

Pancreatic disorders (islet cell disease, diabetes mellitus or diabetes)

The islets are scattered groups of hormone-producing (insulin and glucagon) cells scattered throughout the pancreas. Lack of production or lack of utilization of insulin results in **diabetes mellitus or diabetes**—doubtless the most common of all endocrine disorders. Approximately 10 million Americans, or about 5 percent of the population, have diabetes to some degree.

Types and causes of diabetes

Two main forms of diabetes are identified, and a hereditary factor appears to exist in both. Children of both types of diabetics have a greater-than-usual susceptibility of developing the disease.

Insulin-dependent diabetes (type I, juvenile-onset) results from an inadequate production of insulin by damaged or defective beta cells. Actual damage to the beta cells in the pancreas appears to be caused by an autoimmune response, possibly triggered or augmented by a viral infection (flu, bad cold, chickenpox). This form of diabetes develops in children between five to thirteen years of age, but also occurs at older ages. Once developed, it persists throughout life. By far the more serious form of the disease, it fortunately accounts for only 10 percent of the diabetic population.

Non-insulin-dependent diabetes (type II, adult-onset), usually developing in those of mature years (four out of five are over forty-five), results from over-burdening the body's energy-producing mechanisms by overeating. The obese are particularly susceptible. Interestingly, 85 percent of diabetics were at some time overweight. In this type of diabetes the output of insulin is generally insufficient to handle the surplus glucose in the blood from excessive food intake.

However, it now appears that another factor, at least in some, may be an insulin resistance rather than an insulin deficiency, since many such diabetics produce as much or even more insulin than do nondiabetics. The problem may lie in abnormal insulin receptors. In some diabetics of this type, insulin production gradually diminishes; such would eventually require insulin administration.

Symptoms

When diabetes begins in childhood **(type I),** the condition develops rapidly, and the symptoms, appearing in weeks or months, include increased production of urine, excessive thirst, dryness of the

1013

mouth and skin, a desire to void at night, bed wetting, an increase in appetite in spite of a loss in body weight, weakness and fatigue, and itching of the skin.

The symptoms of diabetes beginning in adulthood **(type II)** often develop slowly, sometimes over a period of years, and include excessive production of urine, increased thirst, weakness, fatigue, and itching of the skin. Sometimes early signs of the disease consist of blurred vision (excess sugar in the fluid of the eye), boils and other infections (urinary tract), and tingling in the hands and feet (see under "complications").

The physician will find sugar in the urine, higher-than-normal sugar levels in the blood (200 mg/dl or more), and evidence that the individual is not using up the blood sugar as quickly, following a meal, as does a nondiabetic. In other words, glucose is accumulating in the blood and being eliminated in the urine instead of being used in the body for production of energy.

Complications

Besides the problems of diabetes itself, the risks, after fifteen to twenty years, of complications and many other serious diseases are greatly increased.

Diabetics are much more likely than the average person to experience heart disease, kidney disease, blindness, and gangrene. Given a normal person's chance of succumbing to one of these conditions as "1," the chart above shows the diabetic's chance of succumbing to these same conditions.

Nondiabetic 1	
Diabetic	
Heart disease 5	
Kidney disease 17	
Blindness 25	
Gangrene 50	

Diabetics are more prone to **infections,** because the disease lowers the body's natural defense mechanisms. Elevated blood sugar levels appear to hinder the white blood cells, which are part of the body's defense force, from engulfing invading germs. Infections of the gums, pharynx, urinary tract, and vagina occur more frequently and are more difficult to cure than among nondiabetics. Minor injuries to the skin, especially of the feet, may develop into serious problems.

Infections make diabetes itself worse, especially if the illness involves nausea, vomiting, and diarrhea. The altered food intake makes the control of blood sugar more difficult.

Disease of the **heart and blood vessels** accounts for more than 75 percent of deaths among diabetics. High levels of cholesterol and blood fats are much more common among diabetics than among the general population. Atherosclerosis occurs at an earlier age and progresses more rapidly, resulting in more high blood pressure, coronary heart attacks, and stroke. Decreased circulation in the lower limbs often results in ulcers in the lower leg and gangrene of the toes.

Atherosclerosis affects the small

blood vessels of the **kidney** filters, resulting in gradual kidney failure. The kidneys of diabetics also appear to be more susceptible to infections. Among diabetics, damage to many areas of the **eye** occurs over a period of years. The retinas of well over half of all diabetics develop serious problems, such as hemorrhages and patches of deterioration, that cause varying degrees of visual loss. Cataracts are common and appear at an earlier age than in the general population.

The diabetic is susceptible to various kinds of **nervous ailments.** The symptoms of nerve degeneration (diabetic neuropathy) include tingling and loss of sensation in the hands and feet, pain in the limbs, muscular weakness, and, not infrequently in men, sexual impotence. Both decreased circulation and loss of sensation in the feet often allow minor injuries to develop into serious infections.

Emotional problems are much more prevalent among diabetics, especially those with poorly controlled blood sugar levels. As sugar levels go from high to low, mood changes occur—the person swings from being anxious or irritable to being happy or depressed. A prolonged illness is, in itself, depressing, especially one requiring constant awareness of virtually all activities— what and how much is eaten, how much exercise is taken, and whether the person is contented or stressed. Even in healthy people stress triggers the "alarm reaction" that raises blood sugar levels. In diabetics the situation is much worse.

Interestingly, a well-controlled blood sugar level reduces or eliminates all these potential or real problems, making the importance of good management in diabetes obvious.

Treatment

General principles. Since the goal of treatment is to maintain the level of blood sugar (glucose) within desirable limits, factors increasing or decreasing blood sugar must be carefully and understandably monitored. For example, food intake increases blood glucose while exercise decreases blood sugar by using it up. Thus those who exercise require less insulin than do sedentary individuals. On the other hand, stress, infections, the later months of pregnancy, the days before menstruation, and the adolescent growth spurt all increase blood sugar and therefore require increased insulin intake.

Recent research has shown that a **diet** rich in dietary fiber and low in fat can control non-insulin-dependent diabetes or greatly reduce the insulin needs, and that such diets make insulin-dependent diabetes much easier to control. In order to obtain such a diet one must avoid or reduce the intake of highly refined foods (which have lost all or part of their fiber) such as refined sugar and sugar-containing products; refined cereals and refined cereal products (which have lost most of their fiber); refined animal or vegetable fats and oils together with animal foods (which contain no fiber) such as dairy products, meat, fowl, and fish. Besides, sugary drinks and alcoholic

1015

beverages are also devoid of fiber. (For details see under "nutrition," page 92.)

Regularity in life's activities, eating, exercising, and sleeping, along with minimum exposure to emotionally charged situations and stressful recreational programs will greatly aid in providing a lifestyle best suited for one who suffers from diabetes.

Insulin-dependent diabetes. Since these diabetics fail to produce sufficient insulin for their needs, the necessary insulin must be supplied. And since insulin does not cure diabetes, the hormone must be taken for a lifetime.

Insulin is a protein, and if taken by mouth would be digested. For this reason it must be administered by injection, and diabetics soon learn to inject themselves at regular intervals. Small insulin pumps that fit into one's pocket are now available. They deliver insulin through a catheter to a needle placed beneath the skin of the abdomen. The insulin delivery is programmed to meet the individual's precise needs. The person whose diabetes is difficult to control can override the program should the need arise.

Insulin comes in three types: fast acting, intermediate acting, and long acting. In each case, the rate at which the insulin begins to work determines the duration of its effect. In other words, rapid-onset insulin has a short duration; slow-onset insulin has a long duration. The physician will determine which type or mixture of insulins best suits the diabetic's needs.

Since the food eaten is the only source of glucose or calories (fuel), the diabetic must learn to understand the various food groups, and what each contributes in the way of carbohydrate (sugars and starches), fat, and protein—the calorie or "sugar" carrying nutrients. Carbohydrate, fat, and a portion of protein can be converted to glucose or sugar. Nutritionists divide foods into groups: milk and milk products; starchy and non-starchy vegetables; fruits, berries, and fruit juices; and meats and protein foods, which are further divided into low, medium, and high fat. Charts are available listing the carbohydrate, protein, and fat content of each food based on its caloric content. A physician or nutritionist will help the diabetic determine his diet and explain how to substitute and exchange calories in and between food groups, enabling him to maintain a rather constant intake of calories.

Non-insulin-dependent diabetes. The majority of type II diabetics can maintain desirable blood sugar levels with a proper diet and regular exercise. The principles of a good diet, high in dietary fiber and low in fat, have been described above. The requirements may not have to be as rigorous as for a type I diabetic, but the total calorie intake should remain as constant as possible. Body fat makes one insulin resistant, so overweight people should make every effort to normalize their weight. If, over a period of time, the blood sugar rises above the desired level, the physician may recommend one of several hypoglycemic drugs which lower blood sugar. Eventually he may prescribe insulin should the condition so indicate.

Special concerns

Despite a carefully regulated program, situations may arise in which the blood sugar rises too high (hyperglycemia) or falls too low (hypoglycemia). Both of these conditions may result in unconsciousness.

Hyperglycemia develops slowly. Inadequate insulin causes fat to be burned, resulting in acidosis. Symptoms consist of an acetone smell on the breath (a sweetish, fruitlike odor), nausea and vomiting, dryness of the mouth and skin, thirst, weakness, increasing lethargy, and unconsciousness (diabetic coma). Untreated, death will ensue. Mild cases can be handled by restricting food or increasing the insulin intake. Severe cases are a medical emergency and should be cared for in a hospital.

Hypoglycemia comes on fairly rapidly and may be due to too much exercise, skipping or delaying a meal, too much insulin, or too large a dose of hypoglycemic medications. Because of inadequate glucose in the blood, the body runs out of fuel or energy. Serious problems may occur if one is driving a car, working with heavy machinery, or swimming.

The individual becomes ill at ease, breaks out in a sweat, and feels weak and shaky. Other symptoms include headache and hunger, slurred speech, hazy vision, confusion, and irritability. If untreated the individual may become unconscious (hypoglycemic coma). Drinking a glass of sweet fruit juice or eating a candy bar should relieve the problem. Drinking a glass of milk and eating a slice or two of bread will release the glucose into the blood more slowly. If one is in a medical facility he may be given an injection of glucagon to raise the blood sugar. However, when a hypoglycemic attack occurs, it indicates a poorly regulated diabetic.

Other conditions that may predispose toward hypoglycemia include fasting, congestive heart failure, certain types of cancer, chronic kidney failure, excessive alcohol intake, high fevers, stomach surgery, and emotional problems. Everyone developing hypoglycemia should be carefully evaluated by a physician.

Pregnancy. A pregnant diabetic mother and her child face many risks to their well-being. Some women develop a diabetes during pregnancy that disappears after delivery **(gestational diabetes)**. Whatever the form of diabetes, experience has shown that careful regulation of the mother's blood sugar levels, to maintain them as close as possible to those of nondiabetic pregnant women, can avoid many problems for both mother and child.

The mother self-monitors her blood glucose levels several times a day, and closely controls her diet and insulin intake, adjusting them as needed to appropriately control her blood sugar concentrations. Her insulin needs increase as pregnancy advances. Many mothers are now using insulin pump systems.

Since the mother's insulin does not pass through the placenta to the fetus, but the glucose from her blood does, the fetus is adversely affected.

1017

When her blood sugar is too high, the baby's blood sugar also becomes too high. This triggers the baby to make its own insulin, which, in turn, accelerates its growth while weakening its muscles. Such a baby is too big and flabby at birth.

It is wise for every diabetic woman who plans to become pregnant to be carefully managed by a knowledgeable physician before she becomes pregnant, and then throughout pregnancy and lactation. Dealing with a diabetic's existing problems before pregnancy will enhance the likelihood of having a healthy, full-term baby.

Tobacco. The evidence that smoking is harmful to health is well established. But smoking is especially harmful to a diabetic mother and her baby. Diabetics have an increased risk of circulatory disorders: atherosclerosis, coronary heart disease, chronic kidney failure, retinal disease, ulcers of the lower leg, and gangrene of the toes. Smoking further increases these risks. Besides, smoking affects the baby of a smoking mother, causing more premature births, lower birth weight, and slower growth.

Alcohol. As mentioned above, it is very important for the blood sugar levels of diabetic pregnant women to be maintained as close as possible to those of non-diabetic pregnant women. Alcohol blocks the production of glucose by the liver, and as a result blood sugar levels may drop, precipitating insulin reactions. It is therefore extremely unwise for pregnant diabetic women to use beverage alcohol.

Besides alcohol's effect on the mother's liver, alcohol passes from the mother's blood via the placenta to enter and circulate in the baby's blood. The alcohol contained in two drinks of beer, wine, or whiskey (30 ml or 1 oz) a day can result in smaller babies at birth and more frequent spontaneous abortions. Larger intakes increase the risk of partial or total fetal alcohol syndrome. This disorder causes deformities of the head and face, small brains and mental retardation, and retarded growth before and after birth. Heart defects and other anomalies occur frequently.

Monitoring your diabetes

Because of advanced testing methods, a diabetic can now analyze his urine for sugar and ketone bodies, and his blood for sugar levels. While urine tests give some indication of the diabetic's status, two more precise tests for determining the blood glucose level exist. One can be done in a few minutes by the diabetic himself, using a couple of drops of blood, a strip of chemically reactive paper, and a meter to measure the level of glucose. He can then modify his diet, exercise, or insulin intake.

The other test is done in the laboratory. Researchers have found that the amount of glucose that attaches to hemoglobin (called hemoglobin A1c), as compared to the total hemoglobin, depends on the prevailing level of glucose in the blood. The normal level is 4 to 7 percent. In mild hyperglycemia the level increases to 8 to 10 percent, while in severe hyperglycemia it may rise to 20 percent. The test need be done only about once a month and provides the physician a useful guide as to how uniformly the blood sugar level is being maintained.

What you can do. Having diabetes is, in itself, a serious handicap to a long and healthy life. However, by wisely monitoring the disease and carefully observing good health habits, you can enjoy life and outlive many who are careless in their lifestyle. (See "a healthy lifestyle," page 124.)

You should at all times wear or carry on your person **identification** giving your name, address, and telephone number; stating that you are a diabetic; and indicating the name, address, and telephone number of your physician. The identification should also request that should you be found acting strangely or become unconscious, medical help be obtained immediately.

Sex related disorders

The male and female sex characteristics, together with many of the sexual activities, depend on the action of hormones. While the influence of one may predominate, generally the response results from many hormones working together. Some of the problems resulting from malfunction of certain of the sex organs are discussed under "disorders of male sex organs," page 1091, and "disorders of female sex organs," page 1096.

Male disorders

Testosterone is the masculinizing hormone produced in the testes, responsible during fetal life for development of the external sex organs, and from adolescence onward for the growth and maintenance of the male secondary sex characteristics. Problems arise when there is too little of this hormone. The body rarely produces too much, but problems are often seen in athletes and others who take testesterone and other anabolic steroids.

Hypogonadism (male). In this condition production of testosterone is diminished or absent, due to a lack of stimulation by the luteinizing hormone of the pituitary (LH), or to a malfunction of the testes. When this occurs prior to adolescence, the boy fails to become a man. He remains slender, his arms and legs are relatively longer than his height, his voice stays high-pitched, his beard does not grow, and his external sex organs remain infantile. In adulthood, the lack of testosterone causes the secondary sex characteristics to regress and impotence to develop. A physician can determine the precise cause and administer the appropriate hormone: either luteinizing hormone (LH, chorionic gonadotropin) or testosterone.

Male sexual precocity. In this disorder, excessive production of testosterone causes a boy to develop adult male characteristics at an earlier age than normal. Possible causes include premature activation of the testes by the pituitary hormone (LH), overproduction of male hormones (overactivity of the pituitary, adrenals, or testes), or a tumor within one testicle producing excessive amounts of testosterone. The physician (endocrinologist) will attempt to determine the cause and prescribe appropriate therapy, which in the case of a tumor will require surgical removal.

Female disorders

Estrogens are the feminizing hormones produced by the ovaries under the stimulus of the luteinizing hormone of the pituitary (LH). They are responsible for the development and maintenance of the secondary sex characteristics of women: the enlargement of the breasts, and the body features and functions of womanhood.

Hypogonadism (female). In this disorder the ovaries fail to produce estrogens (especially estradiol).

This failure results when the ovaries are malformed, function poorly, are missing (from surgical removal), or lack stimulation by the pituitary hormone (LH). When this disorder occurs prior to adolescence, the girl's sex organs, both internal and external, fail to mature beyond childhood status: her breasts fail to develop, her figure retains childhood configurations, and she does not menstruate.

Should the loss of estrogens occur after womanhood has been attained, as by removal of the ovaries or at menopause, certain of the feminine characteristics wane: monthly menstrual cycles cease, pregnancy is no longer possible, the uterus and vagina become smaller, and the breasts tend to droop.

A physician (gynecologist or endocrinologist) will determine the appropriate replacement of the missing estrogens, taking into consideration the interrelationship of other endocrine glands.

CHAPTER 18

The nervous system

The human body is like a large industrial plant in which each department works harmoniously with every other. To accomplish this, effective communication must be maintained between the head office and all suboffices, and between the suboffices and the workers. It is unnecessary, and would be inefficient, to have all communications go directly from each worker to the chief. In a similar way, the nervous system with its vast and complex network of nerves, rclay stations, and head office make up the highly sophisticated and beautifully integrated communications system of the human body.

Neurons and nerves

The nervous system has two types of cells: nerve cells and supporting cells. The support cells do not conduct impulses, but hold the nerve cells and their axons in place.

The primary unit of the nervous system is the **nerve cell** or **neuron.** A typical nerve cell has a cell body with its nucleus, several short processes (projections) with branches called **dendrites,** and one long, relatively unbranched process called an **axon (nerve fiber).** Nerve cells link a receptor (a unit that receives) with an effector (a unit that activates). Nerve impulses pass from nerve cell to nerve cell in only one direction, entering through one of the dendrites and passing via the cell body to the axon. At the end of the axon the impulse is transferred to another nerve cell or to some functioning tissue (muscle, gland cell) that the nerve cell influences. Some axons are short and only carry impulses to another nerve cell close by. Others are long, extending great distances throughout the body.

The point at which the axon of one neuron contacts the dendrite of another is called a **synapse.** In traveling from its starting point to its terminal point, a nerve impulse may cross several synapses, and thus pass through more than a single neuron. Most neurons are linked together in

1021

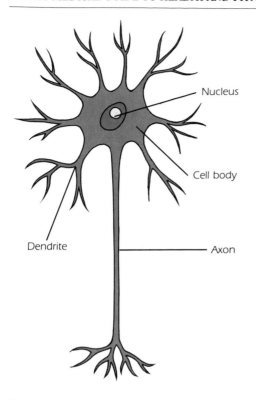

Nucleus

Cell body

Dendrite

Axon

Nerve cell (neuron) and its parts.

chains or rings, often interconnecting with other chains and rings. The impulse or stimulus is transmitted through these extremely complex circuits or "nerve pathways," and

transmission of the resulting response is varied to some degree.

The speed of a nerve impulse as it travels along a nerve fiber (axon) is called the **conduction time,** and varies with the diameter of the fiber—from about 120 thousandths of a second in the large to 0.3 thousandths of a second in the smallest. Each synapse slows the rate of conduction.

Nerve cells carry impulses either toward or away from the spinal cord or brain, or from one part of the spinal cord or brain to another. Thus impulses coming from outlying areas of the body (skin, muscles, glands), are processed, and the responses are transmitted back out to the same or other structures or organs.

The nerve fibers going to or from a certain part of the body are bundled together to form a **nerve,** just as single telephone wires are bundled together to form a cable. Thus at any given moment in any nerve, impulses may be coming toward the brain in certain fibers and going away from the brain in other fibers.

The central nervous system

The **central nervous system** consists of the **brain** and **spinal cord.** The brain is encased within the bones forming the skull, while the spinal cord lies protected in a bony canal within the vertebral column.

The brain

The brain is the highest communication center in your body. It receives nerve impulses from all parts of your body, including your sense organs. Thus it keeps constantly informed of conditions within and without your body, and it uses this information to wisely control all of your body's activities. The brain has four principal parts: the brainstem, the cerebellum, the interbrain, and the cerebrum.

The brainstem connects the spinal cord to the brain, and is made up

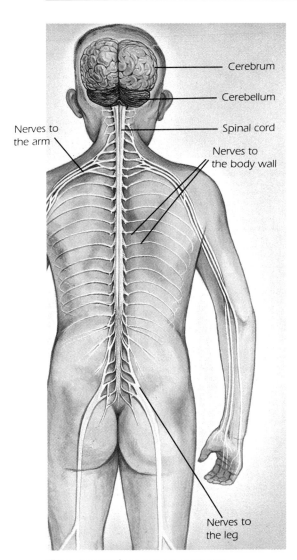

The central nervous system.

conscious, but as soon as conscious control ends, you will begin to breathe automatically again.

The cerebellum consists of two hemispheres behind the brainstem. It automatically coordinates muscular movement, equilibrium, and balance. For example, note the two primary movements of your forearm at the elbow—bending (flexing) and straightening (extending). Each of these movements is coordinated in the cerebellum by the shortening (contraction) of a certain group of muscles. As the flexors contract, the extensors relax or let go to the same degree, allowing your arm to bend in a perfectly smooth motion. To straighten your arm, your cerebellum reverses the process.

The interbrain (hypothalamus) is located at the top of the brainstem, at the center and base of the brain, just above the pituitary to which it is attached. The hypothalamus is an automatic endocrine control center and, with the pituitary, regulates sleep, appetite, and sexual desires. It controls body temperature and coordinates the autonomic nervous system that governs the functions of the body's organs, glands, and blood vessels. Working in conjunction with certain parts of the cerebrum, emotions are formed that influence your thoughts, feelings, words, and actions.

The cerebrum, the largest portion of the brain, comprises the right and left hemispheres, each of which is divided into a number of lobes. The surfaces of the lobes are folded into many large "wrinkles" and clefts, which greatly increase its surface

of the medulla, the pons, and the midbrain. Within these structures reside the automatic control centers of the vital functions of breathing, heart rate, blood pressure, swallowing, coughing, sneezing, vomiting, eye and tongue movements, and balance. Higher levels of control can, within limits, overrule the brainstem. For example, you can hold your breath to the point of becoming un-

1023

area (cortex). The cortex is packed with neurons (nerve cells) whose color in the fresh state gives this part of the brain its popular name, **gray matter.** Deep within the gray matter are accumulations of axons (fibers) which, covered with a fatty sheath (myelin), appear white; hence the term **white matter.**

The cortex of the cerebrum serves as the control board of the nervous system. Each area of the cortex has a separate function and each receives nerve impulses from different parts of the body. The sensory cortex receives input from the skin, eyes, ears, nose, and tongue. The awareness of touch, pain, sight, hearing, smell, or taste, and their significance to our minds, constitutes consciousness.

Another area of the cortex, the motor area, controls the muscles that provide voluntary movement of the arms and legs, hands and feet, and the lips and tongue. Interestingly, the motor areas on the right and left sides of the brain control the muscles on the opposite sides of the body. An adjacent area makes possible the development of patterns of muscle control. Thus the sequential and precise movement of the fingers and hands permits the development of skills to play a violin, to work as a carpenter or dentist, or to run a computer. The complexity of speech is another example. The muscles of the larynx, tongue, face, and jaw, plus those of breathing, must work together. In order to do this, the "speech center" of the cortex must receive nerve impulses from other cortical areas so that what

is said carries the intended meaning.

The brain keeps a record of the sensations and thought processes that occur. This record constitutes **memory.** The highest intellectual functions reside in the cortex: discrimination, judgment, self-control, and willpower. The cortex recognizes moral values, generates ideas, and makes choices and decisions. Here is where life is lived—where we love and suffer, where we draw pictures and make dreams; and where personality itself is formed.

Emotions are attitudes that flavor our thoughts and expressions. Common examples of emotions are fear, anger, love, and joy. The nerve patterns for these were built into the nervous system by the Creator for man's protection and happiness. The emotions influence our conscious thinking, but do not need to control it. Someone strong in character and mature in attitudes can control his behavior in spite of his emotions. Emotions, rightly controlled and properly directed, can be a force for good health and long life; but, uncontrolled, they may weaken or destroy our immunity and the resistance of our bodies, and accelerate the onset of illness and premature death.

The spinal cord

The **spinal cord** consists of many neurons as well as bundles of axons. Thirty-one pairs of spinal nerves emerge at different points along the cord, connecting it to all parts of the body. These nerves are named according to the vertebrae to which they relate: cervical, thoracic, lumbar, and sacral. These connect to all parts of the body. Twelve pairs of cranial nerves pass through holes in the skull and connect the brain to the structures of the head, and those within the neck, chest and abdomen.

The peripheral nervous system

The nerves lying outside the central nervous system, linking it to the organ systems and muscles of the body, are called the **peripheral nervous system.**

The peripheral nervous system is made up of two components: the **voluntary nervous system** and the **involuntary** or **autonomic nervous system.** The involuntary nervous system in turn is divided into the **sympathetic** and **parasympathetic** nervous systems. The neurons of the voluntary nervous system are located within the central nervous system, and their axons go directly from a single neuron in the central nervous system to the muscles they control. These are the voluntary muscles that attach to the bones and that respond when we want to move some part of our body.

The neurons of the autonomic nervous system are located both within the central nervous system, and outside it, as groups of aggregations of neurons, called **ganglia.** Most of these are positioned on the front and sides of the vertebral column (sympathetic chains), around the origins of the large vessels supplying the organs of the body, and in the walls of organs. The fibers originating from neurons within the brain and spinal cord pass to the ganglia via many spinal and a few cranial nerves. When these terminate in ganglia they activate many other neurons whose axons stimulate the responding organs. This is how the organ systems of the body are regulated, such as the beating of the heart, breathing, and the secretions and movements of the digestive tract.

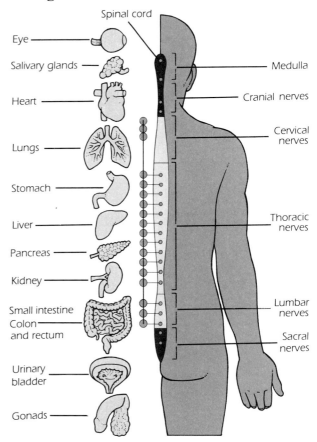

Autonomic nervous system, showing the organs whose functions are regulated by the nerves of the sympathetic and parasympathetic (nervous) divisions.

The **sympathetic nervous system** provides the alarm system of your body. When you are in danger, it prepares you for **fight** or **flight,** whichever seems best under the circumstances. If you are aroused, your heart beats faster, your blood pressure rises, your blood sugar increases, and you breathe more rapidly, providing more fuel and oxygen for your muscles. At the same time, digestion slows down or stops, as does elimination of wastes by your kidneys. Thus all your energy can be mobilized to fight or run for your life.

The parasympathetic nervous system promotes and regulates the major organ systems of the body and assists with maintenance and repair. It stimulates the secretions of the glands, regulates the beating of the heart, and increases the tone and peristaltic activity of the digestive system.

A nervous pathway that operates automatically without having to wait for directions from the brain is called a **reflex.** Suppose, for example, that your finger touches something hot. Instantly, a nerve impulse travels from your finger to the spinal cord, where, through certain connections, it is transferred to nerve cells that control the muscles in your arm and forearm, and you jerk your hand away from the hot object. At the same time, impulses are carried to your brain. These register the sensation of heat from your finger and tell you that you pulled your hand away from a hot object. Many such reflex circuits operate throughout your body, relieving the brain for more important considerations, and thus greatly increasing the efficiency of the nervous system. These reflexes, which vary greatly in complexity, automatically control your balance when you are standing or sitting. They cause you to drive off a fly when it lands on your head and allow you to swallow without thinking.

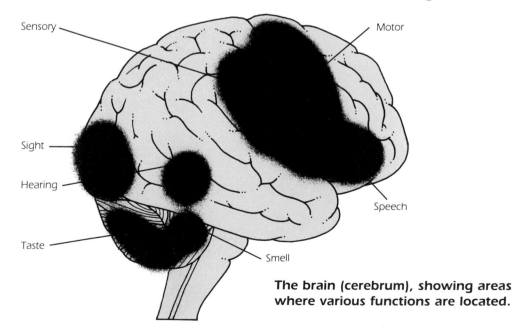

Sensory

Motor

Sight

Hearing

Speech

Taste

Smell

The brain (cerebrum), showing areas where various functions are located.

The brain and nerves

The coverings of the brain and spinal cord (meninges)

The brain and spinal cord are made of fragile tissue. Both are housed in strong bony compartments, one in the skull, the other in the intervertebral canal (within the backbones). Both are surrounded by three membranes called the **meninges.**

The inner covering is thin and adheres to the outer surface of the brain and cord **(the pia mater).** The outer layer is a tough, dense, fibrous covering **(the dura mater)** that lines the inside of the skull and the inside of the bony canal within the vertebrae. The middle layer **(the arachnoid**—Greek "spider") lies within the dura and has hairlike connections (resembling strands of a spider's web) to the pia meter. The space between the arachnoid and the pia meter is filled with fluid **(cerebrospinal fluid)** that surrounds the brain and cord in a jacket of "water," and fills their cavities.

Since the specific gravity of the brain and cerebrospinal fluid is the same, the brain and cord literally float in this jacket of "water," moored, as it were, by the threads of the arachnoid ("the spider"). This protects the central nervous system from all but severe blows.

Breakdown and repair of neurons and nerves

The **body** of a nerve cell (neuron), when injured, cannot regenerate or repair itself. The loss of nerve cells within the central or peripheral nervous systems is irreparable and irreplaceable. Recovery following a loss of function is possible either when the injury is temporary and the nerve cells themselves are not actually destroyed, or when undamaged cells are able to assume the function of those that were destroyed.

Certain peripheral **nerve fibers (axons)** may regenerate. Two forms of injury may occur. In one the fibers are injured but their continuity remains intact. In the other the fibers are severed. In the case of injury, recovery of function is all that is required, and this may take anywhere from a few minutes to several days. When the fibers are actually severed, the part of the nerve fiber that is no longer connected to the cell body dies or degenerates. In order to regenerate, it must have a sheath or tube down which it can grow. In the brain and spinal cord the fiber and its surrounding myelin sheath degenerate together, making recovery impossible. However, in the body's peripheral nerves the fibrous sheath remains even after the nerve itself has degenerated. If the cut ends can be brought together, the portion attached to the nerve body may gradually grow down the sheath, and function may eventually be restored.

The brain—a physical organ

The brain is made up of specialized cells that are designed to carry out

1027

special functions, just as are the specialized cells of the liver, the kidneys, or the heart. The same essential nutrients and the same fuel must be provided for the brain cells as for any other functioning cells. However, the brain is more dependent on receiving oxygen to energize its cells, and for the removal of resulting wastes, than is any other organ or structure in the body.

The production of thoughts is a function of living cells. Thoughts are not something ethereal, but are rather the end product of electro-chemical actions in the neurons. Thus the care of this "master organ of the human body" requires that we follow the same physiological laws as for the care of any other organ or system of the body. You cannot neglect or abuse any of these systems without handicapping the workings of your brain, for they are all interdependent. While the brain is the most important, it is also the most dependent. The welfare of one is the welfare of all.

CHAPTER 19

Disorders of the nervous system

The following general comments will give the reader background information to help him understand the various disorders of the nervous system which will be discussed in this chapter.

Contrecoup hemorrhage in the right frontal region. Result of a left occipital bone fracture.

Cerebral contusion and laceration

ural toma

Arachnoid

Pia mater

ural oma

Common causes of nervous system disorders

When any part of the central nervous system is damaged for whatever reason, other parts of the nervous system, other parts of the body, and even the entire body, may also suffer. The five most frequent problems are listed below.

Vascular disorders. These interfere with the blood supply to a part of the brain and may result in a head-

The brain, from below, having received severe injuries. The three coverings of the brain are indicated: (1) the dura mater, a thick covering on the outside, (2) the pia mater, a thin membrane in contact with the cortex, (3) and the arachnoid in between. Hemorrhages are shown outside the dura, beneath the dura, and in the substance of the cortex.

Extensive hemorrhage in the left basal region as a result of the occipital bone fracture causing the contrecoup hemorrhage.

1029

ache, convulsions, or periods of unconsciousness, but most commonly paralysis.

Injuries. Even though the brain and spinal cord are protected by bony and strong membranous coverings, damage can occur from impact and from shearing forces that disrupt the tissue. Hemorrhage within the brain and cord can cause tearing and pressure injuries. Nerves can be torn apart or crushed. Paralysis, loss of sensation, and even convulsions can result from trauma and unconsciousness.

Degenerative disorders. A number of common nervous problems are caused by a degeneration of the nerve cells in the brain and spinal column. The cause of most of these disorders is not known, though heredity plays a role in some.

Infectious disorders. These may afflict the brain, spinal cord, or nerves. Two examples are encephalitis and meningitis.

Tumors. Benign and malignant tumors can develop within the brain and cord, and malignant tumors (cancers) can be carried to these organs from elsewhere in the body. While benign tumors do not invade surrounding tissues, they still can produce serious and life-threatening problems from damage caused by increasing pressure as they enlarge.

Congenital defects. The results depend on the type, location, and severity of the defect. Hydrocephalus, an enlarged head, for example, is due to increased pressure from too much cerebrospinal fluid within the brain, which is the result of blocked reabsorption.

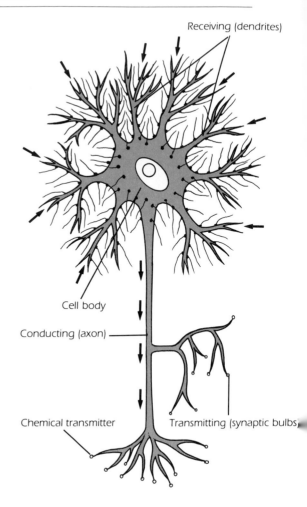

A neuron or nerve cell showing its axon and dendrites, which permit communication with other neurons.

Functional disorders. Some disorders of the nervous system have no apparent structural or chemical cause, so medical authorities classify them as "functional" disorders. As medical science learns more about the workings of the nervous system, some of these disorders may be classified more precisely.

Toxic, metabolic, and nutritional disorders. These disorders of the nervous system are discussed

1030

elsewhere. Toxic disorders are discussed under "Poisons" (see page 519), metabolic disorders are discussed under "Endocrine disorders" (see page 1005), and nutritional disorders of the nervous system are discussed in the chapter, "Nutritional inadequacies and eating disorders" (see page 226).

Common symptoms seen in nervous disorders

The following are a few of the signs and symptoms observed in nervous disorders.

Muscle activity. These include weakness, paralysis, spasticity and rigidity (stiffness), uncontrollable purposeless movements, disturbances in gait, tetany (spasms, cramps), and convulsions.

Speech and swallowing. Speech may be slurred and swallowing difficult.

General sensation. Loss of awareness of pain, temperature, touch, position, equilibrium, dizziness, sight, hearing, taste, and smell.

Headache. An extremely common symptom, from migraine headaches to those from intracranial pressure.

Unconsciousness. Various degrees of impairment of consciousness are dullness, lethargy, stupor, and coma.

Hallucinations and delusions. These symptoms include false sensations of hearing, seeing, smelling, and belief.

Vascular disorders

The brain is dependent on a very rich blood supply, so it is susceptible to diseases that affect blood vessels, such as atherosclerosis. When an artery becomes blocked or bursts (hemorrhages) a stroke occurs. Gradual restriction of blood flow may

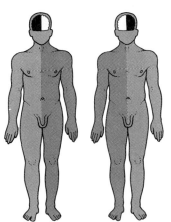

The right and left sides of the brain control opposite sides of the body.

result in senility. The most common problem—strokes—as well as other vascular disorders, will cause various symptoms, depending on the location.

Stroke

A stroke results from damage to some part of the brain because of an interruption in its usual blood supply. While the onset of a stroke is sudden, the underlying cause—typically atherosclerosis—is usually of long standing. The interference in blood supply can have several causes. A clot or thrombus may form on the roughened lining of an artery, partially or completely blocking the flow of blood through the vessel. A fragment of a clot or embolus may break off from a roughened artery elsewhere in the body or from the inner surface of a diseased heart, and carried by the blood, plug an artery in the brain. The wall of an artery in the brain, weakened from atherosclerosis or from an aneurysm, may burst, causing the escape of blood into the tissues of the brain. This hemorrhage is often a complication of high blood pressure.

The brain's demand for blood is so great that it receives one fifth of the blood pumped by the heart! A complete interruption of the blood supply to any part of the brain causes permanent damage to brain cells within about five minutes. About 80 percent of deaths from stroke occur in people sixty to eighty years of age. Four out of five people survive their first attack, but many remain severely handicapped.

Specific areas of the brain control specific functions, such as movement, speech, and sight. Loss of any specific function may indicate which artery is affected. A stroke is extremely alarming. The outstanding symptom—paralysis of one side of the body (hemiplegia)—may be accompanied by loss of feeling (hemianesthesia) in the area of paralysis. Frequently the sufferer has difficulty in speaking (aphasia) and may lose control of the sphincter muscles of the bladder and rectum. Other symptoms include headache, vomiting, and altered consciousness.

A stroke can result from a blood clot (thrombus) or embolus blocking an artery, or from rupture (hemorrhage) of an artery.

What you can do. When a stroke is suspected or has occurred, seek professional advice. Once destroyed, brain cells are not replaced. However, some improvement frequently occurs, mainly by learning to use other nerve circuits, but also by a reduction of tissue swelling at the margins of the destroyed area. Even a mild stroke is a serious matter.

Prevention is of primary importance. To reduce your susceptibility to stroke, you should make every effort to minimize a number of risk factors. These include high blood pressure, smoking, overweight, uncontrolled diabetes, high blood cholesterol levels, sedentary living, and neglected phlebitis (inflammation of the veins).

What your physician can do. Immediate care depends on the severity of the stroke, but generally the sufferer is admitted to a hospital. If the individual is unconscious, circula-

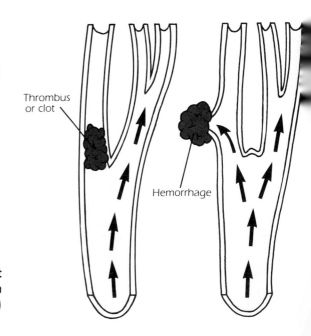

Thrombus or clot

Hemorrhage

tion and respiration must be maintained. Brain scans can pinpoint the exact area of damage. Angiograms of the carotid arteries in the neck can check for atheroma, which may be obstructing blood flow or contributing emboli. Surgical removal of carotid atheroma is generally successful. An anticoagulant (blood-thinning) medication may be used unless a hemorrhage caused the stroke. Trained personnel should provide good nursing care followed by appropriate rehabilitation, possibly including physical and occupational therapy, allowing the sufferer to regain as much activity as possible. A courageous outlook along with mental and emotional support aid recovery.

Transient ischemic attacks (TIAs)

As the name implies, in this condition there are short periods of time, sometimes for only a few seconds, in most cases for five to ten minutes, and never for more than twenty-four hours, when a portion of the brain is deprived of oxygen because of a decreased blood suppply. These episodes are often called **mini-strokes.** The symptoms last only as long as there is a shortage of oxygen, in contrast to a stroke, in which symptoms persist. The cause is a gradual narrowing that leads to an abrupt blocking of an artery to the brain. Typically the blockage occurs when a small clot forms or a small embolus lodges in an artery, restricting its blood flow. The embolus itself is usually a fragment which broke loose from a clot formed on an artery wall

or a defective heart valve, or a detached piece of atherosclerotic plaque.

The symptoms parallel those seen in a stroke and will vary, depending on which particular artery is affected. They may include blackout of vision in one eye (as though a shade were pulled over the eye), weakness and numbness on one or both sides of the body, difficulty in speech, dizziness, and mental confusion. These symptoms are danger signals, since many of those experiencing mini-strokes will ultimately have a major stroke.

What you can do. You should immediately see your physician. However, should your problem be a result of atherosclerosis, you should make every effort to alter your lifestyle to minimize future problems. For suggestions, see page 777).

What your physician can do. The aim of treatment is to prevent future TIAs, and, ideally, to forestall the occurrence of a major stroke. He may prescribe an anticoagulant (blood-thinning or antiplatelet) medication to help decrease further clot formation. Various tests, such as electrocardiograms (EKG) and arteriograms, may aid in determining the source of the problem. The heart will be examined for possible defective valves or abnormal rhythms. Atheroma or clots that narrow arteries outside the brain—carotid arteries, for example—can be surgically removed.

Aneurysm

Aneurysms are localized bulging of arteries caused by a weakness in their walls. Aneurysms in the brain may cause symptoms of headache,

1033

especially on exertion (as when lifting weights), or when the aneurysm presses directly on a nerve. Rupture, causing **subarachnoid or intracranial hemorrhage,** may result in severe headache, unconsciousness, and death (for details see page 799).

Subarachnoid hemorrhage

In this disorder the intracranial hemorrhage is on the outside of the brain, between its middle and inner coverings, the subarachnoid space. The hemorrhage is usually caused by a ruptured aneurysm or a burst blood vessel that has been weakened by atherosclerosis, often combined with high blood pressure. The blood in the arachnoid space, together with the pressure it exerts, causes several symptoms which include sudden, extremely severe headache and stiff neck, accompanied by dizziness, sensitivity to light, nausea, vomiting, mental confusion, and unconsciousness. In this type of stroke—occurring most commonly in middle

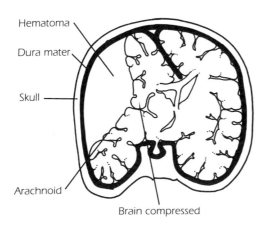

Hematoma

Dura mater

Skull

Arachnoid

Brain compressed

Blood (from a hemorrhage) has accumulated between the dura mater and the cortex, compressing the brain.

age—many of the sufferers die. If you experience a sudden severe headache with stiff neck, see your physician immediately.

What your physician can do. The immediate treatment is to maintain life by supporting the circulation and respiration. The physician will probably order complete bed rest for two to three weeks to help stabilize the patient. He will also attempt to reduce elevated blood pressure. An arteriogram will show the involved area and will also reveal any other aneurysms which are occasionally present. Surgically opening the skull and repairing or obliterating the aneurysms is the best means of preventing further ruptures.

Subdural hemorrhage

The dura is the outermost covering of the brain and spinal cord. When a person experiences a severe injury to the head, such as when an elderly person falls, blood vessels are torn and blood accumulates between the dura and the arachnoid (middle of the three-layer membrane that covers the brain). Since the vessels are veins, the collection of blood or **hematoma** forms slowly, usually over several days. In time, even though bleeding has stopped, the clot degenerates and absorbs fluid, thereby enlarging the hematoma. This increases the pressure on brain structures and the severity of the symptoms.

The symptoms include headache, dizziness, confusion, weakness or numbness on one side of the body, depression, and personality changes, depending on the site of the hematoma. Knowing that a blow or injury was received can aid the physician in making a diagnosis. CT scans or MRI aid in determining the cause and progression. Surgical removal of the clot should bring prompt relief.

Extradural hemorrhage

In this condition blood vessels lying between the skull and the dura (the outermost of the three coverings of the brain and spinal cord) are ruptured by a skull fracture. Since the blood vessel is an artery, blood rapidly accumulates and symptoms from increasing pressure develop within a few minutes to a few hours. These include a sudden, severe headache, nausea, vomiting, confusion, drowsiness, unconsciousness, weakness or paralysis, and even death.

An extradural hemorrhage constitutes a medical emergency. The diagnosis and treatment are similar to those described under subdural hemorrhage. Immediate surgery to release the blood and remove the clots will relieve the pressure. Torn vessels must also be repaired. Recovery is generally prompt.

Injuries to the brain, cord, and cranial nerves

Brain injuries

Accidents are the top-ranking cause of death in the United States for persons under thirty-five years of age, and injury to the head and brain is the major cause of death in 70 percent of these. Several common types of head injuries are discussed below.

Concussion. In a concussion the blow to the head is not sufficient to cause a fracture, but sufficient brain damage occurs to produce some impairment of consciousness. The duration of unconsciousness provides a rough measure of the severity of the damage. A concussion often produces dizziness, headache, inability to concentrate, and memory loss for events just preceding the injury (retroactive amnesia). Unconsciousness may last only a few seconds or minutes in minor injuries, but from hours to days in severe injury. All cases of severe concussion should be hospitalized and carefully observed for several days.

Skull fracture. Three types of fractures may occur: a fracture with no displacement of bones; a fracture in which a fragment of bone is depressed; and a compound fracture in which a piece of bone is driven through the dura into the brain. Besides concussion, the most common complications are torn vessels with accompanying bleeding (see above under vascular injuries). Penetrating fragments of bone can damage the brain and carry the potential of infection.

Symptoms will depend on the area of the head involved and the type and severity of the injury. These include headache, dizziness, confusion, weakness or paralysis of parts of the body, lethargy, unconsciousness, and death. Diagnosis will involve X-rays, electroencephalograms (EEGs), and CT scans. In some skull fractures, cerebrospinal fluid, which is watery in appearance, may escape from the nose or one or both ears. A neurosurgeon will be required to remove any embedded pieces of bone and relieve pressure caused by a depressed fragment. Such injury to brain tissues can result in permanent damage.

Cerebral contusion and laceration. In severe head injuries the surface of the brain may become bruised and torn, and hemorrhaging into the brain substance (**intracerebral hemorrhage**) may occur. Generally swelling of the brain poses a serious hazard because the brain is confined within the skull. Controlling any bleeding or relieving the intracranial pressure may require surgical intervention.

Cranial nerve damage. Fractures of the skull, particularly those involving the base of the skull, may damage certain of the cranial nerves at the site where they exit the skull. The sense of smell, conveyed by the olfactory nerve, may be lost (anosmia) through nerve damage. The optic nerve (conveying sight) and the auditory nerve (conveying hearing) are also frequently injured.

General treatment. Despite successful treatment of the immediate damage resulting from a brain injury, a number of residual problems may persist. These symptoms, spoken of as "post-concussive" or "post-traumatic," include dizziness, headaches, and sometimes personal-

ity changes. The individual may need long-term supportive care and rehabilitation.

Spinal injuries

The spinal cord lies within a canal running the length of the vertebral column or backbone. Thirty-one pairs of spinal nerves emerge from the cord, one on the right and the other on the left, each passing between two adjoining vertebrae (see page 939). While the vertebrae, attached ligaments, and surrounding muscles provide good protection to this part of the central nervous system, severe injuries do occur when the vertebrae collapse from compression, the vertebral processes are fractured, or one vertebra is displaced from another (dislocation). As a result of these injuries to the vertebrae, the nerves can be compressed or torn, the cord squeezed or sheared apart, and the discs between the vertebrae damaged. Four principal types of injuries are seen.

Sprains. A sprain occurs when ligaments attaching two or more vertebrae are stretched or torn by violence or excessive muscle pull. Because the cervical portion of the vertebral column (the neck) is most flexible, it is the part most often sprained. A **whiplash,** for example, occurs when the head is suddenly and violently thrown backward in an automobile accident.

Neck and back sprains cause severe pain, muscle spasm, localized tenderness, swelling, guarding of the injured area, headache (with neck injuries), and difficulty sleeping. Observation of symptoms, together with X-rays of the involved area, will rule out fractures or dislocations. A neck collar limiting the movement of the neck for a whiplash, and a brace for the back may be needed to provide relief and allow healing over time.

Dislocations. A dislocation occurs when one of the bones forming a joint is displaced or pulled out of position, making normal motion impossible. Dislocations in the vertebral column result from accidents, diving into shallow water, or from falling on one's head, shoulder, or even on the feet in a standing position. A heavy blow such as causes the vertebral column to bend sharply in any direction may cause a dislocation. Such an injury often accompanies fractures, torn ligaments, and injuries to the intervertebral discs.

Any shearing movement of one vertebra on another may cause permanent damage to the cord. Immediate care requires the same precautions as when the back is broken. When transporting one so injured, care must be taken to avoid moving the neck and body. Hospitalization under a specialist's care is required. A specialist will order X-rays or a scan to determine whether surgery, in addition to traction, may be necessary.

Fractures. Fractures of the vertebral column are more common in the middle and lower back. They usually result from a fall with forceful bending, from a direct blow on the back, or from the intense pressure produced by sudden strong muscle action as in a convulsion. Forceful bending of the back may also

collapse the body of a vertebra **(compression fracture)** without displacing it—an injury less likely to damage the spinal cord. The symptoms include local tenderness and pain with muscle spasm. After X-rays determine the precise damage, casts and braces are often needed to support the back during the period of healing, and sometimes surgical repair is required.

Herniated intervertebral disc. Twisting movements while lifting or carrying heavy weights will often cause a disk to "slip" or herniate. As it pushes outward, the disk may press against the spinal nerve, causing intense pain. For a detailed discussion see under "Disorders of the joints," page 951.

General problems. When spinal nerves are damaged or torn, muscles supplied by the nerves will be weakened or paralyzed, and the skin overlying the muscles will lose sensation. Since each pair of nerves supplies a certain segment of the body, and there is some overlapping from adjacent nerves, the destruction of a single nerve produces only limited symptoms. But damage to the cord is much more serious. Severe compression or shearing of the cord will cause paralysis of muscular activity and sensation loss below the level of the injury. For example, severance of the cord at the neck level, as sometimes occurs in car accidents, will produce complete loss of function below the site of injury. This condition is called **quadriplegia** because the victim looses all function in the body below the neck, including loss of function in both arms and both

1037

legs. **Paraplegia** results when the injury is below the arms, causing loss of function in both legs and the lower part of the body. When only one side of the cord sustains damage, loss of function will occur on the same side below the level of the injury, causing **hemiplegia** or **monoplegia.**

Degenerative and hereditary disorders

A number of common problems apparently result from a gradual degeneration of nerve cells within the brain and spinal cord. The cause of most of these diseases is not known, although heredity plays a role in some. Symptoms differ widely, depending on the particular area affected.

Multiple sclerosis

This slowly progressive disease involves various parts of the central nervous system. Symptoms may come and go, gradually increasing in severity. Early in the course of the disease the sufferer will appear perfectly normal during periods of remission. The symptoms usually appear between the age of twenty to forty, men and women being affected about equally. In approximately two thirds of the cases the disease progresses slowly so that the person can live out a relatively normal life span, or it may progress rapidly, with an earlier fatal outcome.

The insulating material (myelin) that covers the nerve fibers becomes inflamed and swollen, and gradually degenerates. This deterioration causes the electrical impulses passing along the nerve pathways to short-circuit, thus interrupting normal function. While the cause is not known, an autoimmune response (a condition in which the body's own defense mechanisms turn against itself), triggered by a viral infection, appears likely.

Because this condition can affect any part of the central nervous system, the symptoms differ from case to case and from time to time in the same case. Physical symptoms may include weakness, spasticity, incoordination, trembling, difficulty in walking and talking (scanning speech), double vision, partial blindness, numbness, tingling sensations (paresthesias), and occasionally convulsions. Mental and emotional symptoms include lack of judgment, inattention, and alternating periods of optimism and depression.

Although no known cure exists, those who accept the problem optimistically do better than those who do not. Physical therapy and rehabilitative measures are helpful. Antiimmune and antiinflammatory agents, such as steroids, sometimes slow the disease process, and a nutritious diet will rule out any deficiency. Good nursing care in severe cases is a necessity.

Parkinson's disease (shaking palsy)

This chronic, progressive disorder, usually appearing in middle-aged to elderly persons, is characterized by slowness of movement, rigidity of the muscles, involuntary tremor, and increasing weakness.

The rate of progression varies from person to person, the disability worsening over a period of years. When the muscles of the face become immobile, blinking becomes infrequent, causing the individual to seem to stare, and emotions become difficult to express through facial expression. In advanced cases, saliva may drool from the mouth. The individual takes short, shuffling steps with the body leaning forward and may maintain the same posture for periods of time. The most characteristic feature is shaking of the hands with the tips of the fingers brushing past the ball of the thumb (the "pill-rolling" movement). The tremor worsens as the sufferer becomes tired or excited, but disappears during sleep. The intellect is affected only in terminal stages of the disease.

A deficiency of a nerve-transmitting substance called dopamine, which normally modulates the action of another neurotransmitter, acetylcholine, causes the disease. These chemicals help to regulate the smooth, coordinated movements of the limbs.

What you can do. Attempt to stay in the best physical and emotional health possible by maintaining a regular exercise and rest program, eating a nutritious diet, curtailing emotionally exciting events, and enjoying a cheerful, supportive environment.

What your physician can do. In an attempt to restore the balance between acetylcholine and dopamine, he will probably prescribe a medication that contains L-dopa (which the body converts to dopamine) or agents which might stimulate the production of dopamine. Other agents are used to counter the excess of acetylcholine. Even though side effects can be quite severe, this approach provides the best relief for most sufferers. Rarely, surgery is used to reduce severe trembling.

Amyotrophic lateral sclerosis

This rare, progressive, always fatal disease of unknown origin affects men more commonly than women and typically occurs above age forty. The disease causes degeneration of the nerve cells and fibers that supply the voluntary muscles of the body, with more and more nerve cells and fibers being involved as the disease progresses. The average length of life after onset is about three years.

Weakness and atrophy of increasing numbers of muscles in various parts of the body is characteristic. Most serious problems include difficulty in chewing, swallowing, and breathing. An electromyogram and muscle biopsy will confirm the diagnosis. There is no satisfactory remedy, so the patient should be kept as comfortable as possible.

Combined system disease (posterolateral sclerosis)

This serious disorder causes a degeneration of the posterior and lateral columns of the spinal cord. The degeneration interferes with

1039

the normal transmission of both motor and sensory nervous impulses. Initially one experiences tingling and numbness over the toes and soles of the feet. Later, similar sensations develop in the fingers. If untreated, the troubling sensations spread to the legs, thighs, and hands. Other symptoms include weakness of the leg muscles, unsteadiness and stiffness in walking, and stumbling, especially in the dark. The knees may give way, and the hands become clumsy. Vision may be impaired. After the brain is involved, loss of memory, ideas of persecution, depression, irritability, confusion, and even stupor and coma may occur.

This disorder may develop in the presence of vitamin B_{12} deficiency. The deficiency may result from pernicious anemia, a condition that results when B_{12} cannot be absorbed from the food, or when the diet lacks this vitamin.

What your physician can do. He will do a blood test to determine the level of B_{12}, together with a microscopic examination of the red blood cells. He will prescribe vitamin B_{12} by injection (intramuscular), frequently at first, then less often. If the sufferer has pernicious anemia (see page 815), he will have to take B_{12} for the rest of his life. If a B_{12}-deficient diet was the cause, the diet must be modified to include foods containing B_{12} (meat, fish, fowl, milk, eggs) or a supplement taken regularly. Treatment will bring significant improvement, but often nerve damage may already exist, and a residue of disability may remain.

Wernicke's encephalopathy (Wernicke-Korsakoff syndrome)

This disorder, most common among chronic alcoholics, is due to a deficiency of vitamin B_1 (thiamine). Degenerative changes occur in various areas of the brain (thalamus, hypothalamus, cerebellum) and in the third and sixth cranial nerves (to the eye). Symptoms vary somewhat from case to case, but usually include weakness of the eye muscles (causing double vision), unsteadiness (ataxia), inflammation of the peripheral nerves (neuritis), and mental changes such as apathy, disorientation, and memory loss. Occasionally hallucinations similar to those occurring in delirium tremens are seen.

What your physician can do. Once symptoms have become established, treatment is usually unsatisfactory. However, if the condition is recognized early and adequate vitamin B_1 (thiamine) is administered (preferably intravenously), eye symptoms subside quite rapidly. Ataxia and confusion may improve over a period of months.

Friedreich's ataxia

In this rare hereditary disease—dominant in some families and recessive in others—certain groups of nerve fibers slowly degenerate. Symptoms include failure of muscle coordination, ataxia or a staggering gait, and tremor. Vision is often impaired. A paralysis of certain muscles results in lateral curvature of the spine. No specific treatment exists. Usually beginning in childhood, the disorder progresses slowly, and death occurs as early as age twenty, usually due to involvement of the heart muscle. People with this disorder occurring in their families should seek the counsel of a physician regarding the possible transmission of the disease to their offspring.

Huntington's chorea

Purposeless, jerking, involuntary movements, combined with progressive mental deterioration, characterize this rare hereditary disease that is caused by progressive degeneration of nerve cells in the brain.

The movements consist of grimacing, lurching, and an unsteady waltzing gait. Mental symptoms, not always occurring simultaneously with the physical symptoms, include swings in mood with gradual intellectual deterioration. After onset at thirty to forty years of age, death ensues in about ten to fifteen years. People with this disease occurring in their families should seek counsel from a physician before planning a family.

Dementias

Regardless of the cause, the common feature of dementias is increasing loss of intellectual functions, such as memory, learning, judgment, and reason. Confusion and disorientation as to time and place increase. Eventually the sufferer cannot cope with the simple activities of life. While the cause of the gradual degeneration of nerve cells is unknown, a hereditary pattern appears to exist. Only the most common

forms will be presented.

Alzheimer's dementia (disease). One to two million people in the United States alone suffer from this disease, making it the most common form of chronic dementia in this country. The annual death rate is about 100,000. The disease may begin as early as age forty-five and occurs equally in men and women. The symptoms may include depression, moodiness, lack of sociability and drive. Intellectual functions such as judgment, memory, and decision making steadily decline. An electroencephalogram and a CT scan (computer tomography) will generally help in the diagnosis.

No known treatment exists for this disease, in which life expectancy is reduced by several years.

Arteriosclerotic dementia. In this disease, atherosclerosis occludes the flow of blood in portions of the brain (multi-infarct dementia). It differs from Alzheimer's dementia, in which cerebral blood flow is normal. After an abrupt onset, the course of the disease fluctuates.

Diseases causing dementia. Reversible forms of dementia can result from hydrocephalus and brain tumor (see page 1046), and hypothyroidism (see page 1010).

Neuritis

In neuritis degenerative changes occur in one or more nerves as a result of mechanical injury or metabolic or toxic action. A single nerve (mononeuritis) or many nerves (polyneuritis) may be involved. Depending on the types of nerve fibers carried in the nerve—sensory, motor, or regulatory—the sufferer may experience sharp pains, burning sensations, tingling ("pins and needles"), or numbness. When regulatory or autonomic fibers degenerate, organs of the body may be affected. The skin may be sweaty or dry, hot or cold, pale or flushed, or lesions may erupt.

Mechanical injury can result from penetrating wounds, from fractures in which a nerve is pinched, from a ruptured intervertebral disk, or from pressure against a nerve. Sustained local pressure commonly causes an arm or leg to "go to sleep." If prolonged, such pressure may cause serious damage.

Diabetes, and thiamine deficiency as in chronic alcoholism, may cause polyneuritis. Exposure to toxic chemicals, to germs (such as diphtheria), carbontetra-chloride, and benzene, as well as from heavy metals such as lead, arsenic, mercury, and bismuth may result in polyneuritis.

What your physician can do. Careful examination and laboratory tests can help reveal the cause of the nerve damage. Once the cause has been removed or corrected, prompt recovery usually follows. However, severely damaged nerves will not completely recover.

Neuralgia

In neuralgia, attacks of acute pain occur in areas supplied by a particular nerve, usually one of the cranial nerves, affecting the face, neck, and mouth. Often, in neuralgia, unlike neuritis, no damage to the nerve fibers can be demonstrated.

Trigeminal neuralgia (tic douloureux). The trigeminal (fifth cranial) nerve has three branches that supply sensation to the face. One or more of these branches may be affected, producing excruciating pain in the forehead, eye, cheek, jaw, lip, or chin. Washing or touching the face, exposure to cold, talking, eating, or drinking may trigger paroxysms of lightninglike stabs of pain.

Glossopharyngeal neuralgia. The glossopharyngeal nerve supplies sensation to the tongue and pharynx. In this disorder paroxysms of severe pain involve the back of the tongue, one side of the throat, and the middle ear of the same side. Often brought on by chewing, swallowing, talking, or yawning, the brief attacks are very severe.

Causalgia. This disorder, while not considered to be a true neuralgia, is included here because of the close similarity in symptoms. Excruciating pain follows an injury to a nerve, such as the median nerve in the arm or the sciatic nerve in the hip, thigh, or leg.

Almost any stimulus, such as exposure to air, a sudden noise, a startling experience, or even an emotional excitement, will initiate persistent, severe burning pain. Damage to sympathetic nerve fibers appears to be responsible for the problem.

What your physician can do. Because medications available to give relief have undesirable side effects, they should be carefully monitored by a physician. If the pain persists, offending nerve fibers may be severed surgically.

Infectious disorders

Many organisms, including bacteria, bacilli, fungi, viruses, treponema, and parasites, may invade and cause infections of the central nervous system. Such infections are usually life-threatening and constitute a medical emergency. Only a few of the most common will be presented.

Brain abscess

In an abscess of the brain, a localized infection with destruction of brain tissue is commonly caused by staphylococcus, streptococcus, and pneumococcus. The germs reach the brain through a skull fracture or a penetrating wound, or they spread from an adjacent area, such as the inner ear, nasal sinus, or the mastoid air cells. An infection may also be carried by the blood from the lungs and heart valves.

Symptoms will depend on the location and extent of the abscess. General symptoms include fever, loss of appetite, and debility. Irritation of the brain and its coverings (the **meninges**) results in stiffness of the neck, irritability, and convulsions. Abnormalities in nerve function may be the only symptoms suggesting the presence of an abscess.

A brain abscess is a serious condition with a high mortality rate. An appropriate antibiotic may cure the infection, but often surgical drainage is essential. Early treatment may minimize functional loss.

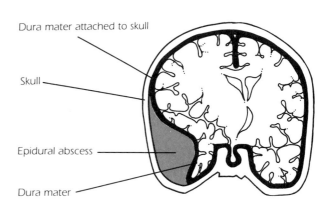

Dura mater attached to skull

Skull

Epidural abscess

Dura mater

An abscess between the skull and dura mater is compressing the brain.

Meningitis

Meningitis consists of an inflammation of the meninges (the covering membranes of the brain and spinal cord). Except for infections spreading from a brain abscess or contaminated penetrating brain injuries, the usual source is an organism carried via the blood from an infection of the middle ear, nasal cavity, nasal sinuses, the tonsils, lungs, or the valves of the heart. Both bacterial and viral meningitis can occur as single cases or in vast epidemics, such as developed in 1917, 1929, 1936, and 1943. Meningococci can, for example, be carried in droplets expelled during coughing and sneezing.

Bacterial meningitis, the most common form of meningitis, is caused in 80 percent of the cases by meningococcus, influenza bacillus,

1043

or pneumococcus. In infants and children the usual bacteria are streptococcus, colon bacillus, and hemophilus influenza.

Symptoms develop rapidly with headache, irritability, nausea, and forceful vomiting. These are accompanied with chills, high fever, rapid pulse, convulsions (especially in children), and rigidity of the muscles (especially those of the neck and back), with pain on bending the neck forward. Confusion and delirium develop, progressing to stupor and coma.

Viral meningitis usually occurs as a complication of a viral infection such as measles, chicken pox, or rubella. The symptoms are similar to, but less severe than, those of bacterial meningitis, except when the brain is involved, as in encephalitis. Then personality changes, impairment of consciousness, seizures, and weakness or paralysis of certain muscles may also occur.

What your physician can do. Diagnosis can be made by evaluating the characteristic symptoms and confirmed by a lumbar puncture—a procedure in which cerebrospinal fluid is removed for laboratory examination. An appropriate antibiotic for the specific type of bacterial meningitis usually cures the inflammation. Viral meningitis is less dangerous, and sufferers generally recover completely without aftereffects.

Encephalitis

In this serious condition the tissue of the brain itself becomes inflamed, usually as a complication of a viral infection—chicken pox, measles, mumps, or the cold sore virus (herpes simplex type 1). It may be spread by contact with a discharge from the nose or mouth (sneeze, cough). In some epidemics insects, including mosquitos and ticks, spread the causative organism. In African sleeping sickness, a form of encephalitis, the bite of the tsetse fly spreads the nonviral organism.

The symptoms resemble those of influenza. In addition, the sufferer may experience sleepiness, severe pain in the neck (especially when the head is tilted sharply forward), coarse tremors, purposeless movements, confusion, delirium, and convulsions.

Residual nervous disorders may follow encephalitis, sometimes appearing many years after the infection. These may include parkinsonism, narcolepsy, unnatural muscle movements (tics, grimaces, and tremors) and personality changes (irritability, hostility).

What your physician can do. Blood tests, a spinal tap (examination of cerebrospinal fluid), and an electroencephalogram will aid in confirming the original diagnosis which was made by observing the symptoms. Since no specific therapy for viral infections exists, the physician will suggest supportive treatment. Certain agents appear to give some success in herpes virus involvement. (For treatment of African sleeping sickness, see page 743.)

Syphilis

Syphilis is a sexually transmitted disease (for additional discussion, see page 1117), often having serious adverse effects on the brain and spinal cord. The two most serious central nervous system manifestations, which occur some fifteen to twenty years after the initial infection, are now considered.

General paresis. In this disease the sufferer has headaches and exhibits unsteady gait, slurred speech, tremor of the hands and tongue, and progressive mental deterioration. This deterioration causes loss of judgment, failure of memory, disorientation as to time and identity, delusions of grandeur (wealth or fame), swings of emotion (from happy to sad), apathy, and complete insanity.

Tabes dorsalis (locomotor ataxia). The affected spinal cord and nerve roots produce numerous symptoms. The individual loses equilibrium and sensation as to the position of the feet. Walking becomes difficult; the sufferer watches each step and slaps his feet on the ground in order to hear each step. Bouts of severe and lightninglike pains in the legs (sharp and jabbing) become progressively worse. Spells of excruciating pains (so called tabetic crises) develop in certain organs, especially in the abdomen. Nausea, vomiting, and diarrhea with a tense abdominal wall may suddenly appear and abruptly stop. Neuralgias, with numbness, prickling sensations, and a feeling of coldness may occur in various areas of the skin. Loss of pain sensation may cause joint destruction.

What your physician can do.

These conditions, appearing in the third and last stage of syphilis, rarely occur today because of early antibiotic treatment of the disease. If however, they do occur, early treatment with antibiotics may halt or slow the progress of the degeneration. Once damage occurs, repair is impossible.

Bell's palsy

In Bell's palsy the muscles on one side of the face are paralyzed, usually temporarily. The ailment comes on suddenly, frequently first observed on waking in the morning. The muscles on the affected side are flabby and sag, while the muscles on the unaffected side (not having a counter pull) draw the face over to that side. There may be discomfort or pain in the region of the jaw and ear on the affected side. Taste, hearing, salivary flow, and tearing may be impaired. While the cause is not known, two possibilities are viral inflammation and reduced blood supply to the seventh cranial nerve as it passes through a bony canal. Recovery usually starts in two to three weeks.

Steroids may be prescribed to reduce inflammation. Since the eye on the affected side does not close completely, it should be protected from injury or drying. Therapy directed toward preserving the muscles on the affected side by electrical stimulation prevents atrophy until the nerve regenerates. Residual problems of weakness, contracture, and spasms occur in cases of permanent nerve damage.

Tumors

Tumors of the brain and spinal cord, whether benign or malignant, are a serious problem. Since bony chambers confine the brain and cord, any increase in the size of a growth brings pressure against the tissues of the cord and brain. Malignant growths cause additional damage by infiltrating adjacent tissues. Both benign and malignant tumors may arise within the central nervous system (primary), while the latter may also invade the brain or spinal cord from other parts of the body (secondary), such as the lungs or breasts. Symptoms result from either pressure upon or infiltration of the brain and spinal cord, and will vary, depending on the location.

A **meningioma** is a benign tumor that develops in the membranes (meninges) surrounding the brain and cord. An **astrocytoma** is a cancerous growth in cells that normally support the nerve cells (neurons) of the central nervous system.

Brain tumors

Headache may be an early symptom of a brain tumor, and it may be associated with nausea and vomiting. Weakness, awkwardness, and convulsive seizures may develop. The sufferer may exhibit drowsiness, changes in personality, strange conduct, or impaired thinking. Vision, hearing, and equilibrium may be involved.

Spinal tumors. The growing tumor affects nerve cells and fibers. Pain may combine with sensation changes in some particular area of the skin—either abnormal sensations or the loss of feeling. Muscle weakness and wasting along with paralysis may result from pressure on nerve fibers or destruction of nerve tissue.

What your physician can do. He may refer you to a specialist. A number of tests are available: an electroencephalogram (EEG), a CAT scan, magnetic resonance imaging (MRI), and X-rays, including the lung, from which a tumor may have spread. Where possible, surgical removal may cure the problem. Where inoperable, radiation and chemotherapy may relieve symptoms for varying lengths of time.

Congenital defects

Congenital defects quite often run in families. It would be wise, therefore, for any couple who are considering having a child and one of them is known to have an inherited abnormality to seek counsel from a well qualified geneticist in order to determine the possible risks to a child.

Hydrocephalus

Cerebrospinal fluid is produced within the internal spaces (ventricles) of the brain and slowly circulates into the space between the exterior of the brain and spinal cord, and the membranes enclosing them.

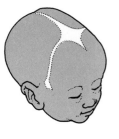

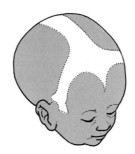

Normal   Hydrocephalic

Normally production and absorption of the fluid proceed at the same rate. In hydrocephalus this balance is destroyed by an overproduction of fluid, a decreased absorption of fluid, or, most commonly, a blocking of its normal flow. As the volume of fluid increases, damage to the brain may occur.

When the problem develops in a growing fetus or in a young infant, the pressure from within the brain causes the bones of the skull to spread apart. The head is enlarged, and the brain may be injured. When it occurs later in life, the skull cannot enlarge, and if the pressure is not promptly relieved, brain damage can ensue. An excessively large head at birth or a head that grows more rapidly than normal are danger signs.

What your physician can do. X-rays and a CAT scan will help reveal the problem. A tube implanted surgically can carry away excess fluid, allowing it to drain into a vein, a body cavity, or the heart itself. Correcting the disorder early enough can avert damage to the brain.

Spina bifida

In spina bifida the vertebral column, which normally covers the spinal cord and terminal spinal nerves, fails to complete its development before birth. The defect, usually on the back part of the lower spine, affects one or more vertebrae. The defect may range from a slight dimple in the skin over the spine to a large opening, covered by a thin membrane, beneath which are the terminal spinal nerves and even the cord.

The least severe cases exhibit no symptoms. As the severity of the defect increases, symptoms include difficulty in walking, weakness and wasting of the muscles of the legs and feet, paralysis of the lower limbs, loss of sensation in the thighs and buttocks, and problems in controlling and emptying the bladder and bowels. Infants with this disorder often have hydrocephalus and may be handicapped mentally. Damage to the covering membrane may allow infection to enter the cerebrospinal fluid, causing meningitis.

Surgical repair is sometimes attempted, but this may in itself cause hydrocephalus. While many infants develop normally, others require extensive rehabilitation to allow for as normal a development as possible.

Phenylketonuria (PKU)

In this hereditary metabolic defect, occurring in one of every 10,000 to 15,000 children, a missing enzyme prevents the amino acid phenylalanine from being converted to tyrosine. Thus phenylalanine accumulates in the blood and spinal fluids, damaging the nervous system. Children untreated in early life display awkward gait, purposeless movement of the hands, and mental retardation. One in four develops seizures.

When the mother is only a "carrier" of the disease, the baby is born normal. If, however, she has the defect, the baby develops as a PKU and is born with a small brain, mental retardation, and other deformities.

What your physician can do. If you know you have PKU, alert your physician. A test called amniocentesis detects genetic defects, such as PKU, if present, from fluid withdrawn from the mother's womb. A newborn infant's urine must be tested to determine the presence of PKU. If present, the infant cannot be breast-fed but must be given a special formula low in phenylalanine. When other foods are added, they, too, must be carefully selected. After the nervous system has matured sufficiently—about the age of twelve—diets higher in phenylalanine can be tolerated. If a woman having PKU desires a child, she should, under the guidance of her physician, go on a diet low in phenylalanine during her pregnancy in an attempt to safeguard her infant.

Myotonia

Some types of myotonia appear to be inherited. In this disorder the sufferer experiences difficulty relaxing the muscles after they have been contracted. Repeated use of the same muscles seems to "warm them up" so they perform virtually normally. Some forms of the disease appear early in life, while others appear later. In some, prolonged rest, exposure to low temperatures, and emotional excitement aggravate the difficulty. Even though no satisfactory treatment exists, the disease is not life threatening, and many sufferers live normally despite their handicap.

Convulsive disorders

A **convulsion** is a violent contraction or series of contractions of the voluntary muscles (those attached to bones), resulting from a sudden and excessive electrical discharge of neurons (nerve cells) in the brain. Children are more prone to convulsions than are adults, but may outgrow the tendency. In children, a very high fever or prolonged holding of the breath (as in a tantrum) may bring on a convulsion. Other causes include low blood sugar, low blood calcium, brain tumor, brain injury, and a brain infection (meningitis or encephilitis). Convulsions may occur when a confirmed alcoholic suddenly stops drinking or when a person addicted to barbiturates abruptly discontinues the drug. They may also occur in eclampsia, a toxicity in late pregnancy, and in tetanus infection **(lockjaw).**

Apart from the excessive electrical excitability in the brain and its abrupt discharge, the cause of most convulsive disorders is often not known. Less than half the cases appear to have an inherited susceptibility. The disorder characterized by recurring convulsions is called **epilepsy (seizure, fit).** Epilepsy may exhibit a variety of forms or groups of symptoms. Some two million Americans suffer from some form of epilepsy (largely controlled by medications). Several procedures can determine the type of epilepsy involved: an electroencephalogram (EEG) generally gives conclusive evidence; X-rays, CAT scan, or MRI may show damage to brain tissue.

Of the many forms of epilepsy, those most frequently seen fall into one of the following types.

Grand mal. A typical convulsion consists of the abrupt occurrence of violent, involuntary muscle contractions, at first tonic and later clonic (contracting and relaxing). The seizure is usually accompanied by loss of consciousness. Often deep sleep, temporary confusion, drowsiness, and headache follow the short attack. Many individuals have a warning sign, called an aura, minutes or hours before the convulsion strikes. These may consist of sensing unusual odors, seeing lights, hearing strange sounds, or being vaguely aware of peculiar feelings. Some learn to prepare themselves for the convulsion by sitting or lying down.

Petit mal. These seizures last only a few seconds. They occur most commonly in children, and most eventually outgrow them. The child suddenly stops all activity (but seldom falls) and stares into space, giving the impression of daydreaming. The muscles of the face twitch, the eyes blink, and the head or arms jerk. When the seizure ends, and the child continues his previous activity, unaware of the interlude. One or many attacks may occur in a day.

Focal (partial) seizures. The attack causes progressive muscular contractions on one side of the body, usually beginning in the area of the face and extending downward to the arms, body, and lower limbs. Sometimes the convulsions move in the opposite direction (Jacksonian epilepsy). Occasionally a grand mal attack may be precipitated.

Psychomotor (partial complex). A seizure may start with a very short aura, followed by loss of awareness of what is happening (amnesia), sudden anxiety or fear, outbursts of laughter or anger, incoherent speech, or other unusual behavior (rubbing or slapping the face). The individual is not aware of what is happening, and is unable to control the events.

What you can do. Regular use of medication is extremely important in controlling convulsive disorders. You must work closely with your physician, make no changes in medication without his knowledge, and promptly report any adverse reactions. Refrain from alcohol and brain stimulants, as they increase the likelihood of a seizure. At all times, carry adequate identification telling who you are, a statement of your problem, your physician's name and address, and what to do in case of an emergency. For information on treating a seizure, see under "emergency managment," page 558.

What your physician can do. He will, of course, determine the type of convulsive disorder you have and will determine which medication best suits your needs. This may require that you try several medications in order to find the one that gives you maximum benefit with minimum side effects. Drowsiness is the most common problem. Your physician will advise you whether you can participate in life-threatening activities, such as driving a car and swimming.

Functional disorders

Headache

Headache is an accompanying symptom of many diseases, and virtually everyone has experienced one at some time or another. Fortunately only a few are serious. The brain itself is insensitive to pain, but the coverings of the brain (meninges) and external structures such as the scalp, the eyes, and the muscles of the head and neck, respond to situations that cause headache. About 20 million Americans seek help from physicians on this account each year.

Indicators of serious headaches. Because a headache may signify the presence of a serious disorder, it is important to analyze the conditions surrounding the headache in order to determine its cause and better select its treatment. For all new, changing, or persistent headaches, see your physician. Watch especially for the following:

1. A headache of sudden onset and great severity may be due to a hemorrhage (bleeding) inside the skull.

2. Severe headache with blurred vision, seizures, clouded consciousness, muscle weakness, or impaired sensation may arise from an expanding blood clot.

3. Headache accompanied by fever and neck stiffness may sometimes be an early sign of meningitis, flu, or some other viral infection.

4. A series of brief headaches, one or more a day with increasing frequency or intensity, is suggestive of an enlarging brain tumor.

5. A persisting headache originating from a particular site may indicate an infection in these organs: Sinusitis in the nose, middle ear infection, tumor of the eye, etc.

In everyday life many situations, singly or in combination, may initiate a headache. These include such things as emotional stress, overwork causing physical or mental fatigue, inadequate water intake (dehydration), overindulgence in food or alcohol, or lack of sleep. The common headaches consist of two main types: tension and vascular headaches.

Tension headaches. Arising from painful contractions of the head and neck muscles, these headaches tend to be steady and non-throbbing, with a sense of constriction or pressure in the head. Anxiety, emotional conflict, pressure of work, or any of the situations listed above may initiate them. They usually come on gradually and disappear gradually.

Correcting the cause, if known, relieves tension headaches. However, heat and massage to the muscles of the neck and scalp may be helpful. A simple procedure, recently developed, gives excellent relief. Sit or stand erect. Then place the right hand on the left side of the scalp and the left hand on the right side of the chin. Twist your head to the left while gently pulling with each hand. Do not bend the neck, but try to tilt the head (the head may not appear to move). Hold the position for ten seconds. Do this three times. Then reverse the procedure to stretch the muscles of the opposite side. Carry out the entire procedure two times a day.

Vascular headaches. Variation in the blood flow through the vessels of the head and neck brings on these headaches, which include **migraine headaches.** The blood vessels of the head and neck first constrict, provoking unusual sensations before the actual headache begins; and then, rather suddenly, the vessels expand, producing pain. The attack is usually preceded (fifteen to twenty minutes) by certain unusual sensations, such as seeing bright or colored lights, which the sufferer learns signals an attack. This pattern of onset may, however, vary widely. Severe nausea and vomiting often accompany the headache. The attack lasts from several hours to several days, and leaves the person exhausted.

A number of trigger factors have been identified, but these vary from person to person. They include dietary factors, such as omitting a meal, use of alcohol, withdrawal of caffeine (once addicted to it), and the use of chocolate; hormonal factors, as when the balance of hormones changes at the time of menstruation or during the use of birth-control pills; emotional factors, such as frustrations occurring in hard-driving persons, or abrupt changes of pace, such as a holiday or vacation; and environmental factors, such as extremes in temperature, exposure to cigarette smoke, exposure to some offensive odor, or sudden exposure to a bright light.

Treatment consists of trying to identify and avoid what triggers an attack. This may require some fundamental changes in lifestyle. Your physician can aid you in finding a medication to relieve the headache, which produces a minimum of side effects.

Dizziness

Numerous factors working together allow one consciously and unconsciously to maintain a state of equilibrium, balance, and movement: the things seen; the direction of the sounds heard; feelings in the feet, hands, and body; the sensations from the muscles, joints, and tendons (proprioception) that help one stand or sit; and sensations from the semicircular canals in the inner ears. Disturbances in any of these functions send conflicting and confused signals to the brain, which are interpreted as dizziness, but which may be lightheadedness or vertigo.

Lightheadedness can occur from changes in blood flow to the brain, as when abruptly sitting up from a lying position (especially in the elderly); or it may be triggered from sympathy or fear when seeing an injury or blood. The person feels dizzy, becomes pale, sweats, feels sick to the stomach, and faints due to decreased blood flow to the brain.

Dizziness may also result from a head injury that damages the semicircular canals. In Meniere's disease, a distressing disorder of the inner ear, dizziness is a prominent symptom (see page 1151). Atherosclerosis may cause dizziness by limiting blood to one set of semicircular canals. Anemia, as well as considerable blood loss from a hemorrhage, can cause dizziness. The toxins of some diseases, drugs taken in excess, and allergies sometimes produce dizziness.

Vertigo is a false impression that the objects around one are revolving, or that the objects are stationary but the person is rotating. The sufferer fears standing, and frequently feels sick to the stomach and may vomit. A viral infection of the semicircular canals and vestibules (labyrinthitis or vestibulitis), or of the nerve leading to the brain from these organs may be irritated or compressed by a tumor. The irritation distorts the impulses, and vertigo results. Overstimulation of the semicircular canals, as in motion sickness, car sickness, or seasickness, is a fairly common problem.

What you can do. When you feel dizzy, sit or preferably lie down until the feeling wears off. If the condition persists, becomes worse, or comes on more frequently, see your physician.

What your physician can do. He will conduct a careful examination and may order some special tests in an effort to determine the underlying cause. If the cause can be cleared up, dizziness will end. Sometimes medication will relieve persistent dizziness.

CHAPTER 20

Mental and emotional disorders

The human brain is undoubtedly the most complex structure known to man. Its capacity to discriminate, judge, exercise self-control, and make choices and decisions gives man preeminence among all that lives. The brain is unique in that it can receive, sort, reject, or store information, which it can later retrieve from the memory bank, and with perspective direct the activities of life. And a person's thoughts can be colored by his emotions; whether a person is calm or worried, happy or sad, peaceful or angry, loving or hateful, confident or fearful, influences his perspective of events.

Countless functions of the brain regulate the physical systems of the body, including many in the brain itself. Even though the electrochemical activities in brain cells can be monitored, the thoughts and emotions they produce can only be evaluated or measured by another mind. Research has revealed that these thoughts and emotions can profoundly affect the physical functioning of the body in general, but can also affect the brain itself, influencing the very production of thoughts and emotions.

In this way a structurally "normal" brain can function in an abnormal manner, for it is the thought patterns directing a person that determine his personality. The way one reacts to the circumstances of his personal experiences has more to do with his state of mental health than do germs or viruses or broken bones. A person's inability to handle the experiences of life, chiefly those that are frustrating or disruptive to his drives, reveal behaviors which are classified as forms of mental illness.

Factors limiting the fulfillment of one's drives:

1. Obstacles in the environment. Many things can occur over which an individual has no control. Examples are an appointment delayed by a traffic jam, bad weather prohibiting an outdoor picnic, financial constraints limiting the purchase

1053

of a home, and a crippling finger injury stifling a career as a musician.

2. Personal limitations. An individual can lack the required capability to accomplish a desired task. Examples are a wife desires motherhood but cannot conceive, a young man's aims for a career in science are thwarted by lack of academic ability, a girl's desire to model are frustrated by physical defects.

3. Conflicts between motives. A person can have two strong drives, one in conflict with the other. Examples might be a young man with limited time and money wishing to marry his sweetheart, yet wanting to complete the requirements for a doctoral degree; someone who yearns to live in the country but finds the only work available requires residing in a city; an individual who has a tendency to be obese but enjoys gourmet foods.

People differ in their capacity to adjust to the impossible or unattainable. One will analyze the situation and, though disappointed, accept alternatives, making the best of the situation. Another blindly persists, and after repeated frustrations, develops a warped personality.

A person with religious convictions has the advantage of confidence in the providential guidance of a Supreme Being. Professional help can also aid in facing limitations. A family physician can objectively discern the series of events which have brought the patient to his present state, and can impartially provide the advice that the patient needs. Sometimes obtaining the counsel of a specialist in this area—a psychiatrist or a psychologist—is desirable.

As we enter the discussion of neuroses and psychoses, the reader might enjoy a humorous, popular definition of these two types of individuals. A radio announcer remarked: "A psychotic believes that two and two makes five; a neurotic agrees that two and two makes four, but doesn't like it."

Neurosis

People with neuroses are not incapacitated, as are those with psychoses, but tend to have pent-up feelings of concern, are irritable and over-sensitive, and allow their beliefs and emotions to predominate over reason.

Anxiety and fear

Anxiety is a type of fear, but functions at a less intense level and tends to be more prolonged. Fear is a reaction to external dangers. It is designed for emergency situations and it triggers the body's alarm reaction (see page 105). This mobilizes the body for fight or flight. Profound changes occur within the major organs systems, but for only a short time, thus doing no harm. But anxiety persisting without an emergency can be harmful. Anxiety is an amplification of worry.

In contrast to fear, which is a response to external dangers, anxiety is a reaction to internal threats. An anxious person may have some or all of the following symptoms. He dreads something intangible, and lives in a state of causeless fear. He is distraught without being able to pinpoint the precise cause; is fearful and nervous. He feels weak, his mouth is dry, his heart beats rapidly, his breathing is fast, shallow, and sometimes difficult, he trembles easily, and he perspires excessively. In long-continued (chronic) anxiety states, the sufferer may experience difficulty sleeping, heartburn, tiredness, diarrhea, frequent urination, and mental abberations.

Conversion reaction (hysterical neurosis)

Hysterical neurosis is an extreme reaction to a situation or experience which the person strongly dislikes or fears. Instead of facing the problem, he escapes from it by developing symptoms of some disorder which will protect him from confronting the reality of the situation (formerly called hysteria). Meanwhile, he is unaware that he has done this. This unawareness stands in contrast to a malingerer who deliberately feigns some disability. The individual with hysteria, his family and friends, believe he has a real illness.

Obviously, a conversion reaction is an unhealthy solution to a problem. Because it imitates many symptoms of disease, such as paralysis, loss of sensation, blindness, loss of memory **(amnesia),** convulsive seizures, or even loss of consciousness, the physician is taxed to tell the difference between the symptoms of hysteria and those of a physical disease. One clue is the person's lack of concern for his seemingly serious problems.

Phobias

Phobias are unwarranted fears that cause the afflicted person to panic, despite knowing his fear to be illogical. Nevertheless, whenever he is exposed to the fear-producing situation, he seems powerless to restrain his dread. Examples are the policeman who becomes afraid of the dark; the businessman who climbs fifteen flights of stairs because he fears riding in the closed elevator **(claustrophobia);** or the person who fears heights **(acrophobia)** even when a fence surrounds the site. Phobias may involve an unreasonable fear of wide-open spaces **(agoraphobia),** restriction of the activities of everyday life because of fear of something happening, of needles, of dirt, of germs, of a certain animal, or of cancer.

Many people can live reasonably normal lives with a phobia. However, others restrict the activities of everyday life for fear of something happening, and some become so unreasonable that their normal behavior is affected, resulting in serious anxiety states.

Depression

Most people have episodes of feeling downcast, sad, or depressed. Major depression, on the other hand, is a state of mind in which the melancholy mood is persistent, pervasive, and constant, continuing for weeks or months.

The symptoms include crying for insufficient cause, a sense of hopelessness, loss of interest in hobbies and achievements, loss of ability to experience pleasure, loss of self-esteem, feelings of guilt and unworthiness to receive help, inability to think, concentrate, and be decisive, and thoughts of suicide or dying. These are accompanied by physical problems, such as the inability to sleep or sleeping too much, a decrease or an increase in appetite, a loss or gain in weight, feelings of weakness and fatigue, and constipation, dizziness, and headache.

Depression—the most common of the major mental illnesses—is estimated to afflict more than 15 percent of Americans at some time in their lives. This disorder appears to run in families and is genetically inherited.

Obsessive-compulsive reaction

An **obsession** is an almost uncontrollable urge to follow the same line of thought over and over. Often the thought is unwelcome, but try as he may, the sufferer finds it virtually impossible to banish it from his thinking. A **compulsion,** by contrast, is an unreasonable urge to do something, even though the act is unnecessary and often unreasonable.

For example, a person becomes obsessed with the thought that he is carrying a germ which could infect other members of his family and even cause their deaths. As a result he develops the compulsion to constantly wash his hands, especially after shaking hands or touching door

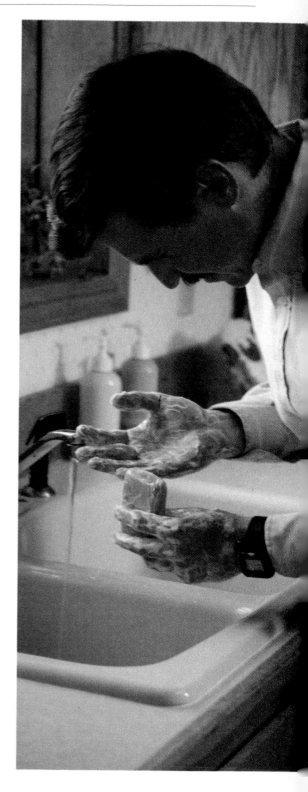

Compulsion is a common form of mental illness.

knobs and before eating. Some people with an obsession are constantly troubled by obscene thoughts that are out of harmony with their standards of conduct. Others feel they must touch all power poles as they pass them on the sidewalk.

Hypochondriasis

In this condition the individual feels depleted of energy, weak, exhausted, fatigued, and abnormally sensitive to pain and other sensations which suggest various body organ ailments. Symptoms often suggest problems in the stomach, the intestines, the heart, and the genitourinary organs. Often the sufferer has a reduced ability to concentrate, is irritable, and sleeps with difficulty.

Suicide

The person contemplating suicide thinks that life is not worth living and believes that no solutions exist to the problems troubling him. He is frustrated and allows his thoughts to center on "ending it all."

Some who attempt suicide do not expect to die, but to be rescued from the endeavor. By this they hope to attract attention to themselves and their plight. Others keep their plans secret and expect to succumb. Anyone who threatens suicide should be closely observed by friends and loved ones, and may require the services of a specialist or even hospitalization.

Unresolved grief

Unresolved grief has two forms: the person may fail to experience grief, or he may continue to grieve for months after the loss. Grief can result not only from the death of a loved one but also from the loss of an arm or leg, or the use of one's limbs.

Normal grief consists of four phases: (1) **Shock** lasts a short period of time, during which the bereaved may be stunned, express an intense wish the loss had not occurred, exhibit few emotions, or behave as if the loss had not happened (denial). (2) **Acute mourning** usually lasts for three or more months. The grieving person now acknowledges the loss but is unreconciled to it. He withdraws from social contacts and experiences waves of intensely sad emotions. (3) **Denial** is often seen when the bereaved denies that the loss has occurred. (4) **Resolution or reorganization** begins when the grieving person reluctantly accepts the loss and begins to plan for the future and resumes his social interests and activities.

Unhealthy complications usually appear during the second phase. The sufferer is unable to cry, bottles up his emotions, and develops symptoms of illness. His friends and loved ones should provide sympathy and understanding and should encourage him to express his emotions and to resume productive activities.

The psychological process of dying and of accepting the death of a loved one is similar: (1) **shock and denial,** in which the person appears numb and unaware of his or her problem; (2) **anger,** manifested by frustration and questions (to God, friends, etc.) about why (3) **bargaining** that includes arguing with others about the reality of the situation, (4) and finally **acceptance**—a gradual reconciliation to the situation and acceptance of the inevitable.

What your physician can do. Since many of the neuroses exhibit physical symptoms, your physician must first rule out any organic disease. Then, with an understanding of the problems which lie at the foundation of the neurosis, he will himself counsel with the individual (psychotherapy) or recommend a well-qualified specialist, such as a psychiatrist or clinical psychologist. Many of the neuroses require time to orient the thinking of the sufferer to realistically face the issues that trouble him. A number of medicinal agents (antianxiety or antidepressant) can be prescribed. These alter the brain chemistry and provide re-lief while the healing process takes place.

Tics

A tic is a spasmodic contraction or twitching of a small muscle or small group of muscles, generally in the area of the face and mouth. This involuntary, purposeless, and unexpected movement includes jerking the head, grunting, clearing the throat, or even pronouncing a word or speaking a short sentence.

Tics, appearing in about 10 percent of children, are often hereditary, and point to a neurotic tendency. Circumstantial evidence suggests that a feeling of personal inadequacy may be a cause. Although most disappear in time, some tics do persist into adulthood. When a tic first appears, professional counsel should be sought.

Psychosis

Psychosis is a form of mental derangement in which the individual's thinking and behavior are irrational and irresponsible. The common term *insanity* applies to any major psychosis. The cause is uncertain. Some believe a hereditary factor exists while others assert that a biochemical imbalance is present in the nerve cells. Specialists generally agree that the psychotic cannot adjust successfully to life's demands and disintegrates under stresses with which he cannot cope. Some persons with a psychosis become difficult to manage and may require professional care or hospitalization.

Withdrawal delirium (delirium tremens, DTs)

Withdrawal delirium is a serious, acute, dramatic condition which affects a habitual user of alcohol when the substance is abruptly withheld. An attack results in mental confusion, delusions, vivid and terrifying hallucinations, tremor, sleeplessness, fear, and profuse sweating, which may cause dehydration. In about 80 percent of sufferers the episode lasts for three days or less and ends suddenly. In the remainder the symptoms persist longer and disappear only to return. Up to 15 percent of delirium withdrawals end fatally.

What your physician can do. He will hospitalize the person and promptly administer medication to control the patient's agitation. He may order fluids or blood by vein to combat shock and prevent dehydration or supplementary B vitamins prescribed as a helpful precaution against a deficiency. He will evaluate the possibility of injury, infection, or inflammation of the pancreas or liver and provide appropriate therapy as needed.

Alcohol amnesia disorder (Korsakoff's psychosis)

This disorder results in a complete memory loss (amnesia) for current and recent happenings. However, older, long-established memories are still available. Other mental processes remain quite normal, so the sufferer hesitates to admit he is out of touch with recent events and makes up imaginary explanations of what has recently occurred.

The psychosis results from damage to that part of the brain in which memory resides. The damage may be temporary when caused by a head injury or a subarachnoid hemorrhage. However, when it results from alcoholism or encephalitis, the memory loss usually remains permanent in spite of treatment.

Bipolar disorder (manic-depressive disease)

This disorder is characterized by mania and/or depression, or a mixed type (mania and depression), in which there are exaggerated mood swings. The irregular shifts in mood range from extreme elation **(mania)** to deep depression. In an attack one mood predominates and shifts to the other, or the mood swings may go back and forth in the same attack. The first attack usually occurs in young adults, and heredity appears to play a role. Between episodes the person is usually normal.

In the **manic phase** the sufferer becomes increasingly excited and combines tireless activities with elation. Judgment and insight are usually poor, and the person may be destructive. Displays of singing, talking, shouting, and delusions of grandeur are common. Any restraint provokes irritation. In the **depressed phase** the sufferer feels downhearted and fearful, developing delusions of self-condemnation and, at times, attempting suicide. He sleeps poorly and in extreme cases may be stuporous.

What your physician can do. He will decide whether hospitalization is necessary, as would be true in any case of suicidal tendencies. Untreated, an attack may last a year or more, but medication usually shortens the attack. He may prescribe agents to alter brain chemistry or he may advise psychotherapy. Most cases respond favorably to kind treatment in addition to a specific program of medication.

Schizophrenia

In this disease the sufferer loses his ability to distinguish clearly between fantasy and reality. Both his ability to think and his emotional responses become confused. The most serious of mental disorders, schizophrenia afflicts more than half of

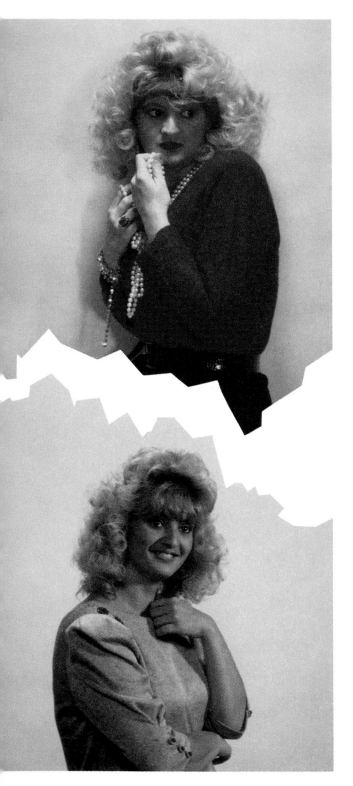

those in mental hospitals.

In schizophrenia, the brain improperly processes information. The disease usually begins in young adulthood, and although the tendency appears to be inherited, only certain individuals exhibit the weakness. Periods of extreme stress and difficult situations appear to trigger the attacks.

The onset is often insidious; the sufferer begins to withdraw and appears preoccupied. His conversations assume an odd pattern, but even if brought to his attention, he remains unconcerned. The schizophrenic may believe he hears voices, often unkind, and that others are listening to him think and stealing his thoughts. As the disease progresses, delusions (such as believing he is being poisoned), hallucinations, odd mannerisms, and sometimes suicidal tendencies develop and may be violent. He lives in a world apart and laughs or smiles at inappropriate times.

While there are many forms of schizophrenia, only the characteristics of the main types are described.

The **catatonic** type may often stand rigidly like a statue (posturing), or do things opposite to those which are requested of him or even opposite to those he himself normally does. He may exhibit apparent stupor or be unwilling to speak. Or again he may become suddenly excited and engage in purposeless activity. At such times he may be dangerous.

The schizophrenic often believes he hears voices, and that others listen to him think and steal his thoughts.

The **disorganized** type is often incoherent, and his thoughts and even his delusions are disorganized, bizarre, inappropriate, and often silly.

The **paranoid** type has delusions, with or without hallucinations, in which he is being persecuted—is suspicious of others, and believes they are out to harm him. Again, his delusions may be grandiose—that he is some notable character, such as the president of a bank, or ruler of a country, or an extremely wealthy individual. At times his delusions may be bizarre, or well organized, or may even appear quite "logical."

The **undifferentiated** type has disorganized thoughts and behavior—his symptoms being a mixture of all three of the above types.

Those with chronic schizophrenia may have periods when they appear relatively normal.

A number of personality traits that are not serious enough to be classified as mental illness may exist throughout life. Two such personality disorders are the paranoid or schizoid. The **paranoid** is generally hostile, irritable, and suspicious. The **schizoid** is withdrawn, shy, and shrinks from social contacts.

What your physician can do. He will determine whether the sufferer needs to be hospitalized. Antipsychotic medications are available to alter the brain chemistry and help relieve the symptoms of disorganized thinking. These, together with psychotherapy and friendly counseling, contribute greatly to recovery. It is extremely important to teach the sufferer how to cope with stressful situations in order to prevent subsequent attacks. Following the acute phase rehabilitation is essential to enable him to regain normal behavior patterns and develop the capacity to carry out the routine activities of life.

Paranoia

Paranoia is identified by delusions in which the individual attempts to bolster his self-esteem by assuming others are plotting against him. He craves recognition, having failed to obtain the acclaim he desires, and contends that the plottings and jealousies of others cause his failures. While the cause is not known, it appears that childhood experiences of not being socially accepted and disappointments in not gaining certain goals cause sullenness and hatred to become exaggerated into a psychosis.

Paranoia often leads the sufferer to imagine himself some great person—a king, a queen, an inventor, or a bank president. He may become dangerous, with a risk of bodily harm to those he feels are plotting against him. He often imagines his mate is unfaithful to him—without any real evidence.

Often paranoid individuals go to court for redress of their imagined mistreatment.

What can be done. Successful treatment consists of sympathetic relationships more than of specific therapy. Many sufferers respond favorably to kindness and sympathy by someone they feel they can trust. But, unfortunately, many paranoid persons never recover.

1061

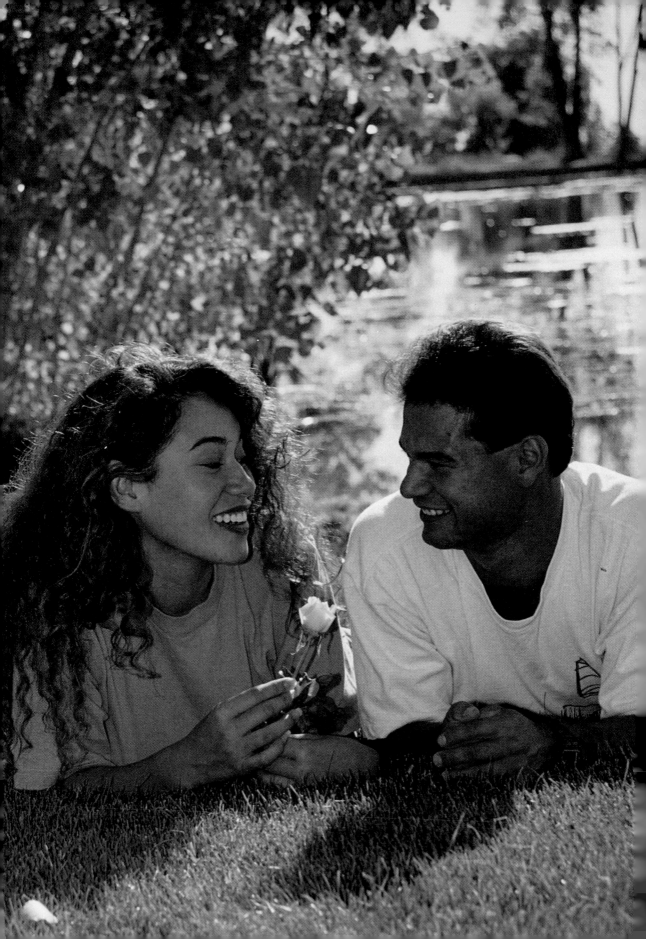

Vol. 3

SECTION 5

THE GENITO-URINARY SYSTEM, THE SEXUAL ORGANS, AND THEIR DISORDERS

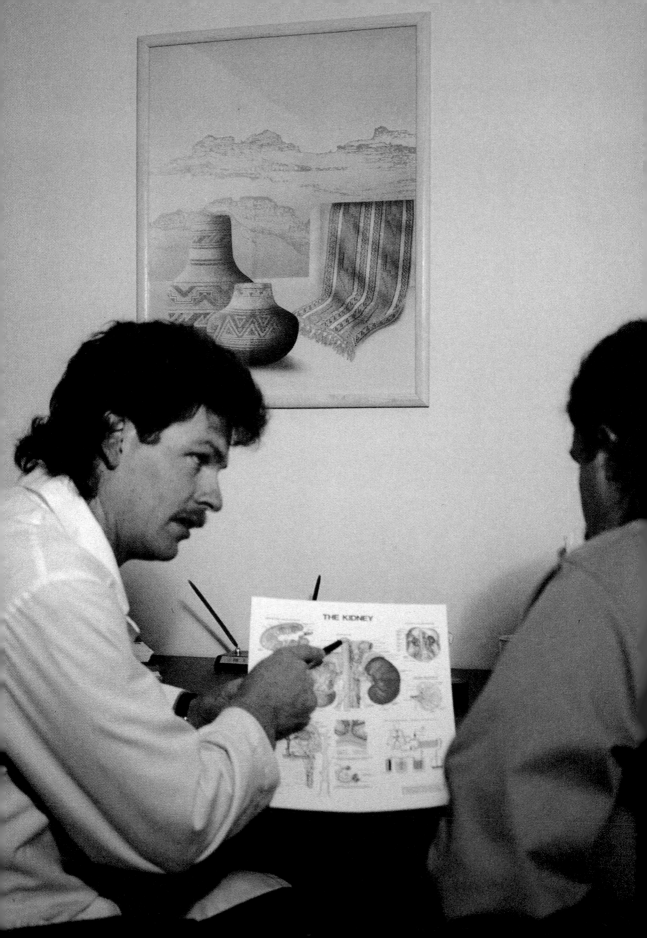

THE KIDNEY

CHAPTER 21

The urinary system and its disorders

The urinary system consists of the right and left kidneys; the right and left ureters (tubes which carry the urine from each kidney to the urinary bladder); and the urethra (a tube which carries urine from the bladder for its discharge outside the body). The kidneys, two brownish, bean-shaped organs about the size of their owner's fists, weigh about 5 ounces (140 grams) each and are located in the upper right and left back part of the abdominal cavity, partially protected by the lower ribs.

Kidney section showing major structures.

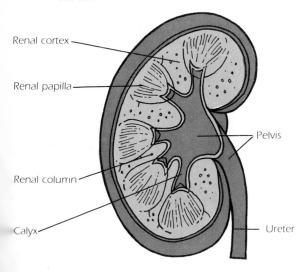

Renal cortex

Renal papilla

Renal column

Calyx

Pelvis

Ureter

The kidneys

The main functions of the kidneys are to maintain the water balance and the levels of the chemical constituents (vitamins, minerals, hormones, blood sugar) in the fluids of the body, help control the alkalinity of the blood, regulate the blood pressure, and eliminate chemical wastes from the body. Every twenty-four hours the kidneys filter approximately 60 quarts of water and then reabsorb about 59 of these quarts. The water and its contents that are not absorbed are passed as urine.

In the average adult, over a quart of blood (1,000 to 1,200 milliliters) flow through both kidneys every minute, or one-fifth of the person's total blood supply.

Each kidney contains about 1,200,000 microscopic filters called nephrons, smaller than the smallest dot. Each **nephron** comprises a glomerulus, surrounded by a hollow capsule (Bowman's), which connects to a tiny tube.

The glomerulus consists of a tuft of

some fifty tiny coiled blood vessels (capillaries) enveloped in an extremely thin and porous sheet of cells, the glomerular membrane, through which are filtered all the constituents of the blood, except the protein and cells. Tiny drops of this filtered fluid enter the Bowman's capsule and flow on down its twisted tube. While each tube is about 2 inches long, the combined length of the 2,400,000 tubes is over 75 miles.

The walls of these tubes absorb back into the blood the needed water and blood chemicals, and secrete into the tube unwanted chemicals from the blood. The unabsorbed chemicals, together with those

directly secreted into the tubes and unneeded water, form the urine, which passes into the ureter and on to the bladder.

The ureters

The right and left ureters are long muscular tubes about 12 inches (30 centimeters) long with a diameter of 2 to 3 millimeters. The ureters connect the pelvis of each kidney (the place at which all the kidney tubules converge) to the bladder. The smooth muscle in the wall of the ureter contracts in waves. Rings of contraction propel about one milliliter of urine toward the bladder with each peristaltic wave. At the point where each ureter passes through the bladder wall a sphincter or valve normally prevents back-flow of urine toward the kidney.

The bladder

The bladder is a muscular sac or holding tank that stores the urine, produced continuously by the kidneys, until the time is convenient for its elimination. It is located in the front of the pelvis, and behind (and when full, above) the pubis. As the bladder fills, its walls stretch, signal-

The urinary system.

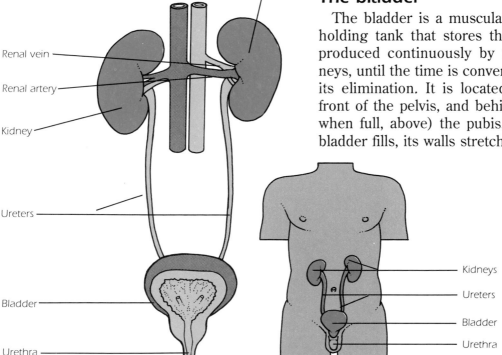

Kidney

Renal vein

Renal artery

Kidney

Ureters

Bladder

Urethra

Kidneys

Ureters

Bladder

Urethra

ling a desire to void. If a person ignores this signal, the bladder will fill still further. Should this sequence be repeated, each succeeding time the urge to urinate becomes more frequent and compelling.

The urethra

The urethra is a muscular tube leading from the base of the bladder to the outside. Several inches long in the male, it travels through the prostate gland (attached to the underside of the bladder) and the entire length of the penis. In the female it is about one inch long and extends from the bladder to the cleft between the labia.

A sphincter or valve in the urethra, under voluntary control, relaxes to allow urine to flow out. Once started, it is possible, though difficult, to stop the flow of urine due to the micturition reflex, which triggers the bladder wall to contract until the organ is completely empty.

Urine

Urine normally consists of sufficient water to carry the chemical wastes of the body, together with excess nutrients. These include urea, creatinine, uric acid, excess vitamins and minerals, and, on occasion, sugar. The color of the urine varies due partly to the volume of water drunk and to certain colors which may be present in the food. For example, the eating of beets reddens the urine. Urine, as it leaves the terminal urethra, is sterile, unless an infection is present somewhere in the urinary tract.

Blood pressure

The kidneys not only handle a large volume of blood, they also regulate its pressure within the body two different ways. The blood vessels provide the space the blood occupies. This space can be enlarged by dilating the vessels, or it can be reduced by constricting them. Enlarging the space drops the pressure; restricting the space raises the pressure. The volume or amount of blood can also be varied—another method of regulating blood pressure. When more water is eliminated, the volume drops and so does the blood pressure. When water is retained, blood volume rises, along with the pressure.

A hormone called **renin** largely controls the size of the blood vessels. A cluster of specialized cells in the nephron gauges the blood pressure and releases the appropriate amount of renin into the bloodstream. Renin triggers the blood vessels to constrict, which raises the pressure. When less renin is released, the vessels relax and the pressure falls.

When needed, renin also prompts the adrenal glands (located on top of the kidneys) to secrete the hormone **aldosterone.** This hormone travels via the blood to the kidney tubules and causes them to absorb more water and salt, thus increasing blood volume and raising the blood pressure.

The kidneys, with their complex functions of controlling water balance, removing body wastes, preserving the alkalinity of body fluids, and regulating blood pressure, are,

1067

like other organ systems of the body, subject to a spectrum of disorders and diseases. One in twenty Americans has kidney disease, and the death rate from many of these illnesses is high.

Problems may arise from exposure to toxic chemicals entering the body by swallowing, absorption through the skin, or inhalation; or they may be produced by bacteria elsewhere in the body. Direct infection can affect the filtering system (as well as other parts of the urinary tract), producing problems throughout the body. Imbalances in chemicals may result in developing stones. Changes in blood pressure affect the kidneys directly and indirectly, and inherited weaknesses and abnormalities may cause diseases. Immunoactive chemicals are found in diseased glomeruli.

Nephritis

The term **nephritis** comprises a number of diseases with similar symptoms. The filters (glomeruli) are damaged, and instead of holding back the blood proteins and the blood cells, they allow one or both to escape into the urine.

Acute glomerulonephritis

The **postinfectious type,** an acute inflammation of the glomeruli, usually results from an infection occurring elsewhere in the body. A streptococcus infection, causing sore throat and scarlet fever, often precedes the nephritis by a week or two. Other common infections which result in nephritis include measles, mumps, chickenpox, malaria, infectious hepatitis, and AIDS.

Acute nephritis may result from chemical poisons, such as phenol (carbolic acid) and turpentine, or they may be a complication of pregnancy (toxemia of pregnancy). Abnormal proteins (such as antibodies) trapped in the glomeruli may also cause acute inflammation.

The symptoms correspond to the amount of blood and proteins that seep through the filters and may include headache, fever, and general lethargy, along with nausea and vomiting. Urine becomes scanty, and fluid accumulates in the tissues (edema), especially in the lower limbs, eyes, and face. The dark-colored, turbid, and sometimes bloody urine contains albumin (the main protein lost from the blood).

What your physician can do. A causative infection should be treated immediately. The susceptibility of the streptococcus to penicillin and other antibiotics has virtually eliminated acute postinfectious glomerulonephritis from this country.

Generally the physician will restrict the intake of salt and water to reduce the high blood pressure and edema (fluid in the tissues). He may prescribe diuretics to increase water loss. A nutritious diet, with possible iron and vitamin supplements for a short period, will aid anemia. Dialysis may be lifesaving in complete renal (or kidney) failure. Many can expect complete recovery. However,

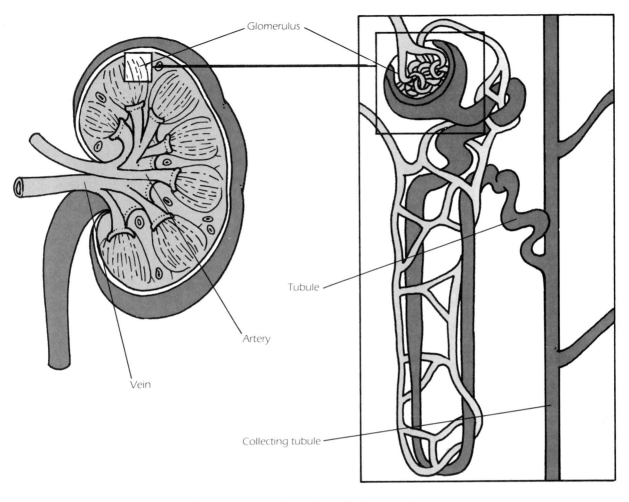

Glomerulus

Tubule

Artery

Vein

Collecting tubule

Kidney section showing cortex and enlarged glomerulus.

in some the disease becomes chronic.

Chronic glomerulonephritis

In this disease a steady, though irreversible, loss in the ability of the glomeruli to filter effectively occurs. It sometimes follows acute nephritis, but usually develops gradually from a low-grade infection, from protracted irritation by chemical substances, or from prolonged overload of urea and salt due to a high-protein, high-salt diet. Toxemia of pregnancy may lead to this condition, as may uncontrolled hypertension.

The damaged filters allow the passage of blood cells and protein. The symptoms will vary, depending on how extensive is the loss of one or both of these blood components. The sufferer may be unaware of any problem for years, and the condition discovered only by a routine physical examination. However, when symptoms of anemia, hypertension, and edema develop, chronic renal failure is imminent (see below).

What you can do. You should be under the care of your physician. The goal in treatment is to reduce the workload of the kidneys so as to maintain their maximum function as long as possible. Following a nutritious diet, low in protein, is imperative, but not easy to achieve because unrefined foods all contain protein. While reducing protein intake to 40 grams per day proves helpful, a diet containing 25 to 30 grams is possible under the direction of a dietician.

Such a diet reduces to a minimum animal foods (milk, eggs, meat, poultry, fish), uses small amounts of legumes, and emphasizes fruits, fresh vegetables, and whole-grain cereals (see page 88).

What your physician can do. With appropriate tests, he can monitor the progress of your disease. If you have high blood pressure, he will care for it. When chronic renal failure occurs, he will determine the time for hemodialysis or peritoneal dialysis (for details, see under "chronic renal failure," below).

Renal failure and uremia

The function of the kidneys is to eliminate waste products from the blood. One healthy kidney can care for all the body's needs with capacity to spare. When the kidneys lose more more than 90 percent of this ability, the wastes, which normally are passed in the urine, accumulate in the blood. This condition, called **uremia,** really means urine in the blood. Sudden damage to the kidney causes **acute renal failure.** Gradual damage results in **chronic renal failure.**

While differences exist between acute and chronic renal failure, the disorders have many symptoms in common, affecting various systems of the body. Some of the following symptoms are seen in every case but not necessarily all. In the digestive system: loss of appetite, nausea, vomiting, and weight loss; in the cardiovascular system: high blood pressure, anemia, and heart failure; in the

respiratory system: shortness of breath; the skin will be pale, dry, and itchy; in the endocrine system: intolerance to glucose; in the nervous system: headache, mental confusion, stupor, and convulsions; and elsewhere: fluid in the tissues (edema).

Acute renal failure

A number of conditions can precipitate acute failure of the kidneys. Among the more common are acute glomerulonephritis (see page 1068). A sudden drop in blood pressure from a failing heart, a massive hemorrhage, or surgery can interfere with kidney function. Protein pigments—released from hemoglobin and myoglobin being broken apart from excessive running (marathons), from acute infections, and from certain drugs of abuse (angel dust)—may block the kidney's filters.

Complete obstruction of the flow of

urine in the ureters or urethra can occur from kidney stones or strictures causing damage to the kidney from back pressure. Toxic chemicals, such as mercury, carbon tetrachloride, phenol (carbolic acid), antifreeze (diethylene glycol), and from certain drugs and mushroom poisoning, may damage the filters and tubules.

Acute kidney failure with uremia and/or oliguria (decreased urine flow) is a life-threatening but generally treatable condition.

What your physician can do. He will determine and treat the underlying cause. If the damage to the kidneys is not too extensive, normal function can be restored. Hemodialysis (removing certain elements from the blood by filtering it through the artificial kidney) relieves the kidney from its work so healing can take place. If the loss of kidney function is not reversible, the condition progresses to chronic renal failure.

Chronic renal failure

Chronic renal failure can result from acute renal failure or from some low-grade but long-sustained destruction of the kidney's ability to function. The causes of such have been described under "chronic glomerulonephritis" (page 1069). Available treatments include hemodialysis, peritoneal dialysis, or a kidney transplant, together with supportive therapy for intercurrent infections, cardiovascular, and other problems.

Other than kidney failure occurring from a sudden and unpredictable problem, one can take steps to protect the kidneys by avoiding exposure to chemicals which must be eliminated, even though no immediate harm can be detected.

The constant use of beverages containing caffeine; the lavish use of aspirin and phenacetin (already shown to damage the kidney) and other headache and pain relievers and sleep producers; the intake in foods and drinks of artificial sweeteners, flavors, colors, and preservatives, place a constant and heavy workload on your kidneys.

The high-protein diet of the Western world, requiring the kidneys to eliminate its many wastes, together with its high salt intake, places on these organs a constant burden. For many, this burden eventually results in premature kidney degeneration and precipitates chronic renal failure.

Nephrosis (nephrotic syndrome)

In nephrosis the damaged filtering membrane allows large amounts of protein (especially albumin) from the blood to pass into the urine. The blood protein is rapidly depleted, and water from the blood passes into the tissues, causing fluid to collect in the tissues (edema), in the abdomen (ascites), and in the chest cavity (pleural effusion). The kidneys also retain salt and water, which furthers the retention of water.

Children, especially between the ages of one and six, are affected more frequently than adults, and boys more commonly than girls. Often associated with some other illness, such as diabetes, nephrosis may develop during nephritis. Recovery generally occurs unless some infection intervenes.

What your physician can do. He can administer corticosteroids, which produce magical improvement in the majority of childhood cases and permit many adult cases to heal. Antibiotics, of themselves, do not change the course of the disease, but usually control infections that often would prove fatal.

Acute pyelonephritis

The terms *pyelo*, meaning "renal pelvis," and *nephritis*, meaning "inflammation of the kidney," specify an infection in the pelvis of the kidney, the enlarged upper end of the ureter that catches the urine coming from the tubules of the kidney. An acute infection here is usually caused by bacteria gaining entrance through the urethra, traveling upward to the bladder, and from there up to the kidney. Sometimes, however, the bloodstream may carry germs from some other part of the body.

The infection is four times more

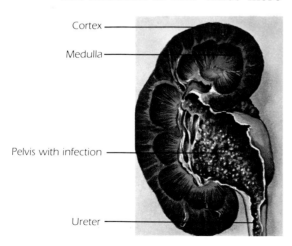

Cortex

Medulla

Pelvis with infection

Ureter

common in women, possibly because women have a short urethra whose opening is close to the opening of the rectum (anus), where germs abound. Anything that tends to obstruct the flow of urine makes this infection more likely to occur. These conditions include an enlarged prostate in men, a stricture in the urethra from a past infection, a stone in the ureter or bladder, a cancer in the urinary tract, and even pregnancy, when the enlarging womb may press on the ureter. An inherited defect in the valves of the ureters (as they enter the bladder) may also allow urine to flow upward to the kidney (reflux).

Regardless of the cause, the symptoms are the same. These usually start with sudden chills, with shivering, then a high fever (up to 104°F), headache, nausea, vomiting, and extreme prostration. Pain, which increases in severity, is over the affected kidney and is constant rather than periodic as with a kidney stone. Painful, difficult urination often is accompanied by a desire to urinate even when the bladder is empty. The urine may be cloudy with pus and tinged with blood.

What your physician can do. An examination will reveal tenderness over the kidney. Examination of the urine will reveal pus and blood. Laboratory tests can identify the precise germ and an effective antibiotic given. Your physician will advise you to rest in bed and drink an abundance of water to aid in washing out the infection. After the acute infec-

Kidney section, showing acute pyelonephritis.

tion is over, he will make every effort to determine the underlying cause and to prevent the infection from becoming chronic. X-rays of the kidney using a dye (pyelogram) and an examination of the bladder will be helpful.

Chronic pyelonephritis

The causes for chronic pyelonephritis are the same as for the acute form of the disease and may result from a carry-over of an acute episode. Often, however, symptoms may be absent (a "silent infection") or so mild that they pass for some other problem and are not identified with kidney disease. The chronic low-grade infection causes slow but progressive destruction of the kidney over a period of years, ending in renal failure. Kidney tissue, once destroyed, cannot be repaired. The first symptoms may include fatigue, frequency of urination (especially at night), swelling of the ankles, anemia, and high blood pressure.

Every effort should be made to find and remedy the underlying cause to prevent further loss of functional kidney tissue. Antibiotic treatment may clear up any infection, but surgical removal of a grossly infected kidney is sometimes necessary. The disease, however, may progress to chronic renal failure (see page 1071).

Kidney stones (renal calculi)

Kidney stones are masses of solid material, the vast majority of which form and enlarge within the kidney pelvis, while about 2 percent develop within the tubules of the kidneys. The common stones are composed of calcium oxalate, uric acid, and cystine—precipitates of chemicals normally held in solution. They occur more frequently in some families and in certain geographic areas.

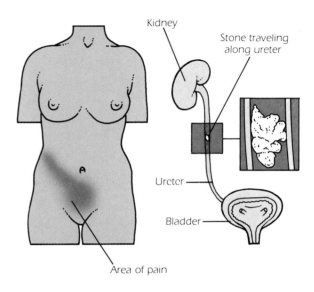

Labels: Kidney; Stone traveling along ureter; Ureter; Bladder; Area of pain

Section through kidney and ureter showing various stones.

Certain factors appear to trigger stone formation, including infections of the kidney; obstructions to the flow of urine due to acquired or inherited defects; metabolic disorders such as gout (increase in uric acid), hyperthyroidism (increase in blood calcium levels), and excessive absorption of oxalate; dietary imbalances (diets high in protein increase excretion of calcium, phosphorous, and uric acid); and not drinking enough water.

Some stones remain in the kidney for long periods without causing symptoms. Usually, however, dis-

1073

comfort ranges from a dull ache in the lower back to extremely severe colicky pain, which comes and goes in waves. Spasm of the ureter muscles causes the pain. As the stone moves down toward the bladder, the pain shifts to the flank, lower abdomen, and then the groin. As the stone passes into the bladder, the pain is relieved. Injury from the stone may cause blood in the urine.

The presence and location of a stone can be determined by means of an X-ray or by X-rays using a dye which is injected into the blood and excreted in the urine (intravenous pyelogram).

What you can do. You should be under the care of your physician. However, you can do a number of things yourself. Drink large quantities of water (enough to produce 4 quarts or 4 liters of urine per twenty-four hours). This may help to flush out a stone, keep it from enlarging, and help prevent the formation of new stones. A low salt intake, and a diet with 30 to 40 grams of protein per day will not only reduce the workload of the kidneys, but also decrease the excretion of wastes which tend to form stones.

What your physician can do. By periodic examinations he can advise as to whether stones are growing or forming. Should you have high levels of uric acid, he may prescribe medications, together with a change of diet, to help correct this situation. The problem of a stone which fails to pass or which blocks urine flow requires treatment.

A stone low down in the ureter can be removed through the bladder.

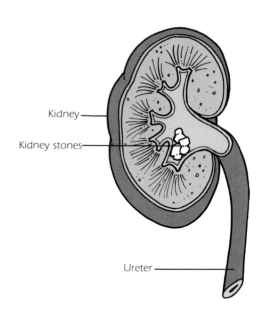

Kidney

Kidney stones

Ureter

Stones in kidney and ureter.

Stones higher up can now be reached using a tube inserted in the side. If not removed the stone can be electrically fragmented and then extracted. Direct surgical removal may be necessary. However, some institutions have an ultrasonic shock wave machine (lithotriptor) which can shatter the stone by directing the shock waves from outside the body.

Floating kidney

The kidneys, surrounded by a thick layer of fat (perirenal fat), are somewhat movable. This surrounding fat helps to loosely hold the kidney below and in the back part of the diaphragm. The right kidney is more likely to move, the prolapse sometimes causing a dull ache or dragging sensation. Only rarely does the ureter become kinked and obstructed.

1074

Most cases need no other treatment than reassurance. Should the problem be severe, careful examination and possibly X-rays can confirm the diagnosis. If the sufferer is thin, gaining some weight often helps. A kidney belt (applied with the feet elevated) may relieve the discomfort. In extreme cases, surgery can anchor the kidney in its normal position.

Inherited disorders and tumors of the kidney

Among the many hereditary diseases and disorders of the kidney that exist, only a few of the more common will be discussed.

Polycystic kidneys

Due to an inherited defect, the tubules of the kidneys fail to develop normally. The blocked tubules fill with urine, forming sacs or cysts scattered throughout the kidney substance. As they continue to enlarge, the pressure gradually destroys normal secreting tissue, and the kidneys become greatly enlarged. If many cysts develop, death may occur in infancy; if only a few, the person may live to an old age. Generally renal failure occurs in mid-life.

Because no cure exists, every effort should be made to prevent complications (high blood pressure, infections, and stones) and deal with them promptly when they occur. When renal failure develops, dialysis and kidney transplantation are available.

Genetic counseling is important. Tests (ultrasound, tomography) can determine the presence and extent of the disease. Then reasonable predictions can be made as to life expectancy, permitting rational decisions as to marriage and professional careers, among other things. Approximately 50 percent of the children of those with the disease will inherit the disorder.

Horseshoe kidney

In this disorder the lower poles of the two kidneys fail to separate during development. The condition generally causes no problems, except increased susceptibility to infections and more likelihood of stone formation.

Alport's syndrome

A defective glomerular membrane causes this inherited glomerulonephritis. In this condition—rarely recognized until the second decade of life and sometimes later—blood and protein are lost in the urine, and the condition progresses to uremia (renal failure).

Cystinuria

In this inherited disorder, cystine, an essential amino acid, is not effectively absorbed from the kidney tubules, causing massive quantities of cystine to be lost in the urine. Stones form, the ureters are obstructed, and renal colic results. If the stones are not passed or removed, renal failure ensues. Cystine is freely soluble only in highly alkaline urine—a pH level difficult to

1075

attain. The drug penicillamine promotes solubility but unfortunately is quite toxic.

Tumors of the kidneys

Cancers developing within the kidney deal with two distinct age groups, infancy and later middle life. **Nephroblastoma (Wilms' tumor)** is the most common renal cancer in children and typically develops before the age of three. The first sign is usually a firm, typically painless mass in the kidney area on one side. Although the growth invades the kidney, blood is infrequently found in the urine, and when present conveys an unfavorable import. Prompt surgical removal of the involved kidney,

combined with possible radiation and chemotherapy, brings chances of survival up to 50 percent.

In adults the cancer **hypernephroma** occurs most commonly between the ages of forty and sixty. The appearance of blood in the urine, loss of appetite and weight, dull pain in the area of the affected kidney, and an accompanying fever are the typical symptoms. A variety of tests such as a CAT scan, ultrasound tomography, or an intravenous pyelogram will reveal the presence of the tumor. The cancer may spread to other parts of the body, typically to the lung and long bones. Surgical removal, followed by radiation and chemotherapy, provide the best results.

Disorders of the ureters and bladder

The right and left ureters carry urine from the right and left kidneys to the urinary bladder (see page 1066).

Ureteral stricture

Occasionally a narrowing or stricture occurs in one of the ureters, interfering with the normal flow of urine. Narrowing may be the result of damage to the lining from the presence or passing of a kidney stone or from some external pressure as from an enlarging tumor. The symptom—pain in the lower back which travels to the region of the groin—may vary from a dull ache to almost intolerable pain.

What your physician can do. He may decide to periodically dilate or stretch the narrowing by passing a

catheter, using a cystoscope, from the bladder up the ureter. When this method is not feasible, he may remove the kidney and ureter on the affected side, but only if the opposite ureter and kidney are functional.

Ureteral calculi (stones in ureter)

See under "kidney stones" (page 1073).

Urinary incontinence

Urinary incontinence is the inability to hold urine in the bladder or release it as desired. A sudden uncontrollable desire to void is called **urge incontinence.** Such loss of control commonly occurs during an infection in the bladder (cystitis) or urethra (urethritis). Other causes of incontinence include spinal cord injury, injury during childbirth, an enlarged prostate, and diseases such as Alzheimer's disease, and multiple sclerosis.

In the case of weakened sphincters and pelvic floor muscles, unexpected vigorous laughing, coughing, and straining (as when lifting something heavy), causes unwilling urine loss called **stress incontinence.**

What your physician can do. He will treat the underlying infection or disease. He may suggest that you strengthen the weak muscles by trying to hold your urine when the urge to urinate comes. Surgical repair may be necessary in some cases.

Urinary retention

Urinary retention occurs in the event of partial or complete obstruction to the outflow of urine. The cause may be a stricture of the urethra, an enlarged prostate gland, a developing tumor within the bladder, or the presence of a bladder stone.

When the obstruction develops gradually, the muscles of the bladder wall enlarge and strengthen, forcing the urine past the obstruction and emptying the bladder only partially. This residual urine decreases the bladder's capacity, often becomes infected, causing inflammation (cystitis), and results in frequent small urinations. The resulting back pressure may damage the kidneys. Eventually, and often quite suddenly, no urine can be passed. As the bladder continues to fill, distention with severe pain results, causing a medical emergency.

What your physician can do. He will drain the bladder with a catheter and then he will determine the basic cause of the problem and treat it.

Cystitis (inflammation of the bladder)

Cystitis is an inflammatory infection of the bladder, rare in men but very common in women. Women are more susceptible because their urethras are short (less than 2 inches or 5 centimeters) while those of men are long (more than 8 inches or 20 centimeters). The opening of the urethra in women adjoins the opening of the vagina, which, in turn, is close to the anal opening (from the rectum). Thus germs can gain entrance to the bladder through the urethra more readily in women.

The symptoms include burning on urination, a desire to void frequently, and urgency to empty the bladder at once (especially in women). There may be fever (usually caused by infections of the kidney or prostate in men) and a dull pain over the bladder. The cloudy urine may contain blood.

Cystitis in men. The cause is an infection of the kidneys (pyelonephritis) or prostate (prostatis), a stricture or some other abnormality in the urinary tract, or a tumor. A culture of the urine will determine the offending organism. An examination of the prostate, kidneys (pyelogram), and bladder (cystoscopy) should establish the cause. An appropriate antibiotic should cure the infection. Other findings will determine additional therapy.

Cystitis in women. While an infection of the kidney or a stricture in the urinary tract may cause the cystitis, the most likely cause is germs entering through the urethra. Many factors may lead to an infection, such as poor hygiene, sexual intercourse, douching, and an improperly placed diaphragm. It is not known why some women are constantly troubled with cystitis.

A thorough examination of the kidneys and bladder (see above), together with a culture of the urine, will confirm the diagnosis. An appropriate antibiotic will generally care for the infection. Any other accompanying problem should be corrected.

To prevent recurrences and to facilitate a cure, women should drink an abundance of water (eight to ten full-size glasses a day) to flush out the bladder. They should avoid drinks such as coffee, tea, chocolate, and soft drinks and should keep the vaginal area scrupulously clean by gentle cleansing with mild soap and water.

Interstitial cystitis

Interstitial cystitis is commonly seen in middle-aged women. It is an inflammatory process in the deep layers of the bladder wall that progressively becomes fibrotic (scarred). The bladder becomes smaller and its walls firmer, with its capacity gradually being reduced. Urination (emptying the bladder) becomes frequent and is painful. Voiding gives only temporary relief. The lining of the bladder (mucosa) becomes thin, and "ulcers" form, which crack and bleed as the bladder distends. The openings of the ureters into the bladder are affected, and remain open or be-

come obstructed. Backflow of urine injures the kidneys (hydronephrosis).

The diagnosis is made by noting the symptoms, by finding that the urine does not contain bacteria, by visual inspection of the bladder lining, and by means of a biopsy of the bladder wall.

While the precise reason for the disorder is uncertain, previous infection in the pelvis, surgery in the bladder area, drug medications, or an autoimmune mechanism are among some of the suggested causes. Since the problem comes on gradually and does not become severe for two or three years, you should see your physician should you observe the above symptoms.

Unfortunately, there is no cure. Taking steroids orally, instilling them into the bladder, or irrigating the bladder with astringents provides some relief, but must be repeated every few months. Sometimes it is necessary to redirect the ureters so that the urine coming from the kidneys is discharged elsewhere.

Bladder stones (vesical calculi)

Stones formed within the bladder are commonly due to obstruction to the flow of urine and to infection in the urinary tract. Twenty times more common in men than in women, they occur in older age groups. A small proportion of stones come from the kidneys, but they are small enough to enter the bladder and are passed in the urine.

The symptoms consist of difficulty in urinating, urgency to urinate, and

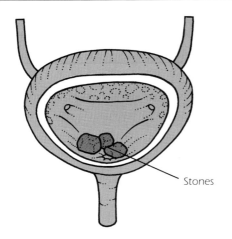

Bladder showing presence of stones.

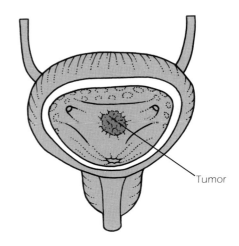

Bladder with tumor on inner wall.

develop so as to block the flow of urine through the ureter, urine will back up into the kidney and cause serious damage (hydronephrosis). Should the growth be near the opening of the urethra, urine will start to flow and then abruptly stop (ball-valve effect). Because most tumors grow inward, cancers may invade the wall of the bladder and spread to distant parts of the body.

spasm of the bladder, with pain which in men may be especially felt in the end of the penis. Some stones act like a "ball valve," intermittently interfering with the flow of urine so that the urinary stream starts and stops. The treatment consists in surgically removing the stone or stones and treating the condition responsible for stone formation.

Tumors of the bladder (benign and malignant)

Both benign and malignant growths develop from the lining cells of the bladder. Almost 50,000 people (three-fourths of them men) get cancer of the bladder each year, of whom more than one in five die from the disease. Those at high risk are smokers (cancer-producing agents absorbed into the blood are eliminated in the urine) and workers in various industries exposed to chemicals or their vapors.

Blood in the urine is the most significant symptom of usually painless bladder tumors. Should the tumor

What your physician can do. You should immediately report any blood in the urine to your physician, who will determine its source by a cystoscopic examination and possibly an intravenous pyelogram (to rule out kidney disease). He will order a biopsy to determine whether the growth is benign or malignant. Benign tumors can generally be removed through a cystoscope. Cancers invading the bladder wall will require resection, and, if they are large, the removal of the entire bladder. When the bladder is removed, an opening in the abdominal wall will

1079

allow urine coming through the ureters to be collected in a bag. Radiation therapy may be necessary both before and after surgery.

Cystocele

A cystocele, a downward protrusion of the bladder into the vagina, occurs when the normal support is weakened from old age or from injury at the time of childbirth. Such weakening of the supportive structures also often causes protrusion of the rectum **(rectocele)** and displacement of the urethra **(urethrocele)** into the lower vagina (space between the labia).

Mild cases of cystocele (and urethrocele) may produce no symptoms. Often one feels a heaviness, especially when straining and after standing for long periods. Retention of urine causes more serious symptoms similar to those of cystitis: frequency of urination, burning on urination, and urgency to void.

What you can do. In less severe cases, the muscular support of the bladder may be strengthened by consistent daily exercise of the sphincter muscles that control the passing of urine and feces. Deliberately contract and relax these muscles for several minutes two or three times a day.

What your physician can do. He will treat your cystitis, and, if deemed necessary, surgically repair the structures which support the bladder and urethra to retain them in their normal positions.

Diseases of the urethra

Because of the distinct differences between the urethra of the male and the female, the diseases involved and their treatment differ somewhat, so will be described separately.

Urethritis in the female. Urethritis, an infection of the urethra, may be a complication of cystitis or an infection of the vagina. The infection—due to some nonspecific organism or to a sexually transmitted germ, such as gonorrhea—often occurs after intercourse and may become chronic.

The symptoms parallel those of cystitis, but generally include discomfort, burning, and mild pain, especially when urine is passed and immediately after.

The physician can determine the specific organism by means of a urine culture and then give the appropriate antibiotic. Recurring urethritis may be controlled by drinking adequate amounts of water, and especially by drinking a glass of water before and following intercourse. Scrupulous hygiene of both partners is important. Should narrowing of the urethra develop, the physician can dilate the opening by inserting probes of increasing size.

Urethritis in the male. Inflammation of the urethra can be caused by the gonococcus, the germ causing gonorrhea, or by some other organism. Transmitted by sexual contact, **gonorrheal urethritis** develops in two to six days after contact with an infected person. The symptoms usually consist of a burning sensation on urination, pain in the urethra, and the discharge of a thick, yellow, puslike fluid.

When treatment is delayed, the infection can extend to the prostate gland, the epididymis, and the bladder. When the disease is untreated, gonorrheal germs may enter the blood and spread throughout the body, affecting the heart, joints, and other organs. Chronic infection can lead to narrowing of the urethra and the formation of strictures.

Nongonococcal or **nonspecific urethritis (NSU)** can occur directly from sexual intercourse or follow gonorrheal urethritis. The organisms vary, but chlamydial microbes cause about half the infections. The ingestion of certain poisons such as turpentine and wood alcohol some-times has this effect. The symptoms may be mild with only a slight watery discharge, or severe with a bloody, pussy emission.

What your physician can do. He will determine the organism causing the infection through laboratory tests, which in the case of NSU may require culturing the organism. Once the organism is identified, an appropriate antibiotic should control the infection. Unfortunately a highly resistant strain of gonococcus has been introduced into the United States, requiring repeated treatments. Your sex partner should receive the same treatment at the same time. Your physician will advise abstinence from intercourse and alcohol during therapy. He can care for strictures in the urethra by using increasingly larger probes.

CHAPTER 22

Sex organs: Male and female

The sex organs enable a man and woman to reproduce themselves by bringing new life into being. The testes in men and the ovaries in women produce the sex cells: the sperm and the ovum. Man's organs are designed to deliver the sperm, while the woman's organs are fashioned to receive the sperm and permit a union of one of them with an ovum. In addition, the reproductive organs of the woman include the uterus or womb, in which the fetus develops for nine months before its birth, and the breasts, which produce milk to nourish the baby after birth.

Besides the above, the testes in the male and the ovaries in the female produce sex hormones, chemicals that stimulate the development of the various sex characteristics and maintain these masculine and feminine characteristics. While the sex organs are not essential for a healthy life, they do make possible the most intimate relations of marriage.

The male organs

The male reproductive organs consist of (1) the two testicles in which the male sex cells and the male sex hormone are produced, (2) the epididymis attached to the back of each testicle, in which the sperm mature and are stored, (3) the vas deferens—a firm, hollow tube that extends from each epididymis and carries the sperm from the scrotum (in which the testicles and epididymides are located) through the lower abdominal wall to the vicinity of the prostate, a gland located just below the bladder, (4) two seminal vesicles, (5) two Cowper's glands, which, along with (6) the prostate, produce secretions that preserve and nourish the sperm, and, finally, (7) the urethra, which runs within (8) the penis, the external male sex organ that serves to introduce the sperm into the vagina of the woman by ejaculating them from the upper end of the vas deferens.

The testicle (testis, plural testes). The testicles make a man a man. Castration—the removal of the

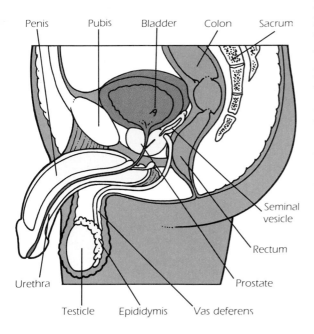

Penis Pubis Bladder Colon Sacrum

Seminal
vesicle

Rectum

Urethra

Prostate

Testicle Epididymis Vas deferens

Section through male pelvis showing male sex organs.

testicles—makes a eunuch. The testicles produce the male sex cells **(sperm)** and the male hormone, testosterone. They enable a man to become a father and to develop the male characteristics of broad shoulders, heavy muscles, a deep voice, and a beard.

The testicles are located in the scrotum, a thin-walled sac that hangs in the midline, below the abdomen, between the upper thighs. Each testicle is an oval-shaped organ about the size of a hen's egg, to the back of which is attached the epididymis. Both are suspended by the spermatic cord, a structure composed of blood vessels, nerves, and the spermatic duct (vas deferens).

Interestingly, because the testicles are outside the abdominal cavity and are therefore cooler than the organs

inside the body, they are designed to function more efficiently at this lower temperature. Muscle fibers in the walls of the scrotum contract when it is cold, drawing the testicles up toward the body where it is warmer, and relax when it is hot, permitting the testicles to hang down where it is cooler. When an individual has a high fever, his testicles no longer produce sperm.

During the early period of development, the testicles develop high up in the abdominal cavity, just below the kidneys. They later descend and enter the scrotum before birth. In a small percentage of boys they descend soon after birth. In a few instances, they remain within the abdomen, a condition called **undescended testicle.** Some can be activated to descend by giving the child a gonadotropic hormone. If this treatment fails, the testicle can be brought down surgically or removed. A testicle left within the abdomen fails to produce sperm and may become cancerous.

Within each testicle are hundreds of tortuous tubules that eventually connect with the epididymis. Two kinds of highly specialized cells line these tubules. One type manufactures testosterone, the male sex hormone, while the others produce 100 million sperm each day. As a sperm matures it develops a tail, which, as it thrashes from side to side, propels it forward.

The **epididymis,** attached to the back of each testicle, is a small, soft-textured organ about the size of a large almond, made up of some twenty extremely twisted ducts, all

1083

leading into the vas deferens. These ducts, if unraveled, would extend some thirty feet (nine meters). In the duct walls are cells that secrete an acid fluid that reduces the activity of the sperm as they await ejaculation.

The **vas deferens,** a hollow tube, extends upward from each epididymis, passing through the abdominal wall, and ending in the urethra, deep within the substance of the prostate. Its walls contain muscle fibers that contract, expelling the sperm during ejaculation.

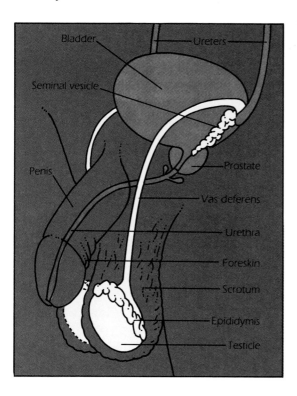

Diagram showing male sex organs.

The two **seminal vesicles** are small, soft, glandular structures that discharge a thick alkaline secretion into each vas deferens at the point at which they enter the prostate. This alkaline fluid neutralizes the acid secretion of the epididymis, activating the sperm to propel themselves with movements of their tails.

Cowper's glands, two in number, adjacent to the lower end of the prostate, secret a thick, sticky fluid into the urethra. This fluid is often released prior to ejaculation and may contain sperm. Thus, withdrawal before ejaculation is not a safe form of contraception.

The **prostate** is a single cone-shaped organ, about 1 inch in diameter (2.5 centimeters), composed of smooth muscle and glandular tissue, with its base attached to the base of the bladder. The urethra, carrying urine from the bladder, passes through its substance. At the time of ejaculation, the prostate's muscle fibers contract, expelling into the urethra a milky fluid that forms about half of the seminal fluid (ejaculate). The secretions of the epididymis, seminal vesicles, Cowper's glands, and prostate together form the ejaculate, which protects, activates, and nourishes the sperm.

The **penis** consists of three parallel tubes (two above and one below) that are packed with blood vessels (erectile tissue) and bound together with a layer of fibrous tissue. In response to sexual desire, the erectile tissues fill with blood under pressure and promptly change the organ from soft to firm, and from small to large. The enlarged head or glans also consists of erectile tissue and surrounds the end of the shaft of the penis.

The urethra runs within the lower of the three tubes of erectile tissue and extends from the prostate to the tip of the penis, where it opens by a cleft in the glans. During intercourse the penis is inserted into the vagina, and on ejaculation, the muscles in the two vas deferens and in the walls of the seminal vesicles and prostate contract rhythmically. The ejaculate, containing the sperm, is thus ejected through the urethra into the depths of the vagina.

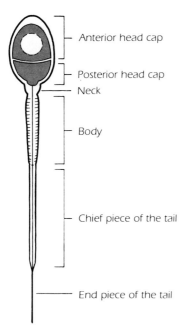

Components of a sperm (male sex cell).

A healthy man in the prime of life discharges, in one ejaculation, about 0.03 oz (3 ml) of seminal fluid containing some 300 million sperm. These are extremely active and can propel themselves through the female reproductive organs (cervix, uterus, and fallopian tubes) at the rate of one inch (2.5 centimeters) in eight minutes.

Normally the glans is covered by the **foreskin,** except at the time of erection, when, as the penis enlarges, this soft, fleshy collar of tissue is retracted onto the body of the penis, exposing the glans. **Circumcision** consists of surgically removing the foreskin. This simple procedure is usually done during the first week of life, and by those of Jewish faith, on the eighth day.

Circumcision is no longer routinely done as it was in the past. Although the foreskin is difficult to retract at birth, it gradually separates from the glans during the first few months of life and can be fully retracted by the age of five. Retraction should not be forced. If it fails to retract, circumcision can be performed. Secretions from glands under the foreskin tend to accumulate and unless removed by washing every day or two become unhygienic. Some evidence suggests that cancer of the penis is more common in those failing to practice proper hygiene.

The female organs

The female reproductive organs consist of (1) the ovaries, in which the female sex cells and the female hormones are produced, (2) the oviducts, each extending from the vicinity of the ovary to the upper part of the uterus on its own side, (3) the uterus, which contains a cavity in which the fetus develops during the nine months prior to birth and which opens below, through its cervix, into the vagina, (4) the vagina, which receives the cervix of the uterus above and opens to the outside of the body below, which provides a space where seminal fluid can be deposited at the time of sexual intercourse, and

1085

which becomes much dilated to form part of the birth canal at the time of childbirth, (5) the vulva, which consists of the several external genital organs, and (6) the breasts, which provide milk for the infant's nourishment following birth.

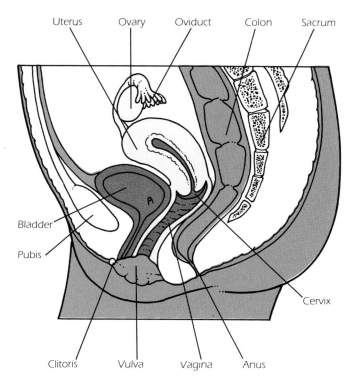

Section through female pelvis showing female sex organs.

The ovary. The ovaries are the essential organs that make a woman a woman. They produce the female sex cells (ova; singular, ovum) and the female sex hormones which are responsible for the secondary sex characteristics of a woman: broad hips, clear skin without coarse hairs, higher pitched voice, and well-developed breasts.

During the early period of development, the ovaries lie high up in the abdominal cavity, just below the kidneys. They then descend and attach themselves to either side of the pelvis. Each almond-shaped ovary is about 1.5 inches (3.8 centimeters) long, 1 inch (2.5 centimeters) wide, and less than half an inch (1 centimeter) thick.

The central portion of the ovary contains blood vessels and nerves. The female sex cells are located near the surface, each sex cell lying at the center of a small group of supporting cells, called a "follicle." At the time of puberty the ovaries contain some 250,000 to 300,000 follicles. Of these, perhaps only about 200 in each ovary develop sufficiently to discharge their ova; the rest regress. Beginning with sexual maturity, a few follicles in both ovaries respond to the hormone that controls the monthly reproductive cycle. Of these, usually only one (in either the right or left ovary) liberates an ovum that is prepared for fertilization, a process called **ovulation.**

Should more than one ovum be released, a twin pregnancy becomes possible. The twins produced in this way are called "fraternal twins", in contrast to "identical twins" originating from a single ovum. The cells forming the wall of the empty follicle now multiply, fill the follicle, become transformed to form a corpus luteum, and produce a hormone that plays a major role during pregnancy.

The oviduct (fallopian tube, uterine tube). The oviduct is a tube about 4 inches (10 centimeters) long. The end nearest the ovary has a funnel-shaped opening with finger-like processes along its margin. These envelop the ovary at the time of ovulation and direct the egg inside the tube. The myriads of microscopic fingers (villi) lining the tube, sweep the ovum into the uterus with a wave-like motion, where the other end of the duct terminates. It is usually within the oviduct that the sperm and ovum meet and where conception occurs.

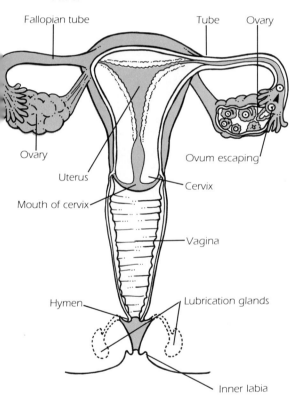

The internal female reproductive organs.

The uterus (the womb). The uterus is a hollow, heavily muscular, pear-shaped organ with the narrow portion directed downward. It receives the oviducts on the upper right and left portions and opens through its cervix into the vagina below. In the nonpregnant state it is 3 inches (7.5 centimeters) long, including the cervix, two inches (5 centimeters) wide at its widest part, and 1 inch (2.5 centimeters) thick, lying between the rectum behind and the urinary bladder in front.

At the time the ovum is released from the ovary, the lining of the uterus becomes thicker, more velvety, and laden with fluid and nutrients—in readiness to receive the fertilized ovum. When the ovum remains unfertilized, the lining and blood vessels break down, and these tissues, together with the unfertilized ovum, are swept out in the menstrual flow (menstruation).

When the ovum is fertilized, the uterus provides for the developing fetus during the nine months prior to its birth, accommodating the rapidly enlarging fetus, together with the amniotic fluid and placenta. It has a rich blood supply to nourish the fetus. At the time of delivery, forceful contractions of the muscular walls of the uterus expel the infant through the birth canal. The uterus also provides a passageway for the sperm to travel from the vagina to the oviducts.

The vagina. The vagina is a soft-walled tube lined with mucous membrane, extending about 4 inches (10 centimeters) from the cervix of the uterus to its opening at the vulva. During intercourse it receives the penis of the male with the seminal fluid. During childbirth it greatly dilates as it forms part of the birth canal.

Its opening at the vulva is often partially closed by a crescent-shaped fold of tissue called the **hymen.** The hymen is frequently absent and becomes stretched or torn by use of vaginal tampons and intercourse.

The vulva (the female external sex organs). The **vulva** consists of several parts. The mons veneris is a pad of fat covered with hair that lies over the pubic bone. The **major labia** are two lips of fatty tissue that enclose the urethral and vaginal openings. The **minor labia** are tissue folds embraced by the major labia, which fuse in front to form the prepuce of the clitoris. The **clitoris,** like the penis in the male, consists of erectile tissue; it is partially covered by the labia minor in front, and becomes enlarged during the sex act. The vestibule is a cleftlike space behind the clitoris in which the urethra opens in front and the vagina immediately behind. The two **Bartholin's glands** in the walls of the vestibule, one on each side, lubricate the entrance to the vagina.

The female breast (mammary gland). The female breast is composed of some fifteen to twenty lobes, each of which is further divided into a number of lobules. Each lobule consists of complicated glandular tissue capable of secreting milk. All the ducts collecting this milk from a single lobe converge to form a common duct. Each common duct enlarges, forming a reservoir for milk, just before it empties through an opening in the nipple.

Dense fibrous tissue interspersed with fat holds the lobes and lobules together. This fibrous tissue connects the breasts to the pectoral muscles of the chest wall. A thick layer of fat overlays the breast tissue and contours its shape, giving the covering skin a smooth and graceful appearance.

The centrally placed **nipple** protruding from the surface of the skin is composed of erectile tissue, which may remain erect or become erect when aroused by sexual activity. The areola, the pigmented skin around the nipple, contains oil-secreting glands that lubricate and protect the nipple while the baby is nursing.

The milk glands are remarkably programmed. Stimulated by the nursing infant and prompted by the hormone estrogen, the cells in the milk glands rapidly increase in size and number. Nutrients are drawn from the blood to manufacture the milk, the precise composition of which changes from week to week, depending on the specific needs of the growing infant.

Richly supplied by highly sensitive nerves, the nipple and breast respond to physical contact, such as caressing or sucking by the infant, or by general sexual arousal.

The monthly cycle (menstruation and pregnancy)

As a girl begins to reach womanhood, her breasts begin to enlarge, and hair starts to grow in her pubic area. A year or two later she undergoes a period of rapid growth, after which she begins to menstruate. At first the intervals between menses are irregular because her ovaries are not producing mature sex cells. However, within a year or so, the time of menstruation becomes regular.

This rhythmic pattern, called the

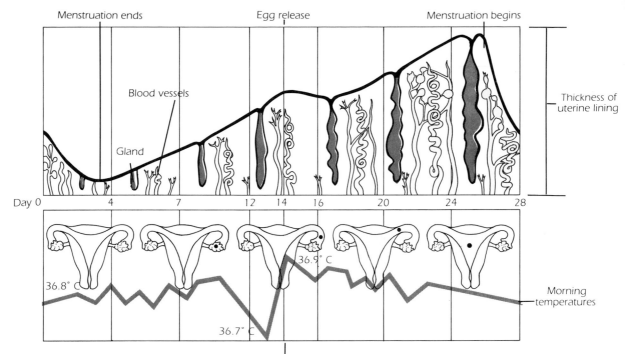

Menstruation ends   Egg release   Menstruation begins

Blood vessels

Gland

Thickness of uterine lining

Day 0   4   7   12   14   16   20   24   28

36.9° C

36.8° C

36.7° C

Morning temperatures

Temperature drop before ovulation (release of egg)

Diagram showing changes in the lining of the uterus (mucosa) and body temperature during a 28-day female sexual (menstrual) cycle. Note the abrupt drop in body temperature at the time of ovulation.

menstrual cycle (more accurately the female sexual cycle) continues throughout the normal reproductive years, and is regulated by rhythmic changes in the female hormones. The ebb and flow of these hormones causes the changes seen in the sexual organs (ovary, uterus, breasts). While the average cycle is twenty-eight days, the interval may vary from as little as twenty days to more than forty days in perfectly normal women.

Stimulated by hormones from the pituitary gland (follicle-stimulating hormone—FSH, and luteinizing hormone—LH), a few mature follicles (up to ten) in each ovary respond, but only one ovary releases an ovum (usually alternating each month between ovaries). This process, called ovulation, occurs fourteen days after

menses begins, in a woman who has a twenty-eight-day cycle.

The cells lining the empty follicle rapidly increase in number and become changed to lutein cells (forming the corpus luteum) which secrete progesterone and estrogen. Under the influence of these hormones, the lining of the uterus, called the endometrium, undergoes considerable change. Blood vessels increase in number, the lining cells multiply rapidly, the endometrium doubles in thickness (becoming 4 to 6 millimeters thick), growing soggy with nutritious secretions known as "uterine milk", and takes on a velvety appearance—all in readiness to receive a fertilized ovum.

When conception does not occur, the level of the ovarian hormones (estrogen and progesterone) drops

1089

suddenly. Without the encouragement of these hormones the endometrium begins to deteriorate. The underlying blood vessels narrow and soon break apart. The lining cells, denied the blood they need, disintegrate. The unfertilized ovum with much of the mucous membrane is shed, accompanied by the loss of considerable blood. Contractions of the uterus (sometimes causing painful "cramps") aid in expelling this blood and tissue through the vagina. This process is called **menstruation.**

Typically, five days after menstruation starts (anywhere from three to seven days is normal), blood flow ceases. A little more than 2 ounces (70 ml) of blood, cells, and tissue fluids are lost. The inside of the uterus is now completely stripped of its lining, and rebuilding of this lining begins again in anticipation of a pregnancy occurring during the next month. The enormous numbers of white cells present in the menstrual flow protect the uterus from possible infection.

When conception does occur, the cells of the endometrium initially act as nursemaids to the fertilized egg when it first arrives in the womb (about four days after conception). A secretion called "uterine milk" provides the rapidly growing embryo the food it needs. After three or four days, the ovum implants itself in the lining. Still later, as the demands of the growing embryo increase, the **placenta** develops. The placenta is an organ which acts as a go-between for the mother and fetus. Oxygen and nutrients from the mother's blood pass to the blood of the fetus, while many of the wastes formed by the fetus move in the opposite direction. These wastes travel through the placenta into the mother's blood, to be expelled by her eliminative organs.

Some of the major events in the calender of a **twenty-eight-day menstrual cycle** are summarized below.

The menstrual flow continues for about five days, following which the rebuilding of the uterine lining begins and continues for eleven or twelve days (proliferative phase). Then, for another eleven to twelve days, the lining cells fill with fluid to nourish the ovum (secretory phase). Fourteen days after the start of menstruation, ovulation occurs. Twenty-six days from the start, if the ovum is not fertilized, the lining begins to disintegrate, and two days later menstruation commences again.

Menopause

Menopause denotes the termination of menstruation and generally occurs between the ages of forty and fifty-five, usually during the late forties. The sexual cycles that have continued since puberty (except during pregnancies) become irregular, and, after a few months or a few years, cease. Menopause may be considered a "burning-out" of the ovaries. By the time a woman reaches the age of forty-five, but few of the viable follicles that can produce an ovum remain, and those that remain are eventually gone. The production of the hormones that control the changes in the uterine lining (endometrium) rapdily decline and finally stop. Menstruation and reproduction can no longer transpire.

Disorders of the male sex organs

A portion of the male sex organs play a dual role, as they are a part of the urinary system. Because of this overlap, the urinary problems of certain of the organs discussed in this chapter have already been dealt with in the chapter, "The urinary systems and its disorders."

The scrotum and its contents

The scrotum is a thin-walled sac suspended below the pubis and the base of the penis between the upper thighs. It is partitioned in the center, each half containing a testicle, epididymis, and the beginning of the spermatic cord (vessels, lymphatics, nerves, and spermatic duct).

Hydrocele

A hydrocele is an excessive accumulation of clear, light-yellow fluid between the two layers of a membranous sac that partially surrounds the testicle and epididymis. This most common scrotal swelling is soft and painless. It may result from an injury or inflammation, but generally the cause is not known. Seen most frequently in men over sixty, it

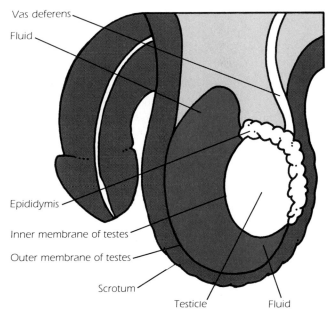

A hydrocele showing collection of fluid in the membranes of a testicle.

1091

causes no harm and needs treatment only if it becomes large and uncomfortable. Tapping the fluid is unsatisfactory since it tends to reaccumulate, so surgical removal of the sac is the preferable treatment.

Varicocele

A varicocele is a mass caused by an abnormal dilatation or swelling of the veins that carry blood away from the testicle and epididymis. Most men have a small varicocele on the left side, especially occurring soon after puberty. The dilated veins feel somewhat like a bunch of earthworms. Large varicoceles may cause a feeling of weight and a mild, dragging pain, but they are not a hazard to health. Although most need no treatment, wearing a support helps if the varicocele is troublesome. In cases of significant distress, a portion of the dilated veins can be surgically removed. Your physician can discuss the possible risks.

Orchitis

Orchitis is an inflammation of one or both testes that is often associated with an infection of the epididymis. Bacteria from chlamydial infection travel from the urethra via the spermatic duct. More commonly a systemic viral infection, especially from mumps, causes the inflammation. Symptoms include severe local pain; the scrotum is red and swollen, and the sufferer feels ill and feverish. A serious complication that causes permanent damage to the cells producing sperm results in infertility.

What your physician can do. He will determine the precise cause and prescribe antibiotic therapy if indicated for bacteria from a chlamydial infection. Bed rest with ice packs to the scrotum will help relieve pain, as will a pillow to support the scrotum. Should an abscess form, surgical drainage may be needed.

Torsion of the testicle

Torsion occurs when a testicle twists on the spermatic cord from which it is suspended within the scrotum. The twisting restricts the blood supply to the testicle (strangulation) and may cause permanent damage to the organ, resulting in infertility. It can happen at any time, even during sleep, but usually occurs during vigorous physical activity. The chief symptom consists of sudden pain in one testicle, followed by rapid swelling and redness. The pain may cause the individual to become sick to his stomach and vomit. Even if the cord untwists by itself, a physician should be consulted because the condition may recur.

What your physician can do. Torsion of the testicle must be distinguished from epididymitis, orchitis, and even cancer, so it is necessary to have the precise diagnosis. Preventing damage to the organ constitutes a medical emergency. Your physician may be able to untwist the strangulation, but it is best to solve the problem permanently by surgical repair, often of both testicles.

Cancer of the testicle

Cancer of the testicle is the most common cancer in men under forty. It occurs more commonly in those whose testicles failed to descend or descended late. Developing in the sperm-producing cells, the cancer is highly malignant, spreading via the lymphatics to other organs, especially to the lungs. It carries a high mortality rate of about 50 percent.

The first sign is a painless swelling of the testicle. If permitted to continue, it will increase in size, produce a feeling of weight, and eventually cause pain. Felt through the scrotum, the tumor is firm and hard.

What you can do. Examine your testicles each month and promptly report any swelling to your physician.

What your physician can do. Surgical removal of the cancerous testicle will provide complete cure if it is discovered early. If the cancer has spread, the surgery will be followed by radiation or chemotherapy, which prove quite effective in treating this type of malignancy.

Epididymitis

Epididymitis is an inflammation of the epididymis, a coiled tube structure attached to the back of each testicle. The infection is usually bacterial (gonococcal) or chlamydial. The organisms travel from the urethra (within the prostate) through the spermatic duct to the epididymis. The inflammation gives rise to swelling, tenderness, pain, and fever, all of which are aggravated by activity.

What you can do. Stay in bed, apply ice packs, and elevate the scrotum to improve drainage and relieve the pain. Your sex partner should also be treated, since the infection is quite often sexually transmitted.

What your physician can do. The prescription of an appropraite antibiotic usually is curative.

Spermatoceles

Spermatoceles, small cysts of the epididymis, are common in those over forty. One or more cysts can be felt through the scrotal wall. They are generally left alone because removal may injure the epididymis.

Disorders of the prostate, seminal vesicles, and urethra

Enlarged prostate

Ten percent of men at age forty have enlarged prostates, and this reaches almost 100 percent by age sixty. As the prostate increases in size, the caliber of the urethra (which lies within the prostate as it leaves the bladder) is narrowed, interfering with the flow of urine. The typical symptoms consist of difficulty in starting the flow of urine, reduced force of the urine stream, and dribbling of urine after voiding. Frequency of urination usually increases, especially at night.

Continued enlargement of the prostate poses several hazards. First, the bladder may not empty completely at the time of voiding, allowing stagnant urine to collect and become infected; second, increasing pressure within

1093

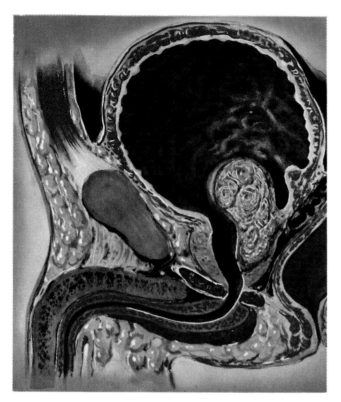

Section showing an enlarged prostate protruding into the urinary bladder.

the bladder to force urine out may cause back pressure in the ureters, thus damaging the kidneys; and third, sudden and complete blockage may prevent the outflow of urine (acute retention). For additional information on problems of the male urethra see page 1080.

What your physician can do. Since the gland enlarges gradually, have your physician determine the best time for prostatic surgery. In the usual procedure—trans-urethral prostatic resection (TURP)—an instrument is passed up the urethra and, with an electric loop, the prostate is removed from within its cap-

sule. The other method is to enter through the abdominal wall, just above the pubis, and remove the gland, passing through or below the bladder. Occasionally removal of the prostate may result in impotence.

Prostatitis

Prostatitis is an inflammation of the prostate that is generally secondary to an infection of the urethra. Since the prostate surrounds the urethra at its exit from the bladder, and many ducts carrying secretions from the prostate open into the urethra, the gland is vulnerable to infection. On rare occasions, germs are carried by the blood to the prostate from an infection elsewhere in the body.

Symptoms of **acute prostatitis** consist of pain at the base or even the tip of the penis, uncontrolled dripping of cloudy fluid, sometimes tinged with blood, from the urethra (originating in the prostate), slowness of the urinary stream, pain on urination, and usually fever. The prostrate is tender on physical examination. **Chronic prostatitis** often follows a bout of acute prostatitis, with symptoms of frequency, urgency, and pain on urination. However, there is no infection. The individual may experience heaviness and discomfort in the pubic and scrotal areas; the prostate may feel boggy and be congested with blood and stagnant prostatic secretions.

What your physician can do. He will prescribe an appropriate antibiotic to treat the infection. Hot sitz baths (see page 597) taken twenty minutes at a time three or four times a day will speed recovery. In chronic prostatitis sitz baths alone may be adequate.

Cancer of the prostate

Cancer of the prostate, the second most common form of cancer in men, is seen mostly frequently in those between sixty and eighty years of age. About 90,000 cases occur each year in the United States, with a mortality of almost 30 percent. Predisposing factors include family background, hormone imbalances, sexual activity, a high-fat diet, and possible viral exposure. The usual type is slow growing.

In its early stages, prostatic cancer produces no symptoms and is only detected by a routine examination of the prostate (palpated through the wall of the rectum), or when an enlarged prostate is being surgically removed, or through a needle biopsy. An enlarged prostate should be examined at least once a year.

The symptoms of cancer parallel those seen in an enlarged prostate, the most frequent being difficulty in passing urine. When undetected, the cancer tends first to spread to the bones of the pelvis and lower limbs, causing pain that may be mistaken for arthritis.

What you can do. Since recent findings suggest that a diet high in fat, especially animal fat, places one at a higher risk for cancer of the prostate, reducing the intake of foods high in animal fat (butter, lard, fatty cuts of meat, cheese) is advised.

What your physician can do. If the malignancy is found early and removed surgically the prognosis is excellent. Complete removal of the prostate carries the hazard of impotence. Other therapies include placing of radioactive iodine in the prostate, general radiation, anticancer drugs, and the removal of the testicles, since the male hormone (testosterone) stimulates cancer growth. Estrogen is also given to counter the male hormone. Removal of the testes and estrogen therapy both have a feminizing effect, together with impotence and a loss of libido.

Seminal vesicle problems.

Since the seminal vesicles are intimately associated with the prostate, infections of the prostate are almost always coupled with infections of the seminal vesicles. Infected urine coming from the kidneys or bladder and passing through the prostatic urethra leads to the invasion of one or both seminal vesicles. For the signs and symptoms of inflammation of the seminal vesicles, see under "prostatitis," page 1094, and "urethritis," page 1080. Other problems of the seminal vesicles are calculi, which occasionally obstruct their ducts, and very rarely, carcinoma.

CHAPTER **24**

Disorders of the female sex organs

Disorders of the ovaries

The ovaries produce the female sex cells (ova) and the sex hormones (estrogen, progesterone, and androgens). Thus they help to regulate the cyclic functioning of the sex organs and assist in the preservation of the female sex characteristics. When the hormones produced by the ovaries are either in short supply or superabundant, problems will arise regarding the menstrual cycle and the female sex attributes. As might be expected, these will differ, depending on the age of the person—before maturity, after maturity, or after menopause.

Hypofunction of the ovaries. In a genetic disorder called gonadal dysgenesis (Turner's syndrome), the ovaries do not develop adequately, thus hindering the transformation from girl to woman. The breasts fail to develop, hair in the pubic and axillary areas is sparse, and the usual monthly cycles are absent, so menstruation does not occur. Treatment

with estrogens will stimulate the development of the secondary female sex characteristics but does not produce ovulation, and therefore, the menstrual cycle does not occur.

The ovaries are interrelated functionally to other endocrine organs such as the pituitary, adrenal, and hypothalamus glands. Normally the hypothalamus activates the pituitary, which, in turn, stimulates the ovary to release an egg. Any factor such as emotional stress, severe illness, severe weight loss, drug abuse, strenuous exercise, or a brain tumor may affect the hypothalamus and thus upset the normal balance and timing of hormonal release. Low levels of thyroid function (hypothyroidism) may also interfere with normal menstrual cycles. The symptoms include irregular menses, infrequent menses, lack of menstruation (amenorrhea), and infertility. After determining the underlying problem, treatment often requires one or more hormones, given singly or in combination.

Hyperfunction of the ovaries. Certain tumors within the ovaries produce excess female or male sex hormones. **Feminizing tumors** can cause puberty to occur at an unusually early age. The breasts develop and menstruation begins at six to eight years of age. Should the tumor form during the child-bearing years, the symptoms are essentially irregular uterine bleeding. When the tumor appears after the menopause, bleeding resumes and is known as "false menstruation." The treatment is surgical removal of the tumor, or the ovary (oophorectomy) with the tumor, or sometimes both ovaries if both are involved. **Masculinizing tumors,** because of excess male hormones, cause the breasts to decrease in size, the voice to deepen, hair to grow on the face and chest, menstruation to cease, and the clitoris to enlarge. After the tumor has been removed, feminine characteristics are reestablished.

Ovarian cysts

Normally when a follicle bursts and releases an ovum, the remaining active follicles that do not rupture, disappear. When these fluid-filled blisters or follicles persist, they are called **follicular cysts.** These cysts may cause aching pelvic pain and occasionally abnormal uterine bleeding. Appropriate treatment with ovarian hormones corrects the problem. Should the cysts continue beyond two months, some other disorder of the ovary exists.

A rare ailment in which multiple cysts develop in both ovaries is called **polycystic ovarian disease.** It typically occurs between the ages of fifteen and thirty, and may result from failure to produce female sex cells. Symptoms include infertility, irregular or absent menstrual periods, and excessive weight gain. Hormone therapy may help to reestablish the normal menstrual cycle and correct the other problems. Sometimes surgical removal of portions of each ovary is helpful.

Ovarian tumors

Both benign and malignant tumors of the ovaries tend to be fluid-filled cavities (cysts). Although not life-threatening, because they do not spread to other parts of the body, **benign tumors** may grow to enormous size if not removed by surgery. One type of benign tumor, a teratoma or dermoid cyst, contains various body structures such as teeth, hair, and bones.

Four out of five **malignant tumors** of the ovary develop within the substance of the ovary. The other spreads from elsewhere in the body. Since they may not produce symptoms early, ovarian cancers are difficult to detect.

Depending on the size of the tumor and whether it is benign or malignant, symptoms result from pressure on the organs in the pelvis. These include a swelling in the lower abdomen, irregularities in the function of the bladder or bowels, a feeling of pelvic fullness, pain on intercourse, and displacement of the uterus. Pressure on the blood and lymph vessels may cause hemorrhoids, varicose veins, and swelling of the legs. As they develop, cancers cause loss of appetite, weight loss, general debility, pain in the pelvic area, and sometimes fluid in the abdomen.

Treatment of tumors is surgical removal, and if malignant, additional chemotherapy (medications which kill cancer cells) and radiation. To provide relief, the physician can draw off any fluid that might collect in the abdominal cavity. Because malignant ovarian tumors are frequently discovered late, the mortality rate is high.

Disorders of the oviducts (fallopian tubes)

Inflammation of the oviducts (pelvic inflammatory disease, salpingitis)

Since inflammation of the oviducts is rarely if ever confined only to the tubes, but involves the uterus, ovaries, and surrounding tissues, it is generally considered under the term **pelvic inflammatory disease** or **PID.** The infection is usually introduced by sexual intercourse, the most common germs being gonorrhea and chlamydia. Other organisms such as streptococcus and staphylococcus may also be responsible. The use of an intrauterine device (IUD), an abortion, or childbirth may initiate an infection. Often the cause is not known.

The infection travels by way of the vagina to the uterus, then through the tubes to the ovaries, and sometimes even into the pelvis (causing peritonitis). An abscess may form in the oviduct. If not promptly treated, the lumen of the oviduct becomes narrowed or even obliterated, interfering with fertilization and causing sterility. On occasion a fertilized ovum fails to pass through the

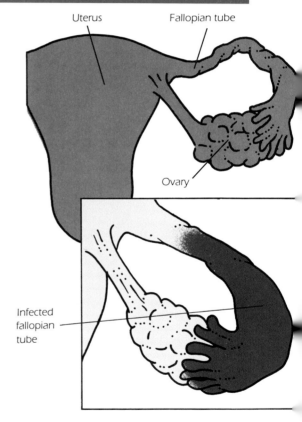

Section showing infection in the fallopian tube (oviduct).

oviduct to the uterus and a pregnancy develops within the tube (ectopic pregnancy). Infections sometimes enter the bloodstream causing blood poisoning. Gonorrheal arthritis and endocarditis are serious complications.

The symptoms vary somewhat with the infecting organism and whether the condition is acute or chronic. An acute infection causes severe pain in the lower abdomen, with tenderness, nausea, vomiting, chills, fever, rapid pulse, and a pussy discharge from the vagina. Symptoms of a chronic infection may include a dull pain in the pelvic area or low back, painful intercourse, irregular periods, and a foul-smelling vaginal discharge.

What your physician can do. In an acute infection he will probably have you hospitalized, where you will be kept in bed for a few days. After determining the infecting germ by culturing the vaginal discharge, he will prescribe the appropriate antibiotic to clear up the infection. Should the problem continue, an instrument is available to examine inside your abdomen for an abscess or other pocket of infection. Sometimes surgery is necessary to relieve the condition.

Resistance to the infection can be promoted by the use of hot sitz baths, in which you sit in hot water with the temperature gradually raised to tolerance. The sitz bath should last about twenty minutes and be repeated two or three times a day.

Ectopic pregnancy (tubal pregnancy)

When a fertilized ovum fails to pass through the oviduct to the uterus, development will begin wherever the sex cell happens to lodge, most commonly in the oviduct. Damage to the tube from a previous infection (see above) usually causes these ectopic or misplaced pregnancies, although previous surgery involving the tubes, the·use of an intrauterine device (IUD) for contraceptive purposes, or a congenital defect of the oviduct may be responsible.

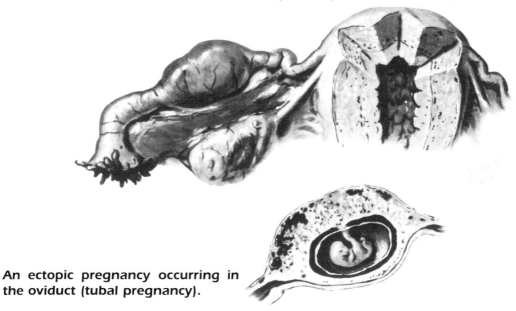

An ectopic pregnancy occurring in the oviduct (tubal pregnancy).

The tissues of the oviduct are not designed to maintain a pregnancy. After about three months the fetus grows to a size sufficient to rupture the tube, producing a life-threatening hemorrhage. Emergency surgery is the only satisfactory remedy, while the fetus perishes.

The symptoms include those of early pregnancy (see page 380), scanty "spotting" through the vagina of dark-colored blood, and cramping pain in one side of the lower abdomen beginning soon after the first menstrual period is missed. Should the tubal pregnancy have gone undetected, the evidences of rupture, besides those mentioned above, consist of marked, sudden, lower abdominal pain, with evidence of sudden hemorrhage. These include fainting, extreme weakness, thirst, profuse sweating, air hunger, failure to pass urine, and shock.

If the tubal pregnancy is detected early, the surgeon will remove the fetus and its membranes and repair the oviduct. It is not possible to save the fetus. After rupture has occurred, the hemorrhage must be stopped and the torn tissues repaired. A transfusion may be essential to restore blood volume and blood pressure.

Disorders of the uterus

Menstrual disorders

From the time a girl reaches puberty to the onset of menopause (termination of the reproductive period), normal cyclic losses of blood, called **periods** or **menstruation,** occur—usually monthly, except during pregnancy, active breast feeding, or use of birth control pills (see page 1088).

Absence of periods (amenorrhea)

In **primary amenorrhea** a girl who has reached the age of puberty fails to have her monthly periods. Possible causes include the failure of the sex organs to develop normally; abnormal functioning of the ovaries, pituitary, thyroid, or adrenal glands; a debilitating illness; excessive dieting (anorexia nervosa); obesity; strenuous exercise; severe emotional stress; and the use of certain drugs.

Secondary amenorrhea is an absence of periods in a woman who has previously menstruated regularly. While many causes parallel those resulting in primary amenorrhea, the most common cause is pregnancy. Adhesions or disease that interferes with the normal passage of the menstrual flow may also be responsible. With menopause, menstruation ceases completely.

What your physician can do. Since amenorrhea is a symptom and not a disease, your physician will determine the precise cause and institute the appropriate treatment. Some girls mature later than others, in which case no therapy is necessary. A pregnancy test will determine whether the individual is pregnant. The physician may prescribe single or multiple hormones to correct an endocrine disturbance. Amenorrhea does not preclude becoming pregnant because ovulation may occur at any time.

Infrequent periods (oligomenorrhea)

In this condition the periods are normal but occur less frequently than the usual eleven to thirteen each year. Low levels of estrogen are thought to cause the condition, which occurs most frequently during early puberty, following childbirth, and prior to menopause. Your physician can determine whether any intervention is needed.

Heavy periods (menorrhagia)

Heavy periods are common with many women, most having them regularly, some occasionally. The condition occurs more frequently when menstruation is being established and when menopause is imminent. Endocrine disturbances generally cause heavy periods in young women. Tumors of the uterus (fibroids, cancer), overgrowth of the lining of the uterus (endometriosis), ovarian cysts, and retention of a portion of the placenta after childbirth may also be responsible.

What your physician can do. He can assess the underlying cause. Hormones (estrogen and progesterone) may alleviate the problem. Other possible causes should be removed. A procedure in which the cervical canal is dilated and the uterine lining scraped away (dilation and curettage or D&C) often provides relief.

Painful periods (dysmenorrhea, menstrual cramps)

Dysmenorrhea is severe pain associated with menstruation. In **primary dysmenorrhea,** which includes the majority of women with painful periods, no actual disease or abnormality of the sex organs exists. Beginning soon after menstruation starts, it may continue throughout the reproductive period, although it frequently disappears following childbirth. Prostaglandins acting on the uterine wall are thought to cause the condition.

Secondary dysmenorrhea begins many years after normal menstruation (usually in the woman's thirties) and is usually caused by some disease such as inflammation of the sex organs, tumors of the uterus or ovary, or obstruction to the flow of menstrual fluid caused by scar tissue or tumor formation.

The symptoms, which vary in intensity, consist of intermittent, sharp, cramping pains that begin in the lower abdomen and extend to the lower back and thighs. In some women, nausea, vomiting, and diarrhea compound the suffering. The symptoms usually peak within twenty-four hours from the beginning of menstruation.

What you can do. You can help relieve the pain by the application of heat, either by fomentations (hot cloths, see page 590) or a heating pad over the lower abdomen and lower back, three or four times each day for twenty to thirty minutes at a time.

What your physician can do.

Your physician can determine what medications may be necessary. Substances that block the formation of the prostaglandins, which appear to cause the problem, usually provide effective relief. The physician must also discover and treat the cause of secondary dysmenorrhea.

Premenstrual syndrome (PMS, premenstrual tension)

PMS refers to a variety of symptoms appearing the week before menstruation. Positive changes include a feeling of well-being and an increase in energy and sexual desire. The negative physical and emotional changes vary widely. Physical symptoms include tenderness and swelling of the breasts, bloating, pelvic pain, headache, diarrhea or constipation, and swollen ankles. Emotional alterations include irritability, anxiety, and depression. With the onset of menstruation, these symptoms subside.

What you can do. You (and your spouse) should recognize the problem. Immediately before and during this period avoid stressful situations, obtain plenty of rest, get regular exercise, and cut down on your salt intake to minimize water retention. Keeping a daily record of your weight and major symptoms during this troublesome period will guide your physician in his efforts to help you.

What your physician can do. If no specific cause can be found, ovarian hormones (estrogen and progesterone) may give relief. Medications are also available to minimize breast discomfort.

Displacements of the uterus

The uterus normally tilts forward and lies above and behind the bladder. Four pairs of ligaments, muscles and fibrous tissue, and the fat contained in the pelvis hold it in position. Even so, the uterus may be displaced backward against the anal canal **(retroversion)** or sideways, or may settle downward **(prolapse).** In an extreme

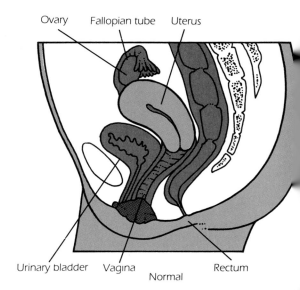

Ovary Fallopian tube Uterus

Urinary bladder Vagina Rectum

Normal

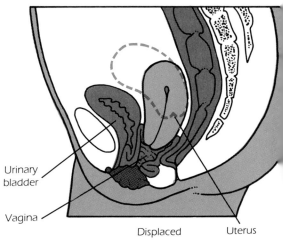

Urinary bladder

Vagina

Displaced Uterus

Positions of the uterus: normal and displaced.

prolapse the cervix may appear in the vulva. Loss of weight, weakening of the ligaments, and unrepaired lacerations due to childbirth are the chief causes of prolapse. Tumors may also push the uterus out of place.

Displacements of the uterus may cause no symptoms, or they may result in pelvic pain, backache, abnormal menstrual bleeding, and an inability to become pregnant.

What your physician can do. He may be able to manipulate your uterus into a more favorable position. If not, the supports of the uterus can be surgically reinforced to retain the organ in a normal position.

Trophoblastic disease

This rare condition in which placental cells grow excessively at the expense of the fetus occurs once in 2000 pregnancies in the United States, while in Asian countries it is ten times more frequent. When the growth is benign—about 80 percent of these cases—it remains within the cavity of the uterus. Called a **hydatidiform mole,** the growth consists of a mass of grapelike vesicles. In about 15 percent of cases, the growth invades the wall of the uterus and is called a **chorioadenoma.** In the remaining 5 percent, the highly malignant cells known as **choriocarcinomas** migrate in clusters to remote parts of the body.

The symptoms, occurring quite early in pregnancy, include excessive nausea and vomiting, very rapid enlargement of the uterus (faster than expected in normal pregnancy), and bleeding from the uterus beginning six to eight weeks after conception.

Often small grapelike fragments of the tumor break away from the larger mass and pass out of the vagina.

What your physician can do. Early diagnosis is important. He will order an ultrasound scan or X-rays, together with a urine test, to determine the presence of abnormal cells. Trophoblastic cells produce large amounts of a hormone HCG (normally made by the placenta), which appears in the urine and allows for monitoring the growths. The physician will remove benign tumors by a D&C (dilation and curettage, see page 1101). For two or more years you need frequent observation to check for recurrence. He will treat malignant tumors with chemotherapy and surgical removal of the uterus.

Endometriosis

In endometriosis, cells identical to those lining the uterus (endometrium) are present in other tissues such as the ovaries, oviducts, uterine wall **(adenomyosis),** vagina, and intestines. These cells respond to the hormones responsible for the sexual cycle and undergo the same monthly changes as does the endometrium.

Endometriosis is seen in women of child-bearing age. The condition may produce symptoms, or symptoms may first appear in the woman's mid-twenties. The most common symptom—pelvic pain during menstruation—appears after years of pain-free periods. Infertility and abnormal uterine bleeding also occur frequently. The isolated masses enlarge and bleed into the surrounding tissue, causing pain and eventually

1103

forming cysts followed by scarring. Over time, the scarring binds the tissues and organs containing the endometrial tissue together. These adhesions may, in turn, cause discomfort and pain.

What your physician can do. He will make a positive diagnosis by obtaining tissues from the uterine lining (by means of a D&C) and by a visual examination using a laparoscope, an instrument that is inserted through a small incision into the abdomen. Treatment with hormones that block the sex cycle may be adequate, especially in older women approaching menopause, when the problem will spontaneously cease. It may be desirable to surgically remove the endometrial tissue or even the organs containing the tissue.

Fibroids

Twenty percent of women over 35 have fibroids, which are the most frequent type of uterine tumors. Fibroid tumors consist of muscle tissue intermingled with varying amounts of fibrous tissue. Benign, round, and clearly delimited from the surrounding tissue, they range from small pea-sized growths to large tumors each weighing several pounds.

Several fibroids are usually present in the wall of the uterus or may even project into its cavity. When they are located in the lower part of the uterus, fibroids may cause problems during childbirth. When in the cervix (outlet of uterus), they may press upon the bladder or the rectum. When located within the body of the uterus, they usually cause profuse and prolonged bleeding, sometimes

menacing life from loss of blood.

The usual symptoms include a feeling of weight in the pelvis and chronic backache. Severe pain during menstruation accompanies excessive bleeding leading to chronic anemia. The tumor may cause a desire to urinate frequently or produce constipation, depending on whether it presses on the blad-

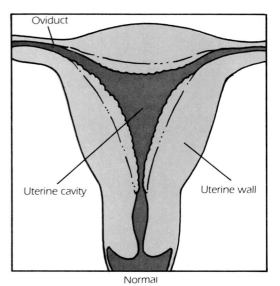

Normal

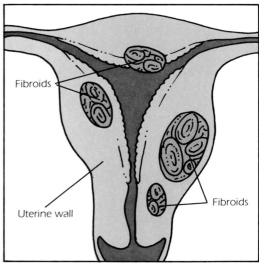

With fibroids

Fibroids in the wall of the uterus.

der or rectum. Fibroids may cause infertility and interfere with pregnancy when conception occurs. They may cause a miscarriage during the early months of pregnancy, or, if carried to term, complicate childbirth, requiring delivery by Caesarean section.

What you can do. Eat a good diet to help prevent anemia due to heavy blood loss. Check with your physician whether you may be anemic and whether you should take estrogens.

What your physician can do. Fibroids without symptoms may not require treatment. Regular checkups (perhaps twice yearly) are important. Following menopause, fibroids shrink and usually give no further trouble. Should your fibroid continue to enlarge and produce other symptoms, surgical removal may be necessary. Many fibroids can be removed without damage to the uterus. In cases of very large or multiple fibroids, depending on your age, the uterus should be removed **(hysterectomy).**

Cancer of the uterus

Cancer of the lining of the uterus (endometrium) is the second most common cancer of the female sex organs, exceeded only by cancer of the cervix. Some 35,000 new cases—most frequently women between the ages of 50 and 70—are seen each year in the United States with a mortality rate of a little under 10 percent.

The risk factors that predispose to endometrial cancer include obesity, never having been pregnant, hypertension, diabetes mellitus, a family history of cancer, late menopause, and long-term unopposed estrogen replacement therapy. Jewish women and women in the higher socioeconomic groups are also at higher risk. Any combination of these risk factors further increases the prospect of developing this cancer.

Abnormal uterine bleeding occurring after menopause or, in younger women, between periods, is the warning symptom of endometrial cancer. The flow may be watery and pink or thick and foul smelling, and may be associated with discomfort and "menstrual" pain.

What you can do. Report any abnormal bleeding to your physician. Seek his advice as to having regular **Pap smears,** a process in which cells shed from the cervix and uterus are examined microscopically. Pap smears are an effective indicator of cervical cancer, and they have also decreased the incidence of uterine cancer by earlier detection.

What your physician can do. He will confirm the diagnosis by a Pap smear or by examining tissue obtained from the endometrium (by means of a dilation and curettage or D&C). The usual treatment of uterine cancer is to surgically remove the uterus (hysterectomy), and, depending on your age and the extent of malignant involvement, the oviducts and ovaries. He may recommend radiation prior to or after surgery and, if the cancer has already spread, chemotherapy. If the cancer is detected early, more than 85 percent can be cured.

1105

Disorders of the uterine cervix

The cervix is the lower end of the uterus that protrudes into the vagina. The chamber of the uterus extends through the cervix as a narrow channel and opens through the cervical opening into the vagina.

Cervical erosion and eversion

Cervical erosion occurs when the epithelium is denuded or destroyed. The squamous cells normally covering the cervical opening are replaced by mucus-secreting cells that line the cervical canal. In some women these cells push out of the cervical opening, and this is known as cervical eversion. These mucus-secreting cells tend to be more susceptible to infection than the vaginal lining cells normally covering the cervix. The precise cause is not known, although childbirth and oral contraceptives seem to predispose to the condition.

What your physician can do. He will do a Pap smear to detect any abnormal change in the cells and a culture of the discharge to determine the type of infection, along with a physical examination. The condition may not require any treatment, or the erosion may be cauterized or frozen. He will prescribe an appropriate antibiotic to treat an infection.

Cervical dysplasia

Cervical dysplasia is an abnormal proliferation of cells at the junction of the mucous-secreting cells of the cervical opening and the squamous cells covering the cervix, which also line the vagina. Seen most often in women between 25 and 35 years of age, it is more common in those who also have cervical erosion. A Pap smear will detect any abnormal cells. If abnormal cells are present, your physician will examine your cervix with a special instrument (colposcope) and take a tissue sample (biopsy). If the cells are non-cancerous, you should have a Pap smear done yearly. If the cells are pre-cancerous, they can be removed by cautery, freezing, laser beam surgery, or occasionally by hysterectomy. A careful follow-up of dysplasia is important. A Pap smear should be done regularly (every six to twelve months) to detect recurrence or abnormal changes.

Cervical polyps

These pear-shaped growths in the cervical canal may result from injury during childbirth or from hormonal imbalance. Small polyps cause no problems. Large polyps may cause bleeding, infection, and infertility by blocking the passage of sperm. They are usually removed surgically on an out-patient basis.

Lacerations of the cervix

Lacerations of the cervix often occur during childbirth, and most such injuries heal without trouble. Extensive lacerations may become infected, causing **cervicitis.** Acute and chronic infections can occur, causing a pus-filled discharge from the vagina. The infection or irritation can spread to neighboring organs, causing itching and burning of the vulva and even cystitis (infection of the bladder). Treatment consists of an appropriate antibiotic and avoiding intercourse until healing has occurred. Old, unrepaired, eroded lacerations predispose to cancer. Problems of this type could be avoided if, following delivery, every mother received a pelvic examination to locate and repair any laceration.

Cancer of the cervix

The most common form of cancer of the sex organs, cervical cancer occurs during the reproductive and postmenopausal years. Of the more than 40,000 new cases seen annually, about one third invade the surrounding tissues, resulting in some 6,000 deaths. Predisposing factors include early teenage sexual activity, multiple sexual partners, multiple pregnancies, and previous pelvic disease, such as cervical dysplasia, genital warts, and herpes.

The symptoms consist of bleeding at times other than menstruation (after intercourse, between periods, and post menopause), an abnormal discharge from the vagina, painful intercourse, and pain in the pelvic region and back. If the cancer is widespread, loss of appetite, weight loss, and general debility may be present.

What you can do. One of the most important preventive measures is to have an annual Pap smear (see page 1105) and a gynecological examination at least every two years during childbearing years, and annually following menopause. Promptly report any abnormal bleeding from the vagina to your physician.

What your physician can do. Should a Pap smear show cancer cells, a tissue sample from the cervix (a biopsy) will be examined by a pathologist. Your physician will arrange appropriate treatment if the cells are cancerous. If the cancer is localized, it may be cauterized, frozen, or removed by laser or regular surgery. This may be followed by radiation. If the cancer has already invaded neighboring tissues, the uterus will be removed (hysterectomy), and possibly the oviducts and ovaries. The surgery will be followed by radiation therapy.

Disorders of the vagina

Vaginal discharge

A colorless and sometimes whitish discharge from the vagina occurs normally at the time of ovulation, during emotional stress, and as a response to estrogens. Blood indicates a more serious condition, such as a cancer. Normally there is an optimal balance between the acid and alkaline fluids in the vagina. Should this balance change appreciably, infections from yeastlike organisms and bacteria tend to develop. Promptly report any abnormal discharge to your physician.

1107

Vaginitis

Vaginitis is an inflammation of the vagina, most commonly caused by an infection. The consistency and color of the normal discharge is altered **(leukorrhea),** causing irritation, with itching and burning and possibly fever. A number of vaginal infections usually responsible for vaginitis are described below. Others are presented under "sexually transmitted diseases" (see page 1115).

Yeast infections (candidiasis, moniliasis). These yeastlike organisms multiply most readily when the acid and alkaline balance of the vaginal fluids is upset, and account for about half of all vaginal infections. Often the infection produces no symptoms; however, these infections appear more frequently in diabetic women and among those using oral contraceptives. Symptoms consist of vaginal burning and itching along with a white discharge. Intense itching of the labia minor, with swelling and redness, is also common.

Trichomoniasis. This protozoan infection constitutes about 10 percent of all vaginal infections. Symptoms are a frothy, yellow-green discharge with a foul smell, with swelling, redness, and itching of the vulva.

Chlamydial infections. These are caused by micro-organisms that are more closely related to bacteria than to viruses. Because the infection is common in men and spread to women through sexual activity, the sexual partner should also receive treatment. An infection of the urethra and vulva frequently accompanies the vaginitis it causes. The symptoms are similar to those of gonorrhea: pain in the lower abdomen, fever, and a thick, foul-smelling discharge. If the infection remains untreated, the ulcers that develop may cause scarring of the vagina.

Nonspecific vaginitis. This bacterial disorder constitutes more than 40 percent of vaginal infections. Typically very few symptoms appear, except for a foul-smelling, grayish, thick, milky vaginal discharge. Both sexual partners should receive treatment, and intercourse is unwise during therapy.

What you can do. Maintain your general resistance with regular exercise, adequate rest and sleep, a nutritious diet, and a generous intake of water. Keep your external genitals clean by washing daily with mild soap and water, and wear clean clothes that will not rub or chafe. Change tampons or pads frequently. Check with your physician regarding douching. The same rules of cleanliness apply to your sex partner. If you are troubled with yeast infections, you may help to restore your bacterial balance by use of cultured milk or yogurt or by taking capsules of *Lactobacillus acidophilus* (available in your pharmacy).

What your physician can do. He can determine by means of a physical examination and appropriate laboratory tests the offending organism and prescribe the specific antibiotic or medication.

Postmenopausal vaginitis. Following menopause the vaginas of some women partially atrophy, possibly due to inadequate estrogen production. The vagina narrows, the secretions diminish, and the lining becomes dry and cracked, often bleeding and even ulcerating. Symptoms include itching, burning, and a pink discharge. Infections may develop (atrophic vaginitis). Intercourse appears to help. In mild cases, vinegar douches may give relief. In severe cases, the physician may prescribe estrogen therapy.

Vaginal fistulas

A vaginal fistula is an abnormal opening between the vagina and the bladder or the urethra or the rectum. These fistulas develop from injuries, infections, radiation burns, or damage at childbirth. They allow urine to pass from the bladder and feces in the rectum into the vagina. Plastic surgery obliterates the opening.

Vaginal cysts

Two types of cysts commonly occur in the vagina. The most frequent are **duct cysts** (Gartner's duct), developing from remains of embryonic tissue, and **inclusion cysts,** occurring at sites of injury (from childbirth or surgery). These nonmalignant cysts can be surgically removed if they are troublesome.

DES therapy

DES or diethylstilbestrol is a synthetic estrogen that was used during the 1940s to prevent miscarriages. Later, evidence indicated that a few of the daughters born to mothers who had received DES during pregnancy showed an increase in the occurrence of vaginal cancer **(vaginal adeno-carcinoma).** Others developed overgrowth of the glandular tissue normally lining the cervical canal but now present in the vagina **(vaginal adenosis).** These women typically experience a vaginal discharge, infertility problems, and more frequent miscarriages. Women who know that their mothers received DES should be sure they have regular Pap smears and a periodic examination by a physician to reduce their risk of developing vaginal cancer.

Disorders of the vulva

The vulva includes the external sex organs: the labia major and minor, the area between the labia (vestibule), and the skin immediately surrounding the labia.

Itching (pruritus)

Itching in the area of the vulva is a common problem. Since it is not a disease but a symptom, the underlying cause must be determined and treated.

Response to irritants. The sensitive mucous membrane and skin of the vulva respond to chemicals that are directly irritant or to which sensitivity has developed (see page 973). These include irritating soaps, detergents, and hygiene sprays. The wearing of tight clothing and contact with synthetic fabrics may also cause problems. The skin itches severely, becomes swollen and inflamed, and later deteriorates and thickens **(vulvitis).** Because continued scratching intensifies the damage, the offending

1109

agent should be identified and removed. Creams containing steroids will provide temporary relief.

Hormonal imbalances. These occur most commonly in post-menopausal women, but are sometimes seen in younger women. The skin at first is thick, dry, and red. Later the tissues become thin, smooth, and shiny and may develop white patches **(leukoplakia).** Scratching aggravates the intense itching, due possibly to a lack of estrogens, and testosterone. Washing with cool water (use mild soap only occasionally), drying gently, and applying a cream or lotion containing these hormones should provide relief. A physician should check periodically that no malignant change in the affected areas is taking place.

Infections. Infections involving the vagina and often the vulva frequently cause itching. Examples are yeast infections and trichomonas (see page 1108). For relief of itching the infection should be treated.

Cancer. Cancer involving tissues of the vulva may cause itching, and may actually be an early symptom. Cancer in this area occurs most commonly between the ages of fifty and sixty. Regular checkups by your physician are important.

Skin disorders. A number of general skin diseases and pubic lice may also involve the vulva and produce itching (see pages 982). Treatment should be directed to the main skin ailment.

Bartholin's gland infection

The Bartholin's glands, one on each side of the vaginal opening, lie within the wall of the vestibule toward the back of the labia minor. Their function is to produce mucus, which moistens and lubricates the tissues of this area. They are vulnerable to infections, especially to gonorrhea, though other bacteria may be involved. The gland becomes red, swollen, very painful, and discharges pus. Should the duct become obstructed an abscess may form.

What your physician can do. He can identify the infecting organism and prescribe the appropriate antibiotic. Hot sitz baths and ice packs will provide some relief. If an abscess has formed, he can drain it by a minor surgical procedure. Should a cyst **(Bartholin's cyst)** later develop and become troublesome, it can be removed surgically.

General disorders

Hot flash

Many women experience a "hot flash" periodically following menopause. The episodes are short, during which there is profuse sweating and a feeling of intense heat. The hot flash may come on at any time, even during deep sleep, leaving the woman hot and awake. In most women, both the frequency and the intensity of the episodes gradually diminish. If they are frequent and severe, see your physician.

CHAPTER 25

Sex problems of men and women

Problems related to successful intercourse can have both physical and emotional causes. The sex act is a highly complex physiological and psychological achievement, and numerous factors may interfere with its desirable performance. Since sexual intercourse normally requires a man and a woman, the physical well-being and emotional state of each of the consenting partners plays a major role in the type of relationship required for a mutually satisfying outcome.

Hormonal influences on sexual desires and activity play an important part in sexual interrelationships. While some problems respond to specific hormones, many do not. Surgical procedures related to the sex organs, a number of diseases, physical and mental fatigue, general debility, the intake of certain medications, the abuse of drugs, and alcohol consumption may have an adverse affect on sexual activity.

At least 50 percent of the time the problem is related to the psychological and emotional attitudes of one or both of the partners. Anxiety (fear of pregnancy, fear of an unsuccessful sexual outcome), insecurity, interpersonal frictions, lack of love and intimacy prior to intercourse—all of these may have a negative influence on one or more phases of the sexual encounter and make the outcome less than satisfactory.

Sex problems of men

The common disorders relate to ejaculation, which is premature or delayed, and to erection, which is weak, too brief, or absent.

Ejaculation. Early or **premature ejaculation** is a very common problem. The man's arousal is such that he is unable to control the time of ejaculation, which occurs prior to or immediately after entry. This is unsatisfactory to both partners, but especially for the woman, who generally requires a longer period for arousal. At the other extreme, delayed or **retarded ejaculation** occurs when the erection is maintained for a prolonged period before ejaculation eventually occurs. Here again, although the man may derive some satisfaction, it is usually distressing to both parties, the moment of climax often having come and gone for the spouse.

While these disorders have no harmful effect on general health, they tend to make the man feel less manly and destroy the pleasure of intercourse. The man becomes anxious to prove himself, and this only compounds the problem. Premature ejaculation can be overcome by cooperative endeavor. The man, by practice, does not allow himself to be aroused too rapidly and suppresses the urge until the appropriate time. The woman restrains herself from arousing her spouse too soon. Both attempt to enjoy lovemaking without too great anxiety for the actual sexual act itself.

In delayed ejaculation, anxiety may hinder the time of release. The pleasure of intimacy should be enjoyed to its height without anxiety as to the point of fulfillment or fear of criticism from the partner. At this time both partners must encourage each other to reach orgasm without allowing thoughts of failure to spoil their pleasure.

Impotence

Impotence is the inability of a man to attain or maintain a satisfactory erection. A number of conditions contribute to this frustrating problem, including surgery of the prostate, endocrine disturbances that reduce circulating testosterone (cirrhosis of the liver, testicular disorders), certain medications (diuretics, tranquilizers), high blood pressure, atherosclerosis (which decreases the blood supply that is needed for erection), certain diseases affecting the spinal cord, the persistent use of drugs, alcoholism, and physical fatigue.

Psychological and emotional factors play an equally important role in causing impotence. These include loss of sexual desire, feelings of insecurity and inferiority, fear of the consequence of intercourse, lack of cooperation by the sexual partner, a recurring sense of guilt over some previous sexual engagement or ongoing infidelity, marital disagreements, disparagement of the man's virility by the woman, family quarrels, and a life schedule so hectic that romance and lovemaking are secondary activities.

What you can do. You should attempt to eliminate those factors which you and your spouse can control. The goal should be closeness and intimacy in an atmosphere of emotional warmth, with all their associated pleasures, not merely a demand for intercourse and physical satisfaction.

What your physician can do. He can determine whether an underlying physical cause exists, and if it does he will provide appropriate therapy. Wise and understanding counsel is often both needed and

1112

helpful to resolve the emotional problems that so frequently exist. Should the cause be solely organic, the doctor may advise the use of an artificial device (requiring surgery) to obtain an erect penis.

Sex problems of women

While many of the factors causing sex problems in men also cause sex problems in women, many distinct differences exist in the types of female sex disorders and in the situations that tend to precipitate them. A woman can passively accept the sexual attentions of a man, making believe that she is responding, but this a man cannot do. Most women appear to have a greater dependence on the male to bring about their sexual arousal and subsequent fulfillment. Given the appropriate circumstances, women will respond more readily than men, both emotionally and physically.

The common sex problems of women are difficulty in arousal, pain during intercourse, and failure to have orgasm (reach the climax of sexual excitement).

Arousal

Ideally, arousal is the response of a person to a person when the union is both intimate and committed. The thoughts should be for each other, the touching and caressing should be pleasurable, and the glance of desire should suggest, "Go on." The emotions aroused are associated with change in the sex organs. Thus, sexual arousal is a response of the organs to the pleasurable thoughts and sensations that are occurring as the couple moves toward the sexual act,

when the body takes control.

The same factors mentioned above that negate orgasm in a woman will also hinder her arousal. These, together with others such as jealousies, resentments, misunderstandings, inattentions, lack of reciprocity and esteem for each other, and the fear of becoming pregnant, all hamper arousal in women.

Pain

Pain during intercourse will seriously affect the prospect of a woman experiencing successful and pleasurable sex. Among the conditions that may cause discomfort and pain are infections of the external genital organs (the clitoris, vulva, labia, and Bartholin glands) and the vagina. Irritations may be caused by contraceptive materials (foams, tablets) and by douching solutions. Occasionally involuntary contraction of the vaginal muscles (vaginismus) will cause pain. In postmenopausal women the labia and vaginal outlet may lose elasticity and become shrunken, and the lining of the vagina itself may become atrophied (senile vaginitis), losing its normal lubrication. In all of these situations, intercourse becomes painful and sexual pleasure is reduced or vanishes altogether.

Other causes of pain during intercourse may be inadequate lubrication, heavy-handed manipulation of the clitoris, masturbation, and a disproportionately long male organ (penis) for the woman's vagina. If any of these problems exist, see your physician.

Orgasm

Orgasm is the height of sexual excitement and fulfillment, at which time the uterus and the muscles in adjacent areas rhythmically contract, and the woman feels a sense of deep satisfaction. Women fall into three categories: those who have never experienced an orgasm; those who have but no longer do; and those who sometimes do and sometimes don't.

When a woman fails to achieve an orgasm, both parties may feel they have let the other down. Anxiety over achievement in itself is self-defeating. The various responses of the sex organs during intercourse are not under voluntary control, but are under the control of the emotional nervous system (autonomic). It is therefore desirable that the partners provide an emotional environment of loving acceptance for each other, each wishing to make the other's enjoyment full. This in itself will help in attaining mutual satisfaction.

Each having a knowledge of his or her own sex organs, as well as those of the other, and sharing with each other the behaviors which each enjoys and responds to the most, are important conditions to successful achievement. Anxieties regarding the other's fidelity, fear of pregnancy, hostile interrelationships, business and family concerns, pressures of life, and fatigue all have a negative effect on sexual fulfillment.

CHAPTER 26

Sexually transmitted diseases

Sexually transmitted diseases are contagious diseases transmitted primarily through sexual intercourse with a partner carrying the infecting organism. These infections may also result from oral or anal sex, or they may be passed by the mother to her infant during pregnancy (syphilis) or at the time of childbirth (gonorrhea).

While somewhat localized, some of these diseases may spread to various tissues and organs of the body and have serious and life-threatening consequences. With prompt and appropriate treatment, gonorrhea and syphilis can be cured, but delay may lead to long-term complications.

The infected person should abstain from sexual activity until his physician indicates otherwise, lest innocent people be exposed and the disease be further spread. Your physician or a special clinic handling these diseases will provide treatment for you and for all those known to have been exposed. All information is held in professional confidence.

The number of people suffering from sexually transmitted diseases has greatly increased in recent years. Several factors contribute to this increase: popular methods of contraception reduce the fear of pregnancy; deteriorating moral standards encourage extramarital and premarital sex; the media (TV, videos, pornographic literature) promote loose sexual behavior; and increased use of drugs and alcohol weakens inhibitions.

Gonorrhea

In the United States, gonorrhea (called the clap) is pandemic. While over two million cases are reported each year, officials estimate that only one in three unmistakable infections are registered. In addition, it is believed that approximately one third of those infected experience such mild symptoms, or no symptoms at all, that they fail to seek treatment, yet are capable of transmitting the disease.

The majority of infections result from sexual intercourse and occur

1115

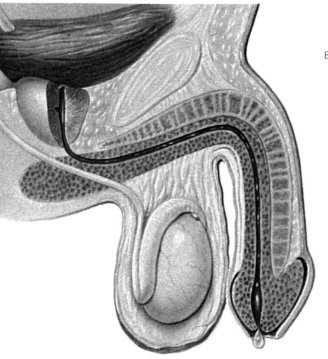
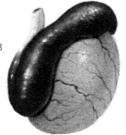
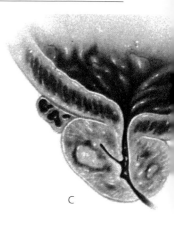

Male sex organs showing inflammation in the urethra, prostate, and epididymis.

most frequently in the urethra of the man and the cervical canal of the woman. Because of anal and oral sex, the rectum and pharynx are also frequently involved. During delivery, a mother may infect her baby. The infant's eyes are most vulnerable, as the disease may cause blindness. Hence the mandatory required treatment at birth.

In men the initial symptoms, typically appearing in two to six days, include itching at the outlet of the urethra, burning on urination, and discharge of thick, yellow, pussy fluid from the urethra. If untreated, frequency and urgency of urination may develop, with the infection spreading to the prostate and epididymis. A long-term complication is urethral stricture.

In women the first symptoms appear usually in three to ten days and consist of pain on urination, pain in the vagina, and a profuse yellow-green, foul-smelling discharge from the vagina. Common complications, infection of the oviducts (**salpingitis**) and pelvic inflammatory disease (see page 1098), may lead to an ectopic pregnancy or to permanent infertility.

Infection in the mouth and pharynx causes sore throat and tonsillitis. In gonorrhea of the rectum the infection produces a constant desire to go to stool and the passing of pussy fluid. Should the germs enter the bloodstream, the disease may affect the heart, joints, bones, and other organs, causing endocarditis, infectious arthritis, osteomyelitis, and meningitis.

What you can do. See your physician promptly should you suspect an infection. Refrain from intercourse until your physician advises otherwise. Practice scrupulous hygiene to prevent towels, toilet seats, or unwashed hands from spreading the infection to infants and children. Refrain from beverage alcohol.

What your physician can do. He will make the diagnosis by both a physical examination and a laboratory test. Antibiotics prove effective in most cases. Unfortunately, resistant strains of gonococcus imported from other countries increase the problem of treating these organisms.

Syphilis

Syphilis is the oldest, and, until the advent of AIDS, the most serious of the sexually transmitted diseases. In the fifteenth century it was disseminated in Europe in epidemic proportions by the soldiers and sailors of that era. Despite the effectiveness of treatment by antibiotics, 100,000 new cases are reported annually in the United States, with more than an another estimated 300,000 untreated cases.

Syphilis is caused by *Treponema pallidum,* a spiral-shaped germ that survives only in human tissues. The bacteria enter the body through the mucous membranes of the urethra (penis), vagina, and mouth, or through broken skin, and are acquired most frequently by sexual intercourse. During the last five months of pregnancy the disease is readily transmitted from the infected mother to the fetus.

When untreated, the disease progresses in three stages. The incubation period, or the time when the

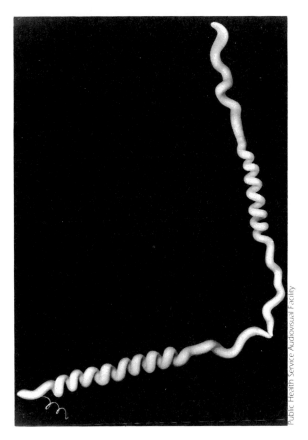

A spirochete (greatly magnified). The germ that causes syphilis.

person is infected to the appearance of the first lesion, averages approximately three to four weeks (but can range from ten to sixty days).

First stage. The first sign of syphilis is the appearance of a papule, which soon becomes a small, painless red ulcer, with raised firm edges. The ulcer is called a chancre (pronounced "shanker"). In men it usually appears on the penis; in women, on the cervix or in the vagina, and occasionally on the breasts. It may occur in the mouth or rectum in either sex. Swollen lymph nodes in the groin, neck, or armpits generally accompany the chancre,

1117

which spontaneously heals in one to six weeks. Because the ulcerated area is filled with germs, the condition is highly infective.

Second stage. From two to six weeks after the chancre heals, a generalized rash develops (on the skin, palms, soles, and membranes) that lasts two to six weeks. The rash consists of small, raised, red, scaling lesions that do not itch. The lymph nodes enlarge, and round, slightly raised, painless gray plaques appear on the lips, in the mouth, and on the skin of the vulva and glans of the penis. The sufferer generally feels ill and has a loss of appetite, headache, and fever. The spleen, liver, eyes, and coverings of the brain (meninges) may become involved. The lesions, which heal in three or four weeks on the average, are filled with germs, as in the first stage, making the sufferer highly infective.

Third stage. The disease becomes quiescent for a variable length of time in the so-called latent or late stage. It may continue to be contagious during the first four or so years of this latent stage, with an occasional return to the mucocutaneous lesions of the second stage. For the most part the person remains symptom-free during this time, which may extend for two years to a lifetime, even though the germs are present in the tissues.

Usually in about twenty years the disease suddenly flares up. While any organ can be affected, the nervous and cardiovascular systems are most often targeted. The effect on the brain can result in paralysis, insanity, senility, and loss of the sense of position and of feeling in the legs. This may be accompanied with sharp, excruciating pains (tabes dorsalis) in the abdomen. Joint surfaces, such as of the knees, may disintegrate. The large vessel that leaves the heart (aorta) weakens and dilates, and the heart valves themselves may be attacked.

Another tragic result of untreated syphilis is the transmission of the disease to the fetus. A fetus carried by a syphilitic mother has a 70 to 90 percent chance of acquiring congenital syphilis during the last five months of pregnancy. The symptoms appear during the first two years of life and include skin lesions, blood-stained "snuffles" (runny nose), hydrocephalus, convulsions, mental retardation, bone changes, blindness, deafness, and malformed teeth. Thus the expectant mother has a compelling reason to submit to tests for syphilis very early in her pregnancy and to receive adequate treatment when indicated.

Tests are available to determine the presence of syphilis. In stage one, the organisms can be seen with a microscope in scrapings from a chancre. In the second and third stages, samples of blood or spinal fluid can be processed to detect the presence of an active syphilitic infection.

What you can do. Should you be infected, you should seek prompt and adequate treatment with a monitored follow-up. You should insist that all sexual partners be notified, examined, and, if necessary, treated.

What your physician can do. Antibiotic therapy with penicillin is

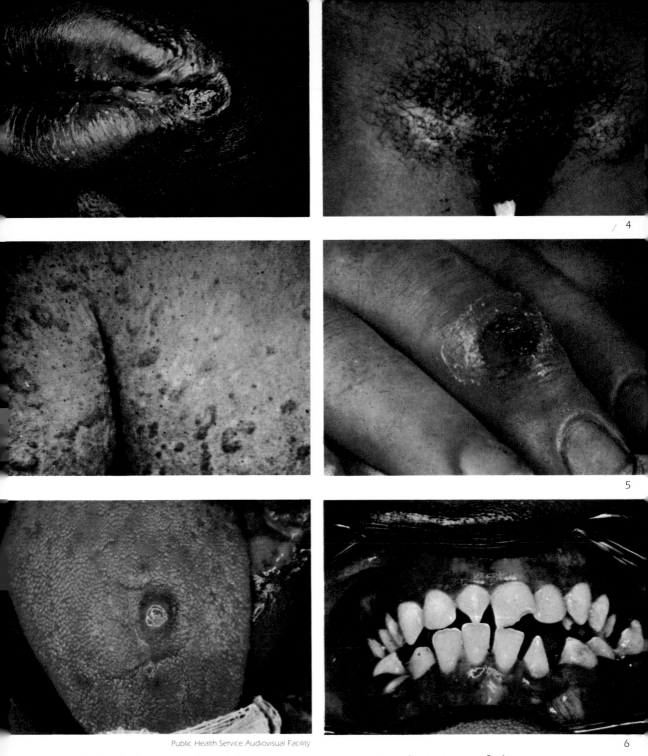

Public Health Service Audiovisual Facility

6

Manifestations of syphilis as they appear on various parts of the body: (1) chancre on the lip; (2) blotches on the skin; (3) chancre on the tongue; (4) swollen lymph nodes of the groin; (5) chancre on the finger; and (6) notched, peg-shaped teeth (the latter a condition typical of syphilis acquired prior to birth).

effective in controlling and eliminating the disease. It may be essential to continue treatment over a period of time.

Chlamydial infections

Chlamydia are microorganisms (not bacteria, viruses, or fungi) most closely related to bacteria since they respond to antibiotics and sulfonamides. Chlamydial infections are increasingly common sexually transmitted diseases that can infect the urethra, epididymis, cervix, anus, and oral cavity, and frequently cause pelvic inflammatory disease (PID). Both a blood test (serum antibody response) and culture method can determine the presence of the infection. The sufferer and all sexual partners should be treated.

Lymphogranuloma venereum has an incubation period of about three weeks. A small papule or painless ulcer develops on the genital organs (penis or labia), which heals rapidly and may even go unnoticed. A general feeling of illness follows, with fever and swollen lymph nodes in the groin of the male and around the anus in the female. The skin turns purplish, breaks down, and forms persistent, painful, draining ulcers. If untreated, healing is slow, and scarring and strictures may develop in the urethra, vagina, anus, and rectum. Infections in the mouth or throat may result in ulcerations of the lymph nodes in the neck. Antibiotic therapy using tetracycline is curative.

Nonspecific urethritis (NSU) or **nongonococcal urethritis (NGU)** is an inflammation of the urethra similar to gonorrhea but with less pain and a more mucous (less pussy) discharge. In women, inflammation of the cervical canal with a discharge of pus and mucus may occur. Sometimes men, but more often women, exhibit no symptoms. Untreated, the infection usually subsides in six to eight weeks. Effective treatment is with antibiotics.

Genital herpes

Genital herpes, an extremely common infection, accounts for 10 to 15 percent of all sexually transmitted diseases. The virus causing genital herpes (Herpes simplex type 2) is very similar to the virus causing cold sores (Herpes simplex type 1).

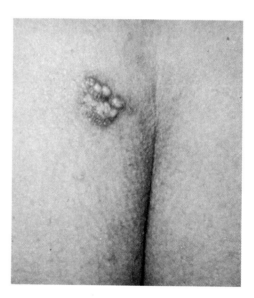

Genital herpes simplex, vesicles occurring on the buttocks.

Spread from a sexual partner during the active phase, the virus enters through any crack in the mucosa. The lesions first develop about a week later (from 2 to 20 days). In men they occur on the penis or scrotum. In women they appear on the labia and the skin around the anus. The skin or membrane reddens, and many tiny vesicles (blisters filled with fluid) erupt. These soon break down to form small, painful ulcers, which later crust and heal spontaneously in about ten days. Headache, fever, and muscle pains accompany the outbreak, and neighboring lymph nodes are tender and swollen. Subsequent attacks become progressively milder.

The virus, however, remains latent in the local nerves. The disease recurs subsequently during times of low resistance, menstruation, pregnancy, local injury, or emotional stress.

In women two serious complications may occur—one to her infant, the other to herself. If the infection is active at the time of childbirth, 10 to 50 percent of infants may become infected from lesions in the cervix or vagina. Of these, some may become blind, develop encephalitis, or become mentally retarded; up to 50 percent may die. It is safest for a mother with active herpes to be delivered by cesarean section. Because a woman with genital herpes has a fivefold higher risk of developing cancer of the cervix, she should have a Pap test at least yearly to detect any early cancerous changes.

What you can do. Bathe the external genital area with mild soap and water, dry gently, and apply a soothing ointment suggested by your physician. Refrain from intercourse from the earliest sign of infection until two weeks after the last symptom has disappeared.

What your physician can do. He can make a positive diagnosis by examining the tissue from a sore or by means of a laboratory culture. Since there is no cure, the treatment consists of relieving the symptoms. He may prescribe a medication (acyclovir) as a lotion, ointment, or capsule. It tends to hasten recovery, relieve symptoms, and prevent recurrent attacks. He may suggest the use of a preparation containing a local anesthetic to relieve severe pain.

Genital warts (condyloma acuminatum)

These soft, pink clusters of wartlike overgrowths develop in the moist areas of the genitalia. Caused by a virus related to those that cause common skin warts, they are transmitted by sexual contact and develop within about three months after exposure to an infected person. In women the cauliflowerlike lesions may become so large as to interfere with childbirth. In rare cases they may become malignant.

What your physician can do. He may paint small warts with a chemical that dries them. He will remove larger warts by freezing, electrocautery, or laser surgery.

Pubic lice
See page 982.

AIDS (acquired immune deficiency syndrome)
See page 830.

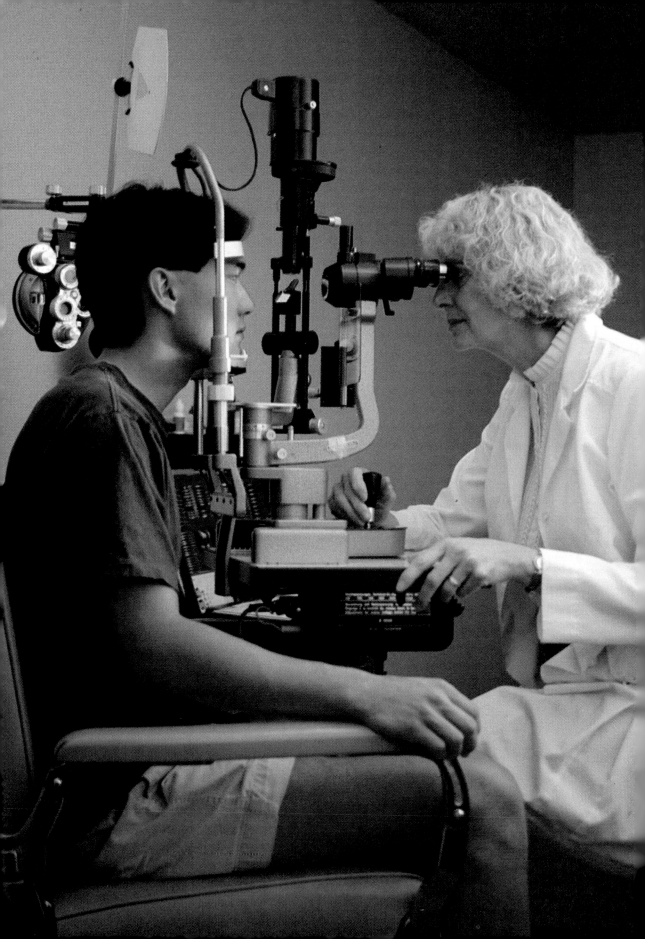

VOL. 3

SECTION 6

THE SENSE ORGANS
AND THEIR DISORDERS

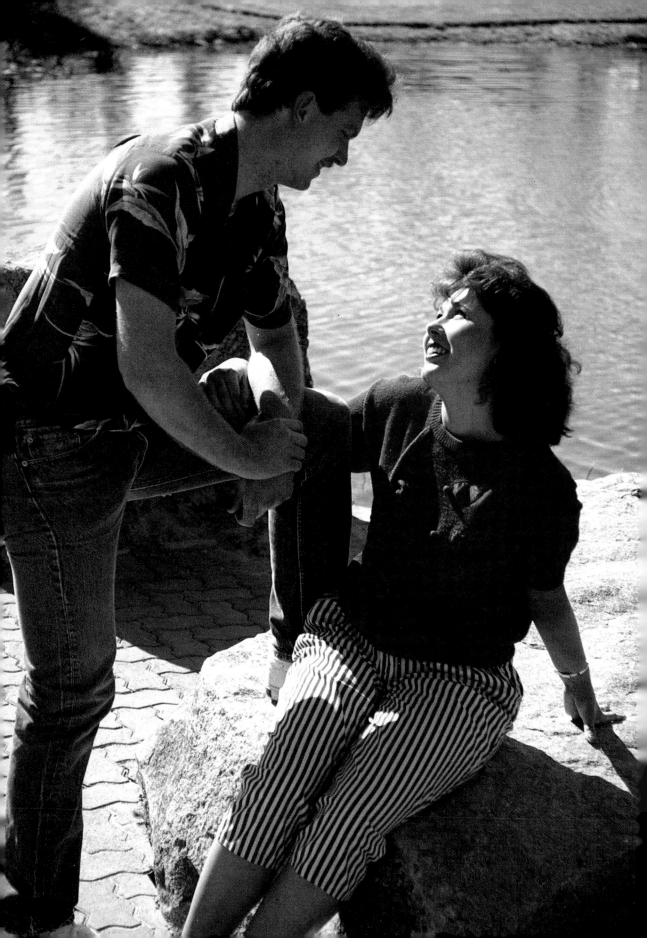

CHAPTER 27

The eye and its disorders

In order to function effectively, the brain must receive information from within the body as well as from outside it. (The brain and its functions have been described elsewhere.) The organs of sensation provide this information by picking up and transmitting to the brain events transpiring in the body's internal and external environments.

Each sense has its own specially designed receptors either scattered widely in body tissues or concentrated in specially designed structures. Each type detects a different signal, converts it to an electric impulse, and transmits it to specific areas of the brain where the particular sensation is perceived. In this way the eyes sense light to see; the ears detect sound to hear; the tongue and nose are sensitive to chemicals for sensing taste and smell; the semicircular canals (part of the inner ear) detect fluid movement for balance and equilibrium; and the skin and other tissues selectively relay signals for touch, cold, heat, position, and pain.

This chapter discusses the eye and its disorders, and subsequent chapters in this final section will discuss the other senses.

The eyes

Of all the senses, sight is the most important, evidenced by the fact that more cortical space has been devoted to vision than to any other sensory function. With normal vision we appreciate the shape, the color, and the movements of the objects and persons around us.

The eye, a highly complex and intricately functioning "camera," operates instantly and automatically, but can, be overridden by the brain. The eyeball itself is a sphere, slightly less than an inch (2.4 cm) in diameter, lying within a bony socket (orbit), well protected against injury. Muscles sur-

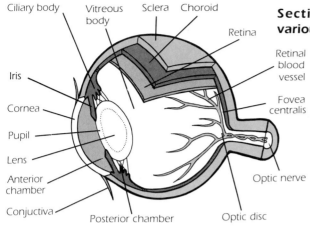

Ciliary body
Vitreous body
Sclera
Choroid
Retina
Retinal blood vessel
Fovea centralis
Iris
Cornea
Pupil
Lens
Anterior chamber
Conjuctiva
Posterior chamber
Optic disc
Optic nerve

Section through the eye, showing its various parts.

blink every few seconds, acting like windshield wipers, keeping dust and other particles from injuring the cornea and preventing it from drying. The "tears" normally drain into two tiny ducts that open on the inner margins of the lids, except when an individual cries, at which time they overflow and run down the cheeks.

The space inside of the hollow eyeball is divided by the lens and its attachments into two compartments. The small **anterior chamber,** lying between the cornea and the lens, is filled with a clear, watery fluid (aqueous humor), which flows from behind the iris out to the pupil. The **iris,** lying in contact with the front of the lens, is a circular structure that consists of longitudinal and circular muscle fiber with an opening in the middle, the **pupil.** The iris appears blue, gray, or brown and gives color to the eyes. The pupil controls the amount of light entering the eye; depending on the intensity of light, it can adjust in size from a pinpoint in bright light to wide open in the dark.

rounding the eyeball move it in whatever direction desired.

In front of the eye the upper and lower **eyelids** act like shutters, closing rapidly to prevent injury, and opening to expose the front of the eyeball and to allow light to enter. **Eyelashes** grow along the margins of the eyelids, improving appearance and acting as feelers that cause one to blink at any closely approaching object. The very edges of the margins are lubricated with an oily substance that prevents the tears from running over on the cheek (except when produced in excess) and seals the eyelids so that no air can contact the eye during sleep.

A smooth membrane, called the **conjunctiva,** covers the underside of the eyelids and folds back on itself to cover the entire outer surface of the eyeball (the sclera) or white of the eye, except at the very front, where it bulges forward to form the transparent **cornea.** Fluid coming from the **lacrimal** or **tear glands,** located under the outer edge of each upper eyelid, constantly moistens the cornea and conjunctiva. The eyelids

The eye showing a dilated and constricted pupil.

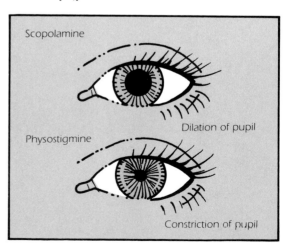

Scopolamine

Dilation of pupil

Physostigmine

Constriction of pupil

1126

The large **posterior chamber,** which lies behind the lens and forms the back three-fourths of the eyeball, is lined by the retina and is filled with a clear, jellylike substance called the vitreous humor.

The **cornea,** really a lens, is a thin membrane, clear and strong. The crystalline **lens,** shaped like a lentil, is located between the cornea and the retina and is composed of translucent elastic fibers. In a camera the lens must be moved forward or backward in order to focus on near or distant objects. But the lens of the eye does this by thickening or thinning, accomplished by the pull of the ciliary muscle located within the eye.

The posterior chamber, filled with a jell-like substance, the **vitreous,** is lined by the **retina,** which corresponds to the film in a camera. The retina consists of ten layers of paper-thin, highly complex nervous tissue. Within these layers, each eye contains some 7 million cone cells and 125 million rods cells. The cones detect both light and color, while the rods discern only light. Because there are fewer cones, as light fails, the ability to distinguish color is lost. Deep in the retina, the choroid, a layer of blood vessels, provides nourishment to the retina. Between these layers is a thin brown-pigmented layer of cells that prevents light being reflected from one part of the retina to another.

In the center of the retina a small depression, called the **fovea** or **macula,** is the point of precise vision, where the object focused on is seen. Color vision resides in the vi-

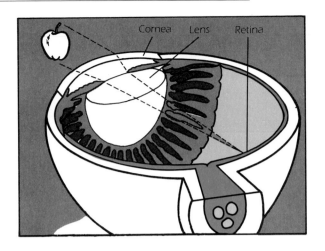

Diagram showing how reflected light from an object is focused on the retina.

cinity of the fovea, where the cones are concentrated. The rest of the retina consists of the area of imprecise vision, which is extremely important because it provides perspective for what is being viewed.

Light, reflected from an object, passes through the cornea and lens, both of which bend or refract the light, bringing it to focus in the fovea. The light now activates a chemical process in the rods and cones, converting the light waves to electrical impulses. These impulses are then carried through each optic nerve to the seeing center of the brain, where what is being viewed is perceived. This image may be acted upon immediately or stored in the memory bank for some future occasion.

Each eye has six muscles located within the orbit and attached to the outside of the eyeball. These muscles are under voluntary control

1127

so the eyes can be moved in any direction. The eyes work in unison so that when the right eye looks outward, the left eye looks inward, both focusing on the desired object. The space between the two eyes (base line) is fixed and is about 2 inches (10 cm). Using the angles made by the line of vision of each eye with the base line, the brain can, by rapid computations, determine the size of an object, whether it is close or at a distance, whether it is moving toward or away from the viewer. The brain can also tell the approximate speed at which the object is traveling. This binocular vision also gives the advantage of depth perception.

Signs and symptoms of eye disorders

The eye is composed of many components, any one of which may be affected by either infections or injuries. Structural abnormalities may be present at birth or may develop over time. Some disorders may be inconvenient, while others may impair vision or even cause its loss. It is extremely important to protect the eyes from harm.

The eyes are unique in that they not only have disorders of their own, but often reveal problems existing elsewhere in the body, such as high blood pressure, diabetes, and jaundice of the liver. The following are common signs and symptoms.

Smarting, burning, and itching. See under "conjunctivitis," "corneal disorders," "eyelid disorders," and "refractive errors."

Pain. See under "injury," "ultraviolet burns," "corneal ulcer," "iritis," and "acute glaucoma."

Light intolerance (photophobia). See under "corneal ulcer" and "iritis."

Color changes (greenish yellow). See under "liver disorders—jaundice," and "excess provitamin A."

Protruding eyes. See under "tumor of the eye" and "hyperthyroidism."

Red eye. See "conjunctivitis," "allergy (hay fever)," "foreign body in eye," "chemical irritants," "corneal ulcer," and "iritis."

Bloodshot eye. See under "hemorrhage (conjunctiva)."

Cross-eye, walleye, squint. See under "strabismus and amblyopia."

Reading difficulties. See under "refractive difficulties."

Blurred vision. See under "glaucoma," "cataract," "iritis," "retinal disorders," and "refractive errors."

Spots. See under "vitreous humor," "retinal detachment," "retinal hemorrhage."

Halos. See under "glaucoma."

Tearing. See under "conjunctivitis," "corneal ulcer," "ectropion," "entropion," "iritis," "lachrymal duct blockage," "allergic reactions," "foreign body," and "chemical irritants."

Safety measures

Some 30,000 to 40,000 injuries to the eyes occur each year, of which 90 percent could have been prevented. Some injuries are temporary, while others may cause partial or total loss of sight.

Well-fitting goggles are without doubt the cheapest and most effective means of protecting the eyes against a wide variety of injuries. When using power tools or walking through brush, one can wear them over one's prescription glasses. Swimming goggles can protect against chemical burn from the chlorine in swimming pools and against infections in open water.

Corneal burn. Excessive exposure to ultraviolet light can cause injury to the cornea. This may occur from the sun's rays passing directly to the eyes or when sunlight is reflected from snow, sand, or water. It may also result from watching arc welding or from exposure to a sunlamp (the rays may pass through the closed eyelids). After a lag period of several hours the sufferer experiences intense pain, inability to open the eyes in light, and the sensation of having sand in the eyes. Your physician may prescribe medication to relieve the pain. Healing will occur in a few days.

Sunglasses are available which limit to various degrees the transmission of both visible and ultraviolet light. "Dark" glasses in themselves may not provide adequate protection, since reducing the intensity of visible light causes the pupil to dilate, thus permitting more ultraviolet rays to strike the eye. The transmission ratio should be 30 percent or less, lower for more intense light (snow, water, and sand). Viewing welding requires special dark glass.

Retinal burn. Looking at a solar eclipse without appropriate glasses (dark smoked glass) may allow enough infrared rays to strike the retina to cause a burn. The result may be permanent vision loss because the lens focuses the sunlight on the point of precise vision, causing this area of the retina to actually be destroyed. Looking directly into the sun's light at midday, as recommended by certain health enthusiasts, may also cause serious eye damage.

Thermal burns. Flash burns caused by the explosive burning of gasoline or some similar volatile substance usually involve the eyelids rather than the eyes proper, for the eyelids close reflexly when the flash occurs. Such burns should be treated as are other burns of the skin. Scarring may distort the lids and require surgical repair.

Chemical burns. The two common types of chemical burns are from alkaline substances (anhydrous ammonia or lye) and acids. Alkali burns are the most hazardous, since the corneal cells can be destroyed in less than a minute, resulting in permanent vision loss. Acid is less damaging, as the tissue cells neutralize the acid more effectively.

Should an accident occur, irrigate the eye with copious amounts of water for at least twenty minutes. Retract the eyelids so the water can wash the entire eye. Be sure to seek expert professional help immediately.

Injuries. Penetrating injuries can damage the cornea, iris, and lens. Corneal injuries will cause tearing and pain. The possibility of infection with resulting inflammation can result in further damage. Nonpenetrating injuries, such as a sharp blow to the eye, can dislodge the retina. If it is not reattached, partial or complete loss of vision will occur. A blow to the eye may also cause hemorrhage in the anterior chamber and predispose to acute glaucoma, or it may dislocate the lens.

Eye injuries justify immediate care by a physician. He may remove foreign objects from under the lids, but continuing pain may indicate corneal damage. Iron and steel fragments can sometimes be extracted by an electromagnet. Your physician will determine whether surgical removal of objects or repair of torn tissues is required.

Eyelid disorders

Drooping or baggy eyelids (ptosis)

In this condition, typically occurring in elderly people, the upper eyelids droop and may even restrict vision. The lower lids may sag and give an unbecoming appearance. Minor plastic surgery remedies the problem and leaves no visible scar.

Blepharitis

Blepharitis is an inflammation of the margins of the eyelids due either to a bacterial infection or to seborrheic dermatitis. Bacteria, usually staphylococci, invade the hair follicles of the eyelashes. The eye margins redden, burn, and itch. Occasional symptoms include scaling and loss of eyelashes.

The treatment consists of thoroughly cleansing the eye margins with a small cotton swab and a mild soap, followed by the application of an antibiotic ointment. Your physician may also recommend eye drops beneath the lids. For seborrheic dermatitis (see page 974) he may suggest the use of an antidandruff shampoo on the eyebrows and scalp.

Sty

A sty is a miniature boil occurring in a hair follicle (eyelash) or in one of the openings of the glands contained in the eyelid. The boil fills with pus (whitehead) prior to bursting, when the pain is relieved, and it heals within a week. Application of hot compresses, alternating with brief cold, for ten minutes four times a day will relieve pain and hasten the spontaneous opening of the sty. Sties should not be squeezed. Should they

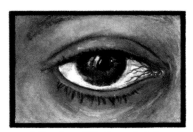

Blepharitis (eyelids).

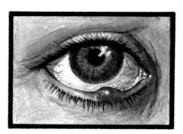

Sty on a lower lid.

recur, your physician may suggest an antibiotic.

Tarsal cyst (chalazion)

A small lump, called a chalazion, develops within the eyelid when the

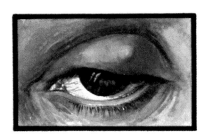

Chalazion (tarsal gland).

outlet to one of the tarsal glands becomes plugged. Secretions from the gland cause the lump to slowly enlarge. Applications of hot compresses three or four times a day for ten minutes followed by gentle massage may clear the duct, and the cyst will disappear. Should the lump persist and enlarge, a minor surgical procedure will drain the cyst.

Yellow patches (xanthelasma)

These soft, yellowish spots or plaques that develop more commonly on the lower eyelids are in themselves harmless and can be removed for cosmetic purposes, but tend to return. These spots usually result from high blood cholesterol or diabetes and should be reported to your physician.

Ectropion

Ectropion is the rolling outward of the eyelid, more commonly of the lower lid. The exposed membrane is usually swollen and red; and, when involving the lower lid, it tends to produce an overflow of tears. It occurs most commonly in elderly people when the muscles holding the lid to the eye weaken. Facial paraly-

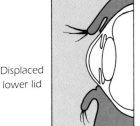
Displaced lower lid

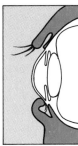
Inturned lashes

Diagram showing eyelashes turned outward (ectropion) and inward (entropion).

sis and contraction of scars in the upper face from injuries and burns may also draw the eyelid downward.

Taping the eyelids together at bedtime is helpful. If the ectropion becomes troublesome, a surgical procedure of loosening the scar or shortening the margin of the eyelid will relieve the problem.

Entropion

Entropion is the rolling inward of the edge of the eyelid and the eyelashes, causing the rough edges of the lids, and especially the lashes, to irritate the cornea **(keratitis)** and endanger vision (see page 1133). Scars from burns, injuries to the lids, and trachoma can pull the tissues out of shape. In the lower lid, muscle spasm or conjunctivitis may cause the condition. Sometimes misplaced eyelashes, directed inward **(trichiasis),** irritate the cornea, despite a normal eyelid.

Plastic surgery can correct en-

1131

tropion by reshaping the eyelid to direct the eyelashes outward. In trichiasis the inwardly directed lashes can be pulled out. If this is unsatisfactory, the hair follicles can be coagulated with electrosurgery.

Tear duct disorder (watery eye)

In this condition tears continually spill onto the cheeks. Normally tears, after moistening and cleaning the eye, are sucked into two small openings at the inner margins of the lids. From there the tears pass to the nasolacrimal tear duct, which carries the tear fluid to the front part of the nose. In most affected infants this disorder is due to the failure of the duct to open at the time of birth. In older children and adults, usually an obstruction caused by an injury, infection, or rarely, a tumor blocks the duct.

In infants the tear duct must be probed, and, in a few instances, reconstructive surgery performed. In older sufferers any infection must be controlled by hot-and-cold compresses or an antibiotic. In some cases, opening with a probe or surgical repair may be necessary.

Disorders of the conjunctiva

Conjunctivitis

Conjunctivitis is an inflammation of the membrane that lines the undersurface of the eyelids and covers the "white" part of the eye (up to the circular margin of the cornea). The cause may be bacterial, viral, or allergic.

Bacterial. A number of germs may cause this highly contagious condition that occurs most commonly in children and young adults (**"pink eye"**). Readily spread by handkerchiefs, towels, washcloths, and unwashed fingers, the inflammation usually involves both eyes, causing them to appear red and swollen. The initial watery discharge turns to mucus and pus, the eyes burn and feel scratchy, and the eyelids tend to stick together. A more serious form, **gonorrheal conjunctivitis,** is carried by fingers or towels contaminated by infectious discharge, or acquired by a newborn at birth from an infected mother.

Viral. These infections tend to produce less discharge, but the eyes are red and feel as if there is sand in them.

Allergic. The eyes are red, itchy, and puffy, with little or no discharge but profuse tearing. Sensitivity to pollens and to chemicals found in soaps, detergents, aerosols, and cosmetics, and often contact lenses produces the reaction.

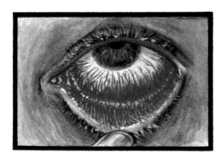

Conjunctivitis (lining membrane).

What you can do. Obtain the advice of your physician. To avoid spreading infectious conjunctivitis, keep your hands scrupulously clean, and do not use common towels, washcloths, or anything that could spread the infection. If you suspect an allergy, try to identify the offending substance and then avoid it.

What your physician can do. He can prescribe an appropriate antibiotic in the form of drops or ointment. The condition should disappear in about ten days and cause no permanent harm. Gonorrheal conjunctivitis must be treated immediately with an antibiotic; otherwise, serious damage and even blindness can result. Allergies may be treated with desensitization (see page 678.

Pterygium

This wedge-shaped fold of membranous tissue containing blood vessels grows from the "white of the eye" onto the cornea. If this tissue, which originates in the inner corner of the eye, grows extensively, it can obstruct vision. Simple eye drops and sunglasses often retard the growth, which occurs more commonly in those exposed to wind and sun. A minor surgical procedure can remove the growth.

Trachoma

A minute intracellular parasite, *Chlamydia trachomatis*, causes this infectious, highly contagious disease. It affects the conjunctiva (the membrane lining the underside of the eyelids and white of the eye) and causes scarring of these tissues. The movements of the lids scratch the cornea, resulting in keratitis and frequently in blindness. The initial symptoms are redness of the membranes, mild itching, the production of a watery discharge, swelling of the eyelids, and sensitivity to light.

Antibiotics provide effective treatment, either in the form of ointments or given by mouth. Cold compresses to the eye relieve the inflammation and provide comfort, but damage to the cornea cannot be reversed.

Hemorrhage

Occasionally, for no apparent reason, a tiny blood vessel breaks, causing blood to flow beneath the conjunctiva. The eye looks red and hemorrhagic but rarely gives pain or discomfort. The problem will disappear spontaneously in about two weeks. Should such hemorrhages become frequent, see your physician, because they may signal the presence of a blood disorder.

Disorders of the cornea

The cornea is the dome-shaped transparent outer layer of the eye, covering the iris and the pupil. It has also been called "the window of the eye."

Keratitis

This is an inflammation of the cornea caused by drying (inadequate moistening with tears), by injury such as scratching or piercing with a foreign object, by excessive exposure to ultraviolet light (sunbathing, sunlamps, or welding arcs), or by contact with volatile chemicals. The symptoms include severe pain, sensitivity to light, tearing, redness of the eyes, and dimness of vision.

Mild keratitis caused by chemicals or ultraviolet light usually heals spontaneously. Anesthetic ointments should be used only on the advice of your physician. Pain relief can be obtained by hot and/or cold compresses or by systemic medication. Should infection occur, immediately consult your physician for appropriate therapy.

Corneal ulcer

One of the complications of keratitis is the erosion of the corneal tissue by the formation of an ulcer. The infection may be bacterial, viral (commonly the herpes simplex virus), or occasionally fungal. Usually an injury occurs first, and then the infection follows. Ulcers may deepen and perforate into the anterior chamber, causing the infection to spread to other tissues. Healing may leave a scar that interferes with vision.

Bacterial ulcers appear as a grayish yellow spot and generate pus.

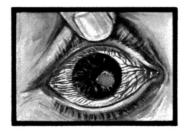

Corneal ulcer.

Viral ulcers (dendritic) can only be seen when stained or with a microscope and do not form pus. The eye is red, sensitive to light, tearing, and very painful.

What your physician can do. A corneal ulcer, a medical emergency, is a serious, sight-threatening condition. Your physician will determine the causative organism and prescribe the appropriate antibiotic, antiviral, or antifungal agent. The medications may be given as drops or ointments or by mouth. Perforated ulcers must receive immediate surgical repair, and severe scarring of the cornea may require a corneal transplant.

Xerophthalmia

In this disorder the cornea and conjunctiva undergo degenerative changes due to a vitamin A deficiency. The condition occurs among confirmed alcoholics and those on an inadequate diet, and is most commonly seen in developing countries. The cornea and conjunctiva appear lusterless. If untreated, the cornea deteriorates, then ulcerates, and finally the eye collapses. If vitamin A is given early, the disease is arrested.

Glaucoma

In glaucoma, pressure builds up within the eye, and damage to the optic nerve results, with partial or complete loss of vision. Normally there is a constant supply of clear fluid (aqueous humor) in the front of the eye (anterior chamber), which drains away as fast as it forms. When the drain becomes clogged, pressure builds up, just as when the drainpipe of the kitchen sink becomes blocked, the sink fills up.

Glaucoma is the leading cause of blindness in the United States, 60,000 Americans being blind on this account. Two of every 100 Americans over thirty-five suffer from this disease, of whom one fourth are unaware of having it. With early detection and proper care, vision can be preserved in 85 percent of those with glaucoma. Three principal types of glaucoma occur.

Congenital. In congenital glaucoma, faulty development prevents adequate drainage of the fluid formed within the eye. Eighty percent of these cases can be recognized within three months after birth. The telltale signs are extreme photophobia (intolerance to light) and a hazy or opaque cornea (the clear structure in front of the colored portion of the eye).

Acute (closed-angle). This type of glaucoma accounts for 10 to 15 percent of total cases. When the iris is pushed forward and protudes into the drainage area, the outflow of fluid is suddenly blocked, causing striking symptoms: sudden blurring of vision with halos around lights, severe pain, and redness of the affected eye. If not treated *promptly*, damage to the optic nerve and retina occurs, with resulting permanent blindness.

Chronic (open-angle). This most common form of glaucoma (85 percent of cases) develops in those thirty-five years of age or older. With age, the drainage system gradually narrows or becomes clogged with deposits. As the pressure builds up imperceptibly over the years, the ret-

ina and optic nerve are injured, often before the disease is recognized. Those over thirty-five should have periodic eye examinations, which include a simple method to determine the pressure within the eye and an ophthalmoscopic check of the interior of the eye. Any vision loss cannot be regained.

What you can do. Should you experience sudden pain in the eye or loss of vision, see your physician immediately. Should you be over thirty-five, have your eyes checked every two or three years. If you do have glaucoma, cooperate with your physician in ongoing treatments.

What your physician can do. Congenital and acute glaucomas require prompt surgical treatment. In the chronic form, appropriate eye drops may prove satisfactory, or these may be supplemented with oral medication. In certain situations laser surgery will relieve the problem. Sometimes a new drainage canal must be prepared surgically.

Iritis

Iritis is an inflammation of the iris (the colored portion of the eye which dilates or constricts) and sometimes the ciliary body to which it is at-

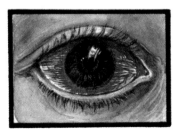

Iritis (iris).

tached. The cause is uncertain in many cases, but it may result from an injury and as a complication of a corneal ulcer. The symptoms include a throbbing pain in the eye, blurred vision, sensitivity to light, and tearing. The iris is usually swollen and dull, and cells float in the aqueous humor. These cells may attach themselves to the inside of the cornea or plug the drainage canal in the front of the eye, causing acute glaucoma with resulting blindness. If untreated, blurred vision and a cataract may develop.

What your physician can do. He will prescribe drops that dilate the pupil and prevent it from sticking to the lens. He may also prescribe steroids to reduce the inflammation.

Disorders of the lens

Cataract

In cataract the lens of the eye becomes progressively cloudy and fogged. Vision continues to fail, becoming fuzzy and blurred; double vision occurs frequently. Typically cataracts develop after the age of sixty and often affect both eyes simultaneously. Besides age **(senile cataracts),** other predisposing factors include injuries **(traumatic cataracts),** diabetes, iritis, infections, long-continued exposure to radiation, as from infrared or heat waves, microwaves, and X-rays **(secondary cataracts),** and inherited tendencies and birth defects **(congenital cataracts).**

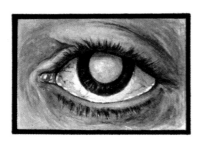

Cataract (lens).

The only effective treatment for cataracts is surgery. Under local anesthetic the surgeon removes the lens (either intact or broken up and evacuated) and replaces it with a new plastic lens. Conventional glasses or contact lenses must be worn if an implant is not deemed suitable.

Refractive errors

The eye is so designed that the entering rays of light normally focus precisely on the retina, where the optical image of the object viewed is produced. In some individuals the light rays fail to focus correctly, thus blurring the image. Four common disorders cause such blurring.

Nearsightedness (myopia). In this condition the light rays from a distant object focus before reaching the retina, but nearby objects can be seen clearly. People with myopia tend to squint their eyes so they can see distant things better. Generally the condition, which results from an elongated eyeball, is inherited and appears in children between eight to twelve years of age and stabilizes at about age twenty. Conditions such as reading a lot or reading in poor light do not cause nearsightedness.

Farsightedness (hyperopia). In farsighted people the eyeball is too

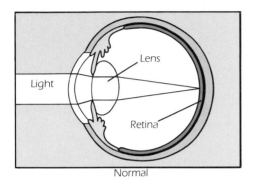

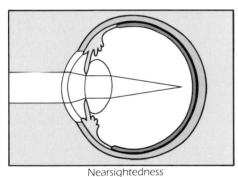

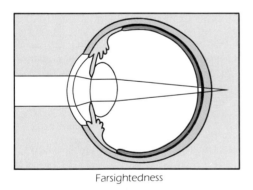

Normal and abnormal refraction.

short, and the light rays focus "beyond" the retina. Distant objects can be seen clearly, but close objects cannot. Sometimes flattening of the cornea or thinning of the lens will cause the problem, which is usually in-

herited and often shows up in children who experience headaches and have difficulty reading.

Aging eyes (presbyopia). Often at age forty-five to fifty the lens loses its elasticity so that it cannot thicken to focus on near objects, causing the individual to hold reading materials farther away from the eyes.

Astigmatism. In this usually inherited disorder, a warped or distorted cornea causes the rays entering in the horizontal plane (or sometimes in any plane) to be out of focus from those entering in the vertical plane. The blurring produced is similar to that seen in a mirror with an uneven surface. On occasion, injury to the cornea causes scarring and results in severe astigmatism.

What your physician can do. Appropriate glasses that correct the focal length of the light rays entering the eyes will resolve the refractive errors of nearsightedness, farsightedness, and presbyopia. Unless the condition is extremely severe, glasses can also correct the distortions of astigmatism. In severe cases of astigmatism (usually due to scarring) the cornea can be "planed," or a corneal transplant may be necessary. For most people, traditional or contact lenses are a matter of choice. Glasses for presbyopia provide focus for a specific distance; hence, bifocals or trifocals may be required for various ranges of vision.

Double vision

Double vision occurs when each eye looks at a different object or sees images of different sizes. In cross-eye and walleye the eyes see different objects, but the child soon learns to ignore the weaker image. In adults it results from the paralysis of the external muscles that move one eye, and may be due to injury, diabetes, brain hemorrhage, or brain tumor. Cataracts may produce a type of double vision. Should you develop double vision, see your physician immediately.

Blindness

Blindness, the inability to see, afflicts an estimated 10 million people in the world. Millions of others are partially blind. Loss of sight can occur from disorders within the eyes, in the nerve pathways that transmit signals from the eyes, and in the visual cortex of the brain.

Faults in the eyes. These can be in either the reception or the transmission of the light rays from the object viewed. Reception disorders include a detached retina, hemor-rhage, inflammation of the choroid, and macular degeneration. Transmission problems may result from scarring of the cornea, an inflamed iris adhering to the lens, a cataract, or a hemorrhage into the vitreous.

Faults in nerve transmission. The optic nerves may be damaged from increased pressure within the eye (glaucoma), from an inflammatory process (optic neuritis), from blockage of the nerve's blood supply due to atherosclerosis, from long use of tobacco and alcohol, from wood alcohol (methanol poisoning), and from severe injury, meningitis, and tumors. Degeneration of the optic nerve may also occur in multiple sclerosis.

Faults in the brain cortex. The visual area of the cortex may be damaged or destroyed by an injury, by a brain hemorrhage, from a vascular occlusion (cortical blindness), or from a tumor.

Disorders of the retina

The retina is the inner lining of the posterior chamber of the eye, the portion of the eyeball located behind the lens. Disorders affecting the retina may cause partial or complete blindness and, therefore, require prompt attention from a specialist.

Retinal detachment

As a person ages, the retina can thin and deteriorate, producing small holes or tears. More frequently the vitreous, which is firmly attached to the retina, shrinks. This pulls the retina away from the choroid, causing it to tear. Fluid from the vitreous passes through the tear and separates or detaches the retina from the pigment and choroid layers, somewhat like loose wallpaper. Retinal detachments can also result from tumors, inflammations, and complications of diabetes.

The first symptoms are usually the "seeing" of floating objects and flashes of light in the affected eye. The vision becomes blurred and, as the retina detaches, a "curtain" or "veil" obscures part of the visual field. Because the detached retina is separated from its blood supply, it must be reattached promptly, or the result will be permanent loss of vision. A detached retina is a real emergency.

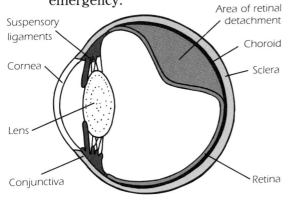

Suspensory ligaments

Cornea

Lens

Conjunctiva

Area of retinal detachment

Choroid

Sclera

Retina

Section showing partial detachment of the retina.

What your physician can do. The methods your physician can employ for reattaching the retina include photocoagulation (with a laser beam), cryopexy (freezing the wall behind the tear), or surgery. He must repair a hole or tear to prevent further seepage of fluid and must sometimes exert pressure to push the retina back against its normal attachment. Treatments are successful in over 90 percent of cases.

Retinal vascular disorders

When either the arteries or veins of the retina become obstructed with a blood clot (thrombosis) or fatty deposit (embolus), the retina is damaged, and vision is partially or completely lost. If an artery is blocked **(retinal artery occlusion),** the area of the retina supplied by it ceases to function, causing blindness in part or all the eye. A blocked vein **(retinal vein occlusion)** generally ruptures into the vitreous, making it cloudy and blurring vision.

One complication of diabetes damages the blood vessels in the choroid **(diabetic retinopathy).** This disorder causes 10 percent of new blindness in the United States each year, resulting in one in every fifty diabetics becoming blind.

What your physician can do. Because the problem occurs more frequently in diabetics whose blood sugar levels are not well controlled, blood sugar levels should be normalized as much as possible. Laser surgery can block the leaking blood vessels. Blood that has mingled with the vitreous and caused it to become cloudy can often, by means of vitrectomy, be replaced with clear fluid, and vision can be restored at least partially.

Retinal hemorrhages

These may be caused by sustained or peaking high blood pressure or hypertension. The arteries supplying blood to the retina become thin and rupture or become thick walled. If objects appear to float before your eyes, report to your physician, who will treat your general high blood pressure with a diet or with medications. This may improve your visual problem.

Macular degeneration

The macula is the point of clear or precise vision in the back part of the retina. At this location the details of what is being observed are "seen." Macular degeneration most commonly develops in the elderly, usu-

1139

ally due to narrowing or blockage of the blood vessels supplying the macula, which, when deprived of its blood supply, thins and degenerates. Less frequently hemorrhage and leakage of fluid from the damaged blood vessels distort precise vision. Macular degeneration may be inherited. It causes partial or complete loss of precise vision while leaving peripheral vision unaffected. There is no known treatment.

Choroiditis

In choroiditis, the choroid layer, made up of blood vessels, is inflamed, and, secondarily, the inflammation may involve the retina and the vitreous humor. After healing, the choroid remains scarred and may permanently impair vision. Generally the precise cause cannot be determined, but sometimes an organism (*Toxoplasma gondii*) spread from the feces of dogs, and occasionally cats, causes the condition. The symptoms include blurred vision, reddening of the eye, and, depending on which part of the retina is affected, loss of peripheral or central vision. Steroids are often used to suppress the inflammation. In children, if only one eye is involved, the child may develop amblyopia.

Strabismus and amblyopia (cross-eye, walleye, squint)

These conditions, in which the two eyes are not directed at the same object, occur in 2 percent of all children. Normally, as growth progresses, the child learns to "fuse" what he sees in his right and left eyes to make a single visual image. Vision with two coordinated eyes provides one with depth perception, the ability to perceive that one object is farther or closer than another, which is a function of the brain.

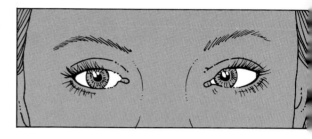

Cross-eye or squint

When one eye focuses on an object and the other looks inward (**cross-eye**) or outward (**walleye**) or up or down (**strabismus**), the cause is generally an imbalance in the pull of the muscles that move the eyes. The brain soon learns to ignore what the wandering eye sees, even though the eye itself is perfectly normal. If the abnormality is not corrected, the sight in this eye will be lost, a condition called **amblyopia.** Amblyopia may also develop when the two eyes do not focus alike, as occurs if only one eye is farsighted or nearsighted or is astigmatic. Any suspicion of strabismus should immediately be reported to your physician.

What your physician can do. He will try to force the weak or lazy eye to work by covering the stronger eye with a patch for several hours a day, or if a refractive problem is the cause, by providing corrective glasses. When correction begins by age two or three, or earlier, the problem should clear up. If the disorder is not discovered till the child attends school (age six or seven), it proves difficult, if not impossible, to retrain the weaker eye, and binocular vision will be lost. Doing exercises to strengthen the weak muscles is essential. In cases of muscle weakness, surgery may be necessary to correct the problem.

Tumors of the eyes

Tumors can be either benign or malignant. **Benign** tumors do not spread but may cause damage from pressure on neighboring structures. **Malignant** tumors may arise within the eye or spread from distant lesions.

Melanoma

A melanoma is a highly malignant tumor (cancer) comprised of melanocytes (cells that produce the brown pigment melanin) in the choroid layer of the eye. Melanomas usually involve only one eye and generally occur in older adults, more commonly those with fair skin and blue eyes. Often they are discovered during a routine eye examination or following symptoms that include the seeing of lights, sometimes colored, and gradual loss of vision.

In young adults the discovery of a melanoma is a medical emergency, because if not removed promptly, the cancer may spread to other parts of the body. In the elderly the tumor generally grows slowly and may be carefully observed before removal.

Retinoblastoma

This malignant, usually inherited tumor of the retina typically occurs before the age of five, developing in one or both eyes. Symptoms include crossed eyes, a whitish reflection behind the pupil, and a family history of the disease. If detected early, the tumor may be destroyed with laser surgery, radiation therapy, or cryosurgery (freezing). In advanced cases, the red, painful eye will have to be removed surgically. Chemotherapy generally proves ineffective.

1141

CHAPTER 28

The ear and its disorders

Hearing

The ear is a remarkable structure consisting of three major parts: the external, middle, and inner ear.

The external ear is composed of what is commonly called the "ear" (auricle) and the ear canal (external auditory canal). The auricle serves as a funnel to direct sound into the ear canal, which is about one inch in length (24 mm) and ends blindly at the ear drum (tympanic membrane).

The middle ear is a space that extends from the inner side of the eardrum to the outer bony side of the inner ear. At the back of the middle ear are the mastoid air cells, and in the upper front is the opening of the auditory tube (eustachian tube), which connects with the nasopharynx (back of the nose and upper part of the pharynx). Through this tube air passes into and out of the hardest bone in the body, the petrous portion of the middle ear that keeps the pressure equal on the inner and outer surfaces of the ear-

drum. When one changes altitude rapidly (as in an elevator), the varying pressure causes the ears to "pop."

The inner wall of the middle ear has two openings into the inner ear: the oval window above, which is covered by the footplate of the stapes, and the round window, which is covered by a thin membrane. Three tiny, jointed bones, the ossicles, span the middle ear. The common names of the little bones are the hammer, anvil, and stirrup. The handle of the hammer (malleus) attaches to the inner side of the eardrum; the foot-piece of the stirrup (stapes) fits against the oval window, while the anvil (incus) lies between the hammer and the stirrup.

The inner ear consists of the cochlea and the semicircular canals (labyrinth). The cochlea for hearing and the semicircular canals are for balance. The **cochlea,** shaped like a snail's shell, lies within the petrous

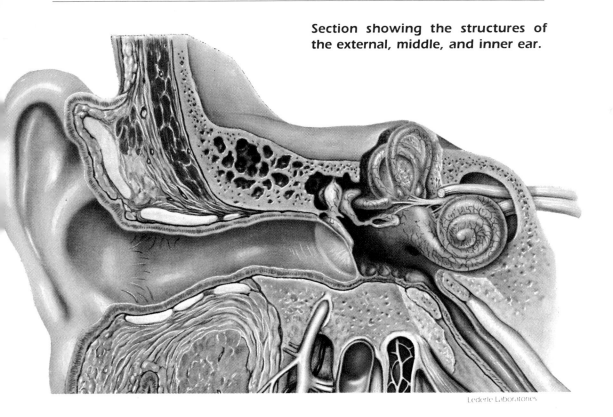

Section showing the structures of the external, middle, and inner ear.

Lederle Laboratories

bone. Comprised of three spiral tubes filled with fluid, the spiral canals begin at the oval window and end at the round window. A tough membrane, called the basilar membrane, runs this spiral course and separates the fluid-filled tubes from each other.

Resting on this membrane are hair cells with nerves that pass to and from them (the organ of Corti). When stimulated by movements of the fluid, these hair cells send nerve impulses to the hearing center of the brain. The cells at the base of the spiral respond to high-pitched sounds while those at the apex, to low-pitched sounds. A grand piano has a range of some seven octaves. This minute "piano" in the inner ear, a million times smaller than a grand piano, has a range of twelve octaves—one lower and four higher than a grand. A grand piano uses some 240 strings, but the piano within the human ear has 24,000 strings!

How do you hear? Sound waves coming over the air are funneled into the ear canal and strike the eardrum. The vibrations of the eardrum activate the ossicles. As the foot of the stirrup moves back and forth, wavelike movements of the fluid in the spiral canals activate the organ of Corti. The mechanical force of these

1143

fluid movements are converted to electrical nerve impulses in the organ of Corti. These nerve impulses are carried by the auditory nerve to the hearing center in the cortex, where they are interpreted. Sound waves conducted through the skull can also actuate the inner ear. This is how the boneconduction hearing aid works.

Hearing safeguards

Within each ear canal are hairs and some 1,000 special glands that produce earwax. Together they impede the entry of most insects. The wax also lubricates the canal, preventing it from drying.

The Creator designed two small muscles within the middle ear to dampen the heavy vibrations produced by loud noises. One, the tensor tympani, tugs the eardrum to keep it from vibrating too violently; the other, the stapedius, pulls the stapes away from the oval window, stifling the movements of the ossicles. When a violent sound enters the ear canal, especially when the noise is anticipated, the muscles reflexly contract to diminish the vibrations reaching the inner ear, protecting it from harm. Unexpected loud noises, such as a gun firing at close range, may rupture the eardrum and damage the inner ear, causing sensory nerve (sensory neural) hearing loss.

Protective rules

Slender or pointed objects (hairpins, pencils, toothpicks) should not be introduced into the ear canal because they may rupture the eardrum.

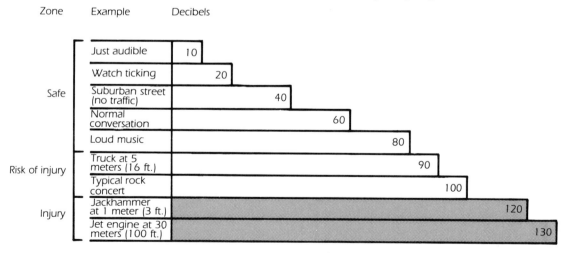

Zone	Example	Decibels
Safe	Just audible	10
	Watch ticking	20
	Suburban street (no traffic)	40
	Normal conversation	60
	Loud music	80
Risk of injury	Truck at 5 meters (16 ft.)	90
	Typical rock concert	100
Injury	Jackhammer at 1 meter (3 ft.)	120
	Jet engine at 30 meters (100 ft.)	130

The intensity of sounds (in decibels).

The smallest thing you put into your ear should be your elbow! For wax accumulating in the ear, see page 1146.

Do not slap someone on the external ear or dive into water with the side of the head directed downward. In both situations, the air within the canal may be sufficiently compressed as to rupture the eardrum.

Persistent exposure to loud noises (din of noisy machinery, hard rock and loud heavy metal bands, jet aircraft) damages the hearing mechanism and reduces a person's ability to hear. Earplugs or insulated ear covers should be worn whenever you are in a noisy environment. Even if traffic noises, airplanes constantly passing overhead, or loud music played do not deafen you, the sounds may exceed your nervous tolerance and make you fatigued, irritable, and inefficient.

Equilibrium

As mentioned earlier, the inner ear contains not only the cochlea but the **semicircular canals (labyrinth),** which are connected to each other. Both ears contain three tiny horseshoe-shaped canals, each placed at right angles to one another. The canals are filled with fluid, and each has a slight bulge containing a tuft of sensitive nerve cells. Turning the head in any direction, or moving it even slightly, sets in motion the fluid in at least one canal of each ear and stimulates the nerve cells in the bulge to send impulses to the brain, indicating the position of the head.

The brain also receives nerve impulses from muscles and tendons, the joints, and the eyes, which it correlates into information about the body's present position and the degree and direction of motion. With this knowledge, the brain, particularly the cerebellum, modifies its control of the muscles so that body parts are moved in harmony with existing circumstances. For example, when a person is standing on one foot, the brain will not direct that foot to be lifted until the weight has been shifted to the other foot. Or, when the body is falling backward, the brain will signal an impulse to step backward.

In some people the nerve cells in the semicircular canals are oversensitive, causing them to suffer from motion sickness. Certain diseases may affect the semicircular canals, making them more sensitive or less sensitive than normal, resulting in a great deal of discomfort.

The two labyrinths are reciprocal to each other. When the head is turned to the left, the discharge from the left semicircular canal is increased while that from the right canal is decreased, and vice versa. When one labyrinth is injured, the unrestrained discharge from the other causes a false sense of rotation called **vertigo,** and a rhythmical, jerky movement of the eyes called **nystagmus.** Many inner ear diseases can cause vertigo.

Disorders of the ear

The ear is vulnerable to many disorders, and these may be associated with pain and/or changes in hearing or equilibrium.

The external (outer) ear

Diseases of the aurical and ear canal may include the skin, cartilage, or bone.

Earwax. Some people produce more wax than others. This wax may accumulate and block the canal, causing temporary conductive deafness, a feeling of fullness, and occasionally earache. Impacted wax may also cause a dry cough. Normally the wax gradually moves outward and can be removed with a finger. Cotton sticks should not be used because they may compact the wax against the eardrum. Soft wax can be gently washed out with warm water, using a rubber bulb designed for the purpose. Hard wax can be first softened with oil or a specially prepared softening agent. Your physician has a special instrument for looking into your ear, and he may use a curette to visually remove the wax.

Foreign body. Small objects often become wedged in the ear canal, usually in children under six years of age. If the object cannot be washed out with a gentle stream of warm water provided by a rubber syringe, your physician may feel it necessary to anesthetize the child to prevent his squirming while the object is being extracted with an ear forceps.

Infections of the ear canal

A **general inflammation (external otitis)** of the skin of the ear canal is commonly caused by bacteria, and sometimes by fungi. Allowing the skin in the canal to remain moist or scratching it while attempting to remove wax initiates the infection. "Swimmer's ear," in which the canal is permitted to remain wet, can cause itching and often severe pain, accompanied by a watery, sometimes pussy, discharge. External otitis may result from a reaction to hair spray or from seborrheic dermatitis.

Otomycosis, a form of external otitis caused by a fungus, tends to resist treatment. The symptoms include itching, stinging, pain, and the presence of black moldy spots.

A **localized infection (boil, furuncle, abscess)** may develop in which a hair follicle becomes infected. The extreme pain is promptly relieved when the boil ruptures.

What you can do. Do not introduce cotton plugs, hair pins, or other similar objects into your ear. Do not scratch your ears, even though they itch. Keep your ears dry by using ear plugs or a shower cap (or swimmer's cap) if you are susceptible to ear infections. If you have an infection, place the affected ear on a heating pad or hot-water bottle. Some people find that an ice pack is more effective than heat. This may provide relief until you can see your physician.

What your physician can do. He will examine your ear through an otoscope and may order a culture to determine the germ causing the infection, or he may have to lance a boil. He may prescribe antibiotics in the form of drops or creams, together with oral medication, depending on the severity of the infection. If the ear canal is severely swollen, a wick may be inserted into the canal. For recurring infections he may prescribe steroid drops or creams. Otomycosis is often treated with a local cleaning and antimyotic agent.

Tumors

Benign tumors do not spread and include sebaceous cysts, which develop from skin glands, usually on the outer "ear." If they enlarge or become infected, they may be removed surgically. Another benign tumor, an osteoma or an exostosis, is an overgrowth of the bone forming the ear canal. These grow slowly and are surgically removed only when they block the canal and impair hearing.

Malignant tumors are generally skin cancers of the outer "ear." The most common type are basal cell cancers, which grow slowly and seldom spread. These should be removed by your physician. He will freeze small tumors and surgically excise others. Other forms of cancer may require surgery, chemotherapy, or radiation.

Disorders of the eardrum

The eardrum forms a wall between the outer and the middle ear, and therefore is susceptible to a variety of problems that can arise in either of these areas.

Rupture

An eardrum can be torn, or it may burst, for a variety of reasons, including the passage of hairpins, pencils, and toothpicks through the ear canal;

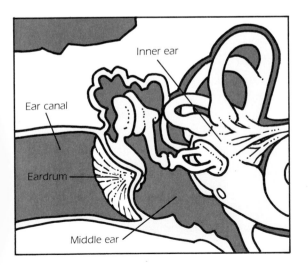
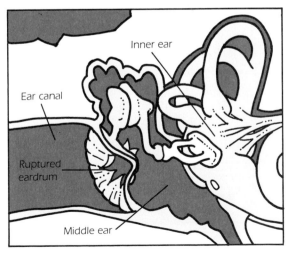

Rupture of the eardrum.

sudden air pressure or a loud noise, such as a slap on the ear or the firing of a gun at close range; or an inflammatory process. The symptoms include mild pain, slight loss of hearing, and possibly a discharge of blood, or, if from an infection in the middle ear, pus.

What your physician can do. He will determine the extent of the injury. A small rupture may heal by itself. He may prescribe an antibiotic to prevent infection. If the rupture is due to an inflammatory process, the underlying infection must be treated with antibiotics. If the ear has a persistent discharge, your doctor will treat it with antibiotics, ear drops, or surgery. If a hole remains, it must be surgically repaired.

Retracted eardrum

The eardrum is pushed inward, or retracted, when the pressure on the outside of the eardrum is greater than that in the middle ear. The cause is blockage of the auditory (eustachian) tube, which normally allows free passage of air between the middle ear and the back of the nose. Infections in the posterior nose (nasopharyngitis), enlargement of lymphoid tissue (adenoids), or allergies which involve the nasal mucosa may close the auditory tube. When the auditory tube is temporarily blocked, a sudden change in atmos-

pheric pressure **(barotrauma),** as when rapidly descending in an airplane, or when scuba diving, forces the drum inward. Again, if there is prolonged closure of the tube, the air in the middle ear is absorbed, and the drum, because of the vacuum formed, is retracted. On occasion, blockage of the tube causes the middle ear to fill with fluid. A retracted drum causes pain, a feeling of fullness or heaviness in the ear, and loss of conductive hearing.

What you can do. Chewing gum or swallowing hard will often clear up the condition. Usually you will hear a popping noise in your affected ear, indicating that the eardrum has resumed its normal position. If neither of these works, and *if you have no infection in your nose or throat,* close your nose with your finger and thumb and gently blow, keeping your mouth shut. This should force air up your eustachian tubes. If you have an allergy or mild infection in your nose or pharynx, and must travel by air, an antihistamine or a decongestant may help. Should the problem persist, see your physician.

What your physician can do. He may make a small slit in your eardrum (myringotomy) and insert a ventilating tube to allow air in or the fluid out. He may use antibiotics to clear up any infection you may have in your upper respiratory area.

Disorders of the middle ear

Otitis media

Otitis media, or inflammation of the middle ear cavity, is due primarily to infections caused by bacteria or viruses and impairment of the eustachian tube. Otitis media progresses through stages, from acute to chronic, and can be classified according to these stages.

Acute suppurative otitis media results from the spread of an upper respiratory infection, either from a virus or bacteria, into the middle ear through the auditory tube (eustachian tube). It may follow a common cold, bacterial tonsillitis, scarlet fever, or measles. Because the infection inflames the lining of the auditory tube, it becomes partially or completely filled with pussy fluid.

The increasing pressure within the middle ear from accumulating fluid and/or pus causes the eardrum to bulge outward, producing severe pain (earache) that is typical of acute otitis. Other symptoms include ringing in the ear, hearing loss, chills, and fever. An infant or young child will cry constantly, turn his head from side to side, and rub the infected ear with his hand. Should the eardrum rupture spontaneously, blood and pussy fluid will flow from the ear canal, relieving the pain. If it fails to rupture and is left untreated, the infection may spread to the mastoid air cells, resulting in mastoiditis. It may even cause meningitis or brain abscess.

Otitis media with effusion occurs when the middle ear is filled with fluid either from a blockage of the auditory tube or following acute otitis media. The fluid may be thin and watery (serous otitis media) or thick with mucus (mucoid or secretory otitis media). Serous fluid is drawn into the middle ear as a result of the auditory tube becoming blocked (causing a negative pressure). Mucoid fluid collects because of the increased secretion of mucus by glands located in the lining of the middle ear. Typical symptoms of this stage of otitis media are a feeling of fullness in the ear, conductive hearing loss, and a mild, dull headache.

What your physician can do. In accute suppurative otitis media, treatment is directed toward controlling the infection with antibiotics and relieving the pain. In otitis media in the effusion stage, a long-term course of antibiotics may be recommended. Decongestants usually do not help, especially in infants and children. If fluid in the eardrum persists more than three months, the doctor may recommend incising the eardrum and placing a ventilating tube in it for drainage.

Chronic otitis media (suppurative otitis)

This disorder is a persisting inflammation of the middle ear, probably a carry-over from childhood infections, causing progressive destruction of the structures in and around the middle ear. This condition is usually due to an underlying pathology such as granulation tissue, cholesterol granuloma, or cholesteotoma. Partial destruction of the eardrum allows foul-smelling fluid and pus to escape from the ear canal. The ossicles may also sustain permanent injury. Infection frequently spreads to the mastoid process **(mastoiditis),** the projecting bone just behind the ear, which is filled with cells similar to a honeycomb.

Chronic otitis produces a constant discharge of pus through the ear canal. If the infection worsens, pain

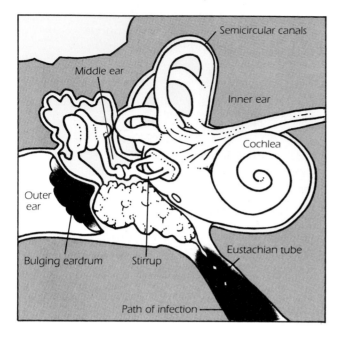

Infection of the middle ear (otitis media).

therapy is not effective because the mastoid has poor circulation, the air cells must be surgically removed because they harbor pockets of pus. Following eradication of the infection, reconstructive surgery in the middle ear may restore partial or complete hearing, depending on the extent of the damage done.

Otosclerosis

In otosclerosis, bone growth around the foot of the stirrup (stapes), one of the three tiny bones in the middle ear, progressively fixes it to the bony wall of the inner ear (oval window). This increasing loss of movement results in gradual conductive hearing loss. There appears to be a hereditary factor predisposing to this disorder, which occurs more frequently in women than men. In the majority of sufferers it occurs in both ears. Surgery to replace the stapes with a tiny prosthetic device (stape-

and fever may result. Acute mastoiditis will cause a fever and intense pain, with redness and swelling of the skin behind the ear.

What you can do. Avoid activities, such as swimming or showering, which might permit water to enter the middle ear through the perforation in the eardrum. You should see your physician as soon as possible.

What your physician can do. He will determine the severity and extent of the infection using an otoscope, to examine the eardrum, X-rays to show bone damage, and a culture to reveal the infecting organism. Appropriate antibiotic therapy will give the best results, even though the infection may be difficult to eradicate, but sometimes areas of infection must be removed surgically. In acute **mastoiditis,** antibiotic

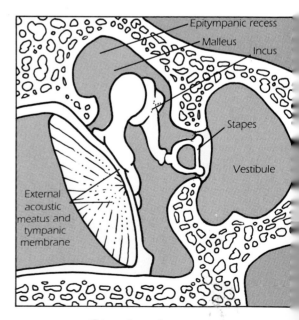

Otosclerosis

dectomy) can restore hearing dramatically. If surgery cannot be performed, a hearing aid can help.

Cholesteatoma

Cholesteatoma is an unusual disorder in which superficial (epithelial) skin cells, commonly arising from the eardrum, begin to multiply rapidly. The lesion may start as a congenital epithelial cyst, from a perforation of the eardrum, or as a complication of a chronic infection of the middle ear. A pocket or sac forms filled with keratin (skin) debris. The invading cells may destroy the eardrum, the bones of the middle ear, and the mastoid air cells, and it may also erode the bones separating the ear from the brain. The facial nerves may be affected. The cells are not malignant (they do not metastasize), but they do secrete a bone-digesting enzyme. The process is made worse if the cholesteatoma becomes infected.

The symptoms include slight to severe hearing loss with earache, headache, discharge from the ear, dizziness, and weakness of the facial muscles. Untreated, the germs may enter the coverings of the brain, causing meningitis or an epidural abscess.

What you can do. If you have any of the symptoms mentioned above, and especially if you experienced ear infections as a child, see your physician.

What your physician can do. He will make a careful examination of your ear—visually with an otoscope, together with X-rays and hearing tests. If there is an infection, he will administer antibiotics. However, it is difficult to get the antibiotic in contact with the germs. Surgery is essential, and if the lesion is small it may be completely removed. Large lesions require extensive surgery, often repeatedly, as any cells that are not removed start a new focus of growth. The bones of the middle ear may require rebuilding. Your doctor may recommend that you use a hearing aid.

Disorders of the inner ear

The organs of the inner ear are the cochlea, for hearing, and the semicircular canals (labyrinth), for balance and equilibrium.

Meniere's disease

In this troublesome illness, attacks of extreme dizziness associated with nausea and vomiting occur periodically. No pain, fever, or disease of the digestive organs accompanies the dizziness. The sufferer usually experiences a more or less persistent ringing in the ear (tinnitus) along with progressive fluctuating nerve-type deafness and fullness or pressure in the affected ear. One ear is affected at first, but later both may be involved.

Attacks of dizziness with nausea and vomiting may last from a few minutes to several days, and may occur at intervals from a few weeks to a few years. Between attacks few if any symptoms may appear. Usually

1151

the attacks of dizziness gradually become less frequent and less severe, but the deafness becomes worse.

The immediate cause of Meniere's disease is an increase in fluid pressure within the inner ear that affects both hearing and balance. Either increased production or decreased reabsorption of fluid causes the increased pressure. Factors appearing to aggravate or even precipitate an attack include emotional stress, allergies, and hypoglycemia.

What you can do. At the time of an attack, lie still with your eyes closed to minimize the dizziness. Discontinuing the use of tobacco and caffeine-containing beverages, together with adopting a low-salt diet, have also been suggested.

What your physician can do. The diagnosis and treatment will require the attention of a specialist, who will use an audiometric test to determine sound conduction through the air and the bones. More sophisticated tests are available if required. He may prescribe medications to decrease nausea, vomiting, and dizziness during an attack. Diuretics may reduce the volume of fluid in the inner ear. Surgery can provide consistent long-term benefits. Making an opening in the sac where the inner ear fluid accumulates, allowing the fluid to escape (sometimes shunting it into the fluid-filled space around the brain), can prevent damage from excess fluid in the inner ear. When severe dizziness persists, the surgeon deliberately destroys the labyrinth (labyrinthectomy) or cuts the nerve to the semicircular canals (vestibular neurectomy).

Labyrinthitis

This infection, involving the semicircular canals and often the entire inner ear, may be caused by pus-producing germs spread from an infection of the middle ear (otitis media) or from a complication of meningitis. At other times it results from a virus infection. In either event, the inflammation causes profound symptoms: extreme dizziness, often with severe nausea, vomiting, and ringing in the ears. The sufferer or the things around him spin in circles. Although the viral infection usually disappears in a few weeks, the more dangerous bacterial form often results in partial or complete hearing loss.

What your physician can do. In both forms, he will prescribe bed rest and medication to reduce dizziness. For the bacterial infections he will give appropriate antibiotics. If the infection persists, he may have to surgically remove infected tissues, resulting in total loss of hearing and equilibrium on the affected side.

Deafness (hearing loss)

The brain is made aware of sounds through the hearing mechanism of the ears. Sound waves or vibrations of the air enter the outer ear and strike the eardrum, setting it in motion. The three tiny, jointed bones carry all back-and-forth movements of the eardrum across the middle ear to the inner ear, where their movements are converted to waves in the inner ear (cochlea). Here the fluid waves activate electrical impulses through hair cells in the organ of Corti, which are carried via the auditory nerve to the hearing center of the brain, where sound is perceived.

Problems of either conduction (mechanical) or transmission (neural) cause hearing loss.

Conductive deafness

Interference in the conduction of sound waves to the fluid in the inner ear causes this form of deafness. Several factors may contribute to this interference: (1) accumulation of **wax** in the ear canal obstructing air waves from reaching the eardrum; (2) fluid in the middle ear (otitis media with effusion) either from a blocked auditory tube or from the aftereffects of acute otitis media; (3) **otosclerosis,** a condition in which the inner ossicle (stapes) becomes rigidly attached to the bone of the inner ear (oval window), preventing vibrations of the eardrum from reaching the inner ear; (4) **chronic otitis media** with a large perforation of the eardrum, fixed ossicles, or destroyed ossicles, all of which interfere with sound conduction; and (5) **tumors** in the ear canal or in the middle ear disrupting proper conduction.

What your physician can do. He will first determine the cause. Wax can easily be removed (see page 1146). Middle ear fluid can be removed by lancing the eardrum or by inserting a ventilating tube. A

stapedectomy will relieve the problem caused by otosclerosis (see page 1150). Chronic infections of the middle ear can be treated with antibiotics (see page 1149). Surgery can repair a perforated eardrum (tympanoplasty) and ossicles can be replaced or realigned (ossiculoplasty). Tumors require surgical treatment.

Nerve deafness

Various conditions can interfere with the passage of nerve impulses between the inner ear and the auditory area of the brain, and most of them are permanent.

The cause of the hearing loss is in either the cochlea, the auditory nerve, or the hearing area of the brain. Several common causes of nerve deafness occur.

Advancing age. With advancing years hearing gradually declines, first the high-pitched sounds, and later at all levels.

Excessive noise. Intense, prolonged noise in excess of 95 decibels (for four or more hours per day), whether from rock music, a pneumatic hammer, a jet engine, or a garden mower, and many other sources of very loud sound, can damage the inner ear (see chart, page 1144).

Chemical injury. A number of drugs may injure nerve conduction, such as neomycin (an antibiotic that causes severe damage), aspirin, and quinine (causes both ringing in the ears and hearing loss), and streptomycin (an antibiotic that affects equilibrium more than hearing).

Other causes. Other causes of partial or complete hearing loss include Meniere's disease, certain viral

1153

infections (herpes zoster and German measles in the mother during early pregnancy), skull fracture involving the inner ear, tumors, especially an acoustic neuroma, which may, because of nerve injury, cause partial or complete hearing loss.

What your physician can do. In most of the situations listed above where partial hearing loss has been sustained, providing a suitable hearing aid is all that he can do. **Hearing aids** must be tailored to the individual's need. Some require a hearing aid that increases the level of all frequencies, while others—commonly those with hearing loss due to aging—need only the high frequencies. An acoustic neuroma can be removed surgically. In selected cases of total deafness an electronic device, called a cochlean implant, can be inserted into the inner ear. This will restore some hearing.

CHAPTER 29

Other special senses

Taste and smell

Taste is the sense that allows us to select and enjoy foods in harmony with our desires and preferences, but it is closely associated with the sense of smell, which greatly aids the perception of taste. Most of the receptors or "taste buds" are located on the surface of the tongue and are particularly numerous at the tip, along the side, and near the back. Taste buds are also found in the membranes of the palate and pharynx. Each taste bud—a tiny, microscopic (0.002 in. or 0.05 mm) rounded structure—is located just beneath the membrane but connects with the surface by a minute opening that permits fluid to enter.

While people generally classify tastes into four primary categories—sour, sweet, salty, and bitter—combinations of these permit us to enjoy literally hundreds of different tastes. Beyond this, in a broader sense, flavor evaluates the color, texture, odor, and taste of a food, to determine whether it is acceptable or not. The sour taste is triggered by acids, the salty taste by salts, the sweet taste by sugar and a number of other organic compounds, and the bitter taste by alkaloids and other organic compounds. Saccharin, though not a sugar, is some 600 times as sweet as table sugar (sucrose).

Each taste cell in a taste bud has several microscopically small taste hairs that protrude through the opening of the taste bud into the mouth. At the bases of the hairs—which appear to act as receptors—are a network of taste nerve fibers that activate the taste cells. In general, sweet taste is perceived at the front surface and tip, salty and sour tastes along the sides, and bitter at the back of the tongue. Interestingly, four pairs of nerves carry the impulses from the taste buds to the taste perception area of the brain (the fifth, seventh, ninth, and tenth cranial nerves).

Smell provides the sense which allows us to distinguish odors (see page 1156). Food particles, volatile oils, and other substances carried in the

1155

air reach the olfactory membrane in the upper recesses of the nose. Here receptors are excited to carry nerve impulses to the area of the brain that interprets odors. Along with the taste buds, the sense of smell aids us in appreciating flavors. It is reported that 50 percent of the enjoyment of drinking a cup of coffee is from its aroma rather than from its taste. In fact, smell has been called "the better half" of taste. That is why, when our noses are congested with a cold, our food does not taste as good.

Disorders of taste and smell

Taste loss. Injuries to the surface of the tongue and mouth cavity from excessively hot food and drink or from caustic chemicals will destroy the sense of taste. If the taste nerves are not destroyed, the taste buds will recover and taste will be restored. When a nerve conveying taste is destroyed, the taste buds supplied by that nerve completely deteriorate. If, interestingly, the nerve regenerates, the cells of the mucous membrane rearrange themselves and develop into a new taste bud.

Taste alterations. People with cancers often have changes in their ability to taste. They are less sensitive to sweet, so foods have to carry higher concentrations of sugar to taste sweet. On the other hand, their ability to detect bitter increases. Meat is often said to have a rotten or foul taste.

Anosmia. Anosmia is the loss of the sense of smell (see page 1155). Those who have lost this sense often report that no food tastes good.

Sensations of temperature, touch, pressure, and pain

While the senses of sight, hearing, equilibrium, taste, and smell have their receptors grouped into rather compact organs or areas, as in the eyes, ears, semicircular canals, tongue, and nose, the specific receptors for the sensations of temperature, touch, pressure, and pain are scattered throughout the body structures. Impulses carried to the brain provide information, moment by moment, as to what is occurring in any part of the body.

The sense of touch helps one in handling objects, while the sense of position allows one to know the exact location of any part of the body. The musician depends on his senses of touch, position, and hearing to know just how to produce the most pleasing sounds on his instrument. Touch helps the surgeon to know how firmly to grasp his instruments and how much to stretch the tissues with which he is working. A blind person develops his sense of touch to tell him his whereabouts, and even to read.

Pressure receptors tell the brain how much the tissues are being compressed when a person sits too long in the same position or when the foot is crowded into too small a shoe. Other receptors respond when stretched. They signal that one is bloated or that the urinary bladder needs emptying.

Perhaps a few extra words regarding **pain** may be of interest. More pain receptors are scattered throughout the body than all the receptors for all the other sensations combined. And why is this? At first thought it might seem a mistake for the Creator thus to have made us. The excruciating pain of a coronary attack, the agony of a kidney stone, the intolerable throbbing of a toothache, the suffering of an extensive burn. You legitimately ask, Why?

But another side to this question exists. The diseases most dreaded are those that do not produce pain, or fail to produce it early enough. Leprosy destroys the sense of pain, and the poor leper, unaware that he has stubbed his toe or burned his finger, disregards his injuries. Minor damage develops into serious problems. In time he may lose his finger and toe. If the very first cancer cell that developed in the body sent a pain signal to the brain, few, if any, would die of cancer. Thus pain can be a blessing rather than a curse, for it works as the alarm call of the body, crying out that something is wrong and needs to be treated. How many of us would rest the torn ligaments of a sprained ankle if it did not hurt? We would merrily go on our way. The ligaments would not heal, the ankle joint would become weak, the bones, in time, would erode, and we would lose the use of that joint.

The words written by the apostle Paul, and found in the New Testament, express most beautifully how remarkably every part of the body contributes its share in enabling the body to function as a whole:

"Now the body is not one member but many. If the foot should say, 'Because I am not a hand I don't belong to the body,' does that alter the fact that the foot *is* a part of the body? Or if the ear should say, 'Because I am not an eye I don't belong to the body,' does that mean that the ear really is not part of the body? After all, if the body were all one eye, for example, where would be the sense of hearing? Or if it were all one ear, where would be the sense of smell? But God has arranged all the parts in the one body, according to his design. For if everything were concentrated in one part, how could there be a body at all? The fact is there are many parts, but only one body. So that the eye cannot say to the hand, 'I don't need you!' nor, again, can the head say to the feet, 'I don't need you!' On the contrary, those parts of the body which have no obvious function are the more essential to health; and to those parts of the body which seem to us to be less deserving of notice we have to allow the highest honor of function. The parts which do not look beautiful have a deeper beauty in the work they do, while the parts which look beautiful may not be at all essential to life! But God has harmonized the whole body by giving importance of function to the parts which lack apparent importance, that the body should work together as a whole with all the members in sympathetic relationship with one another. So it happens that if one member suffers all the other members suffer with it, and if one member is honored all the members share a common joy" (1 Corinthians 12:14-26, Phillips).

The charts on the following pages may be photo-
copied for use by family members.

FAMILY MEDICAL RECORDS

Biographical information useful to a physician and others in dealing with a family member's illness and in outlining an individual health-protection program.

HUSBAND

NAME _____ Date of Birth _____

CHILDHOOD DISEASES RECORD

Disease	Approximate age at time of illness	Aftereffects	Doctor
Whooping cough			
Chicken pox			
Measles (rubeola)			
German measles			
Mumps			

IMMUNIZATION RECORD

Disease	Date of immunization	Repeat date	Repeat date	Repeat date	Doctor
Smallpox					
Diphtheria					
Tetanus					
Polio					

DISEASE AND ACCIDENT RECORD

Disease or accident	Date	Approximate duration of illness	Aftereffects	Doctor	Hospital

SURGERY RECORD

Type of surgery	Date	Doctor	Hospital	Length of hospitalization	Results

PERIODIC MEDICAL EXAMINATIONS

Date	Doctor	Significant findings

Biographical information useful to a physician and others in dealing with a family member's illness and in outlining an individual health-protection program.

WIFE

NAME _____ Date of Birth _____

CHILDHOOD DISEASES RECORD

Disease	Approximate age at time of illness	Aftereffects	Doctor
Whooping cough			
Chicken pox			
Measles (rubeola)			
German measles			
Mumps			

IMMUNIZATION RECORD

Disease	Date of immunization	Repeat date	Repeat date	Repeat date	Doctor
Smallpox					
Diphtheria					
Tetanus					
Polio					

SURGERY RECORD

Type of surgery	Date	Doctor	Hospital	Length of hospitalization	Results

DISEASE AND ACCIDENT RECORD

Disease or accident	Date	Approximate duration of illness	Aftereffects	Doctor	Hospital

PERIODIC MEDICAL EXAMINATIONS

Date	Doctor	Significant findings

RECORD OF PREGNANCIES

Beginning date	Periodic prenatal care (Yes or No)	Delivery date	Unusual circumstances	Hospital	Doctor

Foundations of health are laid in childhood. Keeping a detailed record of significant happenings in the child's life will enable parents to maintain careful supervision of factors contributing to normal development.

CHILD

NAME OF CHILD _____ Date of Birth _____

IMMUNIZATION RECORD

Disease	Doctor	Date of first inoculation	Date of second	Date of third	Date of booster	Repeat date	Repeat date
Diphtheria							
Whooping cough							
Tetanus							
Smallpox							
Polio							
Measles							
Mumps							

DISEASE AND ACCIDENT RECORD

Disease or accident	Date	Duration of illness	Complications or aftereffects	Doctor	Hospital

SURGERY RECORD

Type of surgery	Date	Doctor	Hospital	Length of hospitalization	Results

PERIODIC MEDICAL AND DENTAL EXAMINATIONS

Date	Doctor	Significant findings

Foundations of health are laid in childhood. Keeping a detailed record of significant happenings in the child's life will enable parents to maintain careful supervision of factors contributing to normal development.

CHILD

NAME OF CHILD _____   Date of Birth _____

IMMUNIZATION RECORD

Disease	Doctor	Date of first inoculation	Date of second	Date of third	Date of booster	Repeat date	Repeat date
Diphtheria							
Whooping cough							
Tetanus							
Smallpox							
Polio							
Measles							
Mumps							

DISEASE AND ACCIDENT RECORD

Disease or accident	Date	Duration of illness	Complications or aftereffects	Doctor	Hospital

SURGERY RECORD

Type of surgery	Date	Doctor	Hospital	Length of hospitalization	Results

PERIODIC MEDICAL AND DENTAL EXAMINATIONS

Date	Doctor	Significant findings

Index

A

Abdomen
> Cramps in, **2**-611
> Distension of, **2**-611
> Masses in, **2**-612
> Rigidity of, **2**-612
> Tenderness in, **2**-612

Abdominal injuries, **2**-553
Abdominal pain, **3**-878
Abrasions, **2**-553
Abscess, **2**-702
Accidents
> As leading cause of death in children, **2**-443, **2**-452

Acclimatization to high altitudes
> Graded ascent, **1**-42
> Staging, **1**-42

Acetominophen, **1**-330
Acid rain, **1**-65
Acnc, **2**-489, **3**-982
Aquired immune deficiency syndrome
> See AIDS

Acromegaly, **3**-1006
Actinic keratoses, in the elderly, **2**-500
Actinomycosis (lumpy jaw), **2**-705
Acute epiglottis
> See Croup

Adam's apple
> See Larynx

Addiction
> See Drug abuse

Addison's disease, **3**-1007
Adenoiditis, **2**-470
Adenoids
> See Tonsils

Adenomyosis
> See Uterus, disorders of; Endometriosis

Adolescence, **2**-431, **2**-476
> Changes in female during, **2**-480
> Changes in male during, **2**-479
> Character formation in, **2**-477
> Physical development, **2**-478
> Sexual interaction during, **2**-482

Adrenal disorders
> Addison's disease, **3**-1007
> Adrenal virilism, **3**-1008
> Cushing's syndrome (and Cushing's disease), **3**-1007
> Hyperaldosteronism, **3**-1008
> Pheochromocytoma, **3**-1008

Adrenal gland hormones
> Aldosterone, **3**-1001
> Cortisone, **3**-1001
> Epinephrine, **3**-1001
> Glucocorticoids, **3**-1001
> Hydrocortisone (cortisol), **3**-1001
> Mineralocorticoids, **3**-1001
> Norepinephrine, **3**-1001
> Sex hormones, **3**-1001

Adrenal glands, **3**-1001
Adrenaline, **3**-1001
Adventist health studies
> Comparisons among Adventists, **1**-123
> Health habits of Adventists, **1**-122
> Observed health advantages, **1**-122
> Studies done outside the United States, **1**-123

Aerobic exercise, **1**-38
African sleeping sickness (trypanosomiasis), **2**-743
Age
> As risk factor in heart disease, **3**-779

AIDS, **3**-830, **3**-831
> Kaposi's sarcoma and, **3**-831
> Pneumocystis carinii and, **2**-752, **3**-831
> Toxoplasmosis and, **2**-752
> Treatment of, **3**-831

Air
> Composition of, **1**-62
> Ions, positive and negative, **1**-66
> Pollution in, **1**-64

Albinism, **3**-986
Alcohol
> As risk factor in diabetes, **3**-1018
> Content of, in standard alcoholic beverages, **1**-287
> Dependence, **1**-293
> Delirium tremens (DT's), **1**-293
> Tolerance for, **1**-292
> Use of that develops cross-tolerance, **1**-293
> Withdrawal from, **1**-293

Alcohol, effects of
> On digestive system, **1**-288
> On heart and blood vessels, **1**-290
> On nervous system, **1**-289
> On other drugs, **1**-292
> On sexual behavior, **1**-291
> On the unborn (fetal alcohol syndrome) **1**-292

Alcohol rub, **2**-577, **2**-598
Alcoholic
> Rehabilitation of, **1**-293

Alcoholic beverages
> Economic and social impact of, **1**-286
> Incidence of, **1**-286
> Why people drink, **1**-287

Alcoholics Anonymous, **1**-294
Alkalosis, from hyperventilation, **2**-617
Allergens, **2**-673, **3**-921
> "Germ," **2**-675
> "Injected," **2**-674
> Additives and preservatives, **2**-674
> Drugs, **2**-674

(4)

Asbestosis, **3**-930
Ascariasis
    See Roundworms
Ascites, **2**-613
Aspirin, **1**-330
    Cautions concerning use of, **1**-331, **2**-467, **2**-732
Asthma, **3**-920
    In children, **2**-458, **2**-470
Asthma attack, **2**-529
Astigmatism, **3**-1187
Atherosclerosis, **1**-7, **3**-776, **3**-779
    Angioplasty as treatment for, **3**-790
    Atheroma (plaque), **3**-780
    See also Arteries: arteriosclerosis
    In children, **2**-457
    Increased risk of, in diabetes, **3**-1014
    Plaque (atheroma), **3**-780
    Risk factors in, **3**-776, **3**-777
    Symptoms of, **3**-780
Athlete's foot (tinea pedia), **3**-978
Attention deficit disorder
    See Hyperactive child
Autonomic nervous system
    See Involuntary nervous system
AZT (azidothymidine) as AIDS treatment, **3**-831
Azul
    See Pinto

B

Baby teeth
    See Teeth, Primary (deciduous)
Bacillary dysentery (shigellosis), **2**-712
Back pain, **2**-642
Bacteremia, **2**-703
Bacterial endocarditis
    See Endocarditis
Bacterial infection, **3**-705
Bad breath
    See Halitosis
"Bag of waters," **2**-399
Balantidial dysentery (balantidiasis), **2**-745
Balantidiasis
    See balantidial dysentery
Baldness, **3**-992
    Alopecia areata, **3**-992
    Male pattern, **3**-993
Baltimore College of Dental Surgery, **3**-889
Bandages, **2**-513
Bartholin's glands, **3**-1088
Basic Life Support (BLS) procedures, **2**-508
Bath, **2**-575
    Sun, **2**-600
Bedpan, **2**-574
Bejel

    See Endemic syphilis
Bell's palsy, **3**-1045
Bends, the
    See Decompression sickness
Bile
    Production of by liver, **3**-848

Bilharziasis
    See Flukes: Blood flukes
Biliary cirrhosis, **3**-872
Bilirubin, **1**-72, **2**-418, **2**-627
Biopsy, **1**-18
Birth defects
    Congenital, **2**-374
    Environmentally caused, **2**-377
    German measles as cause of, **2**-377
Birthmarks, **2**-463, **3**-993
Bites
    Animal, **2**-530
    Ant, **2**-533
    Human, **2**-531
    Snake, **2**-531
    Spider, **2**-531
    Tick, **2**-533
Black eye, **2**-533
Black lung (coal miner's disease), **3**-930
Blackheads and whiteheads
    See Acne
Blackwater fever
    See Malaria
Bladder, **3**-1066
Bladder and ureter disorders
    Bladder stones (vesical calculi), **3**-1078
    Cystitis (inflammation of the bladder), **3**-1077
    Cystocele, **3**-1080
    Interstitial cystitis, **3**-1078
    Tumors, **3**-1079
    Ureteral calculi (stones in ureter), **3**-1076
    Ureteral stricture, **3**-1076
    Urinary incontinence, **3**-1076
    Urinary retention, **3**-1077
Bladder stones, **3**-1078
Blastomycosis, **2**-739
Bleeding, **2**-614
    From an injury, **2**-614
    From the bladder, **2**-614
    From the lungs, **2**-614
    From the mouth, **2**-615
    From the nose, **2**-615
    From the rectum, **2**-615
    From the skin, **2**-615
    From the stomach, **2**-615
    From the vagina, **2**-614, **2**-615
Bleeding, as early medical practice, **1**-3
Bleeding, severe (hemorrhage), **2**-614, **2**-624
    What to do in event of, **2**-517, **2**-541

(8)

See Cardiovascular disease
Corpuscles
 See Blood cells
Cortisone, **3**-1001
Cough, **2**-453, **2**-618, **2**-648
Coughing, **3**-905
Cowper's glands, **3**-1084
CPR
 See Cardiopulmonary resuscitation
Cramps, muscle
 See Muscles, disorders of
Cretinism, **2**-423, **3**-1010
Crohn's disease (regional ileitis), **3**-859
Cross-eye (Squint), **3**-1140
 In children, **2**-469
Croup, **2**-458
Cryptococcosis (torulosis), **2**-740
CT scan
 See CAT scan
Cushing's disease
 See Cushing's syndrome
Cushing's syndrome, **3**-1007
Cutaneous leishmaniasis
 See Leishmaniasis: Oriental sore
Cuts, **2**-554
Cyanosis, **2**-619
Cystic fibrosis, **2**-461, **3**-922

D

D&C
 See Dilation and curettage
Dandruff, **3**-974
Deafness (hearing loss), **2**-620, **3**-1152 Conductive
deafness, **3**-1153
 In children, **2**-469
 In the elderly, **2**-503
 Nerve deafness, **3**-1153
Death, process of accepting
 Acceptance, **3**-1058
 Anger, **3**-1057
 Bargaining, **3**-1057
 Shock and denial, **3**-1057
Decision making
 Discrimination, **1**-102
 Judgment, **1**-103
 Self-control, **1**-103
 Willpower, **1**-103
Decompression sickness, **2**-559
Deformities
 Congenital, **2**-426
Dehydration, **1**-80
Delhi sore
 See Leishmaniasis
Delirium, **2**-558

Delirium tremens, **3**-1058
 In alcohol withdrawal, **1**-293
Delivery
 Date of, **2**-384
 Signs of, **2**-399
 See also Labor
Delivery, complications of, **2**-401
 Abnormal presentations, **2**-403
 Birth injuries, **2**-404
 Caesarean section, **2**-402
 Episiotomy, **2**-402
 False labor, **2**-401
 Forceps delivery, **2**-402
 Hemorrhage following delivery, **2**-403
 Multiple births, **2**-404
 Premature birth, **2**-401
 Premature rupture of the membranes, **2**-402
 Respiratory distress syndrome, **2**-404
 Retained placenta, **2**-403
Dementias
 Alzheimer's dementia (disease), **3**-1041
 Arteriosclerotic dementia, **3**-1041
Dengue (breakbone fever), **2**-724
Dental caries
 See Tooth disorders
Dentist
 Training of, **1**-9
Dentistry
 Endodontics, **3**-890
 History of, **3**-889, **3**-890
 Orthodontics, **3**-890
 Periodontics, **3**-890
 Prosthodontics, **3**-896
Dentures, **3**-896, **3**-897
Deoxyribonucleic acid
 See DNA
Depression, **3**-1055
 In the elderly, **2**-502
Dermatitis
 Allergic, **2**-464, **2**-678, **3**-973
 Atopic, **2**-678, **3**-971
 Atopic, in children, **2**-462
 Atopic, in infants, **2**-421
 Chronic, **3**-974
 Contact, **3**-972
 Contact, in children, **2**-470
 Dyshidrosis, **3**-974
 Irritant, **3**-972
 Nummular, **3**-975
 Seborrheic, **3**-974
 Stasis, **3**-975
 Xerotic eczema, **3**-974
DES therapy, and increased disease incidence, **3**-1109
Detached retina, **3**-1138
Diabetes, **3**-1013
 Adult-onset (type II), **1**-6, **3**-1013

F

See Esophagus
Hiccup, **2**-560, **2**-624
High blood pressure
See Hypertension
Histamine, **2**-675
Histoplasmosis, **2**-740
Hives (urticaria), **2**-676, **3**-989
In children, **2**-471
Hoarseness, **2**-624, **3**-915
Hodgkin's disease, **3**-832
Home patient care, **2**-572
Administering enemas, **2**-574
Alcohol rub, **2**-598
Bedsore prevention, **2**-577
Counting respiration rate, **2**-574
Determining pulse, **2**-573
Food and drink, **2**-577
For contagious diseases, **2**-580
Giving baths, **2**-575
Importance of good nursing in, **2**-582
Medications, **2**-579
Patient bowel movements, **2**-574
Prevention of stiff joints, **2**-578
Taking temperature, **2**-573
Use of bedpan, **2**-574
Home treatments, **2**-585
See also Dry heat applications
See also Hydrotherapy
See also Thermotherapy
Homeostasis, **1**-30, **2**-587
Homosexuality, **2**-483
Hookworms (ground itch), **2**-752
Hormones, **3**-999
"Hot flashes," **3**-1110
Hot-water bottle, **2**-599
Hunger, **1**-226
Huntington's chorea, **3**-1041
Hyaline membrane disease, **2**-404
Hydatid disease
See Tapeworms
Hydatidiform mole
See Trophoblastic disease
Hydrocephalus, **3**-1046
Hydrocortisone, **3**-1001
Hydrophobia
See Rabies
Hydrotherapy, **2**-589
Alcohol rub, **2**-598
Cold compress, **2**-593
Cold mitten friction, **2**-592
Fomentations, **2**-590
Heating compress, **2**-593
Hot and cold to the chest, **2**-592
Hot foot bath, **2**-589
Hot half-bath, **2**-597
Hot mitten friction, **2**-593

Hot-and-cold immersion baths, **2**-589
Ice water or ice pack, **2**-597
Showers, **2**-595
Sitz bath, **2**-597
Sponge or rub, **2**-598
Steam inhalation, **2**-594
Tub bath, **2**-596
Hymen, **3**-1088
Hyperactive child, **2**-449
Hyperglycemia, **3**-1017
Hyperkinetic child
See Hyperactive child
Hypertension, **1**-7, **1**-32, **1**-778, **3**-785
In children, **2**-457
In the elderly, **2**-496
Hyperthyroidism, **3**-1009
Hypochondria, **3**-1057
Hypoglycemia, **3**-1017
Hypotension, **1**-32, **3**-904
Hypothermia, **1**-32, **2**-555
Hypothyroidism, **3**-1010
Hysterectomy, **3**-1105
Hysteria, **3**-1055

I

Ichthyosis (fishskin), **3**-988
In children, **2**-465
IgE
See Immunoglobulin E
Illness, **2**-367
Illusionary drugs
See Drugs of abuse
Immunity (defenses), **2**-605, **2**-760, **3**-828
Immunizations, **2**-407
Immunoglobulin E, **2**-675
Impetigo, **3**-975
In infants and children, **2**-422, **2**-465
Impotence, male, **3**-1112
Incontinence, **2**-624
Indigestion (dyspepsia), **2**-621, **2**-625, **3**-853
Infancy, diseases and disorders of
Atopic dermatitis (eczema), **2**-421
Bronchiolitis, **2**-422
Cerebral palsy, **2**-427
Congenital deformities, **2**-426
Congenital glaucoma, **2**-427
Congenital rubella (German measles), **2**-421
Down's syndrome (mongolism), **2**-428
Hemolytic anemia of the newborn (Rh disease), **2**-426, **3**-818
Hypothyroidism (cretinism), **2**-423
Impetigo, **2**-422
Infant colic, **2**-424
Infectious diarrhea, **2**-424

Jaundice, **1**-72, **2**-418
  Pyloric stenosis, **2**-425
  Respiratory distress syndrome (RDS), **2**-422
  Rickets, **2**-426
  Sudden infant death syndrome (SIDS), **2**-423
  Whooping cough (pertussis), **2**-42()
Infancy, general problems of
  Diarrhea, **2**-417
  Drooling, **2**-417
  Excessive crying, **2**-416
  Fever, **2**-417
  Jaundice, **2**-418
  Spitting up (regurgitation) and vomiting, **2**-419
  Teething, **2**-418
  Thumb sucking, **2**-418
  Umbilical hernia, **2**-419
Infarct, **3**-783
Infection, **2**-700
  Contagious, **2**-703
  Generalized, **2**-702
  Localized, **2**-702
  Prevention of, **2**-704
  Therapy for, **2**-704
Infectious mononucleosis
  See Mononucleosis
Infuenza
  In children, **2**-458
Influenza (flu), **2**-725
Inner ear
  Cochlea, **3**-1142
  Organ of Corti, **3**-1143
  Semicircular canals (labyrinth), **3**-1142, **3**-1145
Insomnia, **1**-57, **2**-633
  See also Sleep disorders
Insomnia (sleeplessness), **1**-57
  Causes of, **1**-58
  Cures for, **1**-59
Insulin, **3**-1003
  Discovery of in 1921, **1**-6
Intercourse, **2**-625, **3**-1111
Intestinal hernia, **3**-862
Intestinal infarction, **3**-861
Intestinal obstruction, **3**-860
  Adynamic ileus, **3**-860
  Mechanical blockage, **3**-860
Intoxication, alcoholic, **1**-288, **1**-290, **2**-560, **2**-626
Intrauterine device, **3**-1098, **3**-1099
Involuntary nervous system
  Ganglia, **3**-1025
  Parasympathetic nervous system, **3**-1025
  Sympathetic nervous system, **3**-1025
Ions
  Positive and negative, **1**-66
Iron
  Storage of in liver, **3**-843
Islet cell disease

  See Diabetes
Islets of Langerhans
  See Pancreas
Itching, **2**-626, **2**-660
IUD
  See Intrauterine device

J

Jaundice (icterus), **2**-627, **3**-869, **3**-873
  Of the newborn, **1**-418
Joints, disorders of
  Ankylosing spondylitis, **3**-956
  Bunions, **3**-956
  Dislocations, **2**-548, **2**-549, **3**-950
  Gouty arthritis, **3**-955
  Herniated disk (slipped disk, prolapsed disk), **3**-951
  Infectious arthritis (septic arthritis), **3**-954
  Osteoarthritis (degenerative joint disease), **3**-954
  Pain, **2**-662
  Rheumatoid arthritis, **3**-952
  Stiffncss, **2**-578

K

Kala-azar
  See Leishmaniasis
Kaposi's sarcoma
  See AIDS
Keloid, **3**-995
Kidney diseases and disorders
  Inherited disorders, **3**-1075
  Nephritis, **3**-1068
Renal failure and uremia, **3**-1070
Tumors, **3**-1075, **3**-1076
Kidney stones, **3**-1073
Kidney tumors
  Hypernephroma, **3**-1076
  Nephroblastoma (Wilms' tumor), **3**-1076
Kidneys, **3**-1065
  Floating, **3**-1074
  Nephrons, **3**-1065
Kidneys, inherited disorders
  Alport's syndrome, **3**-1075
  Cystinuria, **3**-1075
  Horseshoe kidneys, **3**-1075
  Polycystic kidneys, **3**-1075
Kissing disease
  See Mononucleosis
Knock-knees, **3**-945
Korsakoff's psychosis
  See Psychosis: Alcohol amnesia disorder

L

Labor
  "Breaking of the bag of waters," **2**-399
  "Show," **2**-399
  False labor, **2**-401
  First stage, **2**-399
  Second stage, **2**-400
  Signs of, **2**-399
  Third stage, **2**-400
Lactose intolerance, **2**-454, **3**-858
  In teenagers, **2**-493
Large intestine, **3**-841
  Appendix, **3**-841
  Ascending colon, **3**-841
  Cecum, **3**-841
  Descending colon, **3**-841
  Sigmoid colon, **3**-841
  Transverse colon, **3**-841
Larynx, **3**-901
Larynx, diseases of, **3**-914
  Hoarseness, **3**-915
  Laryngitis, **3**-915
  Vocal cord damage, **3**-915
Leishmaniasis
  Espundia (American leishmaniasis), **2**-747
  Kala-azar (dumdum fever), **2**-748
  Oriental sore (tropical sore, Delhi sore), **2**-747
Lens, disorders of
  Aging eyes (presbyopia), **3**-1137
  Astigmatism, **3**-1137
  Blindness, **3**-1138
  Cataract, **3**-1136
  Double vision, **3**-1137
  Farsightedness, **3**-1137
  Nearsightedness, **3**-1136
  Refractive errors, **3**-1136
Leprosy (Hansen's disease), **2**-708
  Lepromatous leprosy, **2**-709
  Tuberculoid leprosy, **2**-709
Leptospirosis, **2**-721
Leukemia, **2**-682, **3**-823 - **3**-825
  Acute, **3**-824
  See also Blood, diseases of
  Chronic, **3**-825
  Granulocytic, **3**-824
  Lymphocytic, **3**-824
Leukoplakia, **3**-850, **3**-916
Lice
  Body, **3**-982
  Head, **3**-982
  In children, **2**-464
  Pubic (crab), **3**-982
Life
  Defined, **1**-23
  Relation of health to, **1**-23

Life expectancy, **1**-24
Life, dimensions of
  Breadth (quality), **1**-26
  Depth (love for God and man), **1**-27
  Length, **1**-25
  Length (life expectancy), **1**-24
Lifestyle
  As consideration in establishing a home, **2**-365
  Healthful, **1**-124, **1**-125
  Influence of on health and disease, **1**-117
  Westerner's, **1**-124
Lifestyle diseases, **1**-8, **1**-29
Lipids, blood
  See Cholesterol
Lipoproteins, **3**-777
Lips
  Cracking of (cheilosis), **3**-846
Lister, Dr. Joseph
  Control of wound infection pioneered by, **1**-5
Little's disease
  See Cerebral palsy
Liver, **3**-842
  Abscess of, **3**-873
  Cancer of, **3**-873
  Cirrhosis of, **3**-871
  Functions of, **3**-843
Liver rot
  See Flukes
Liver spots, **3**-987
Lobar pneumonia
  See Pneumonia
Lockjaw
  See Tetanus
Louse typhus
  See Typhus
Low blood pressure, **3**-804
Low blood sugar
  See Hypoglycemia
LSD (lysergic acid diethylamide), **1**-302
Lump in the throat, **2**-628
Lumpy Jaw
  See Actinomycosis
"Lumpy breasts," **1**-262, **2**-616
Lung abscess, **3**-927
Lungs, **3**-902
  Covering of (pleura), **3**-905
Lupus (SLE), **3**-957
Lyme disease, **2**-720
Lymph, **3**-826
Lymph nodes
  Infection-fighting role of, **3**-827, **3**-828
  Lymphocytes, **3**-827
  Phagocytes, **3**-827
  Swollen (lymphadenopathy), **3**-831
Lymphatic system, **3**-826
  Lymph nodes, **3**-826

R

Rabbit fever
  See Tularemia
Rabies (hydrophobia), **2**-730
Radiation therapy in treatment of cancer, **2**-696
Rape, **2**-492
Rash (skin eruption), **2**-632
  From drugs, **2**-632
  From infectious diseases, **2**-632
  In diseases of the skin, **2**-632
  In infants, **2**-632
  Of pellagra, **2**-632
  Urticarial reactions (hives), **2**-632
Ratbite fever
  Bacillus form, **2**-711
  Spirochete form, **2**-711
Raynaud's disease
  See Arteries, diseases of
RDS (Respiratory Distress Syndrome)
  See Infancy, diseases and disorders of
Recipes, **1**-191
  Index of, **1**-225
Rectum, **3**-842
  Prolapse of, **2**-633
Refined grains, **1**-90
Reflex, **3**-1026
Relapsing fever, **2**-722
Relaxation, **1**-52
  Progressive, **2**-601
Religion
  In the home, **2**-367
Religious beliefs
  Negative, effects of on health, **1**-113
  Positive, effects of on health, **1**-112, **1**-113
Religious faith
  Benefits of, **1**-115, **2**-367
  Influence of on health, **1**-114
Religious responses to adversity
  Fatalism, **1**-114
  Legalism, **1**-114
  True belief, **1**-115
REM (rapid eye movement)
  See Sleep
Renal failure
  Acute, **3**-1070
  Acute pyelonephritis, **3**-1072
  Chronic, **3**-1071
  Chronic pyelonephritis, **3**-1073
  Kidney stones (renal calculi), **3**-1073
  Nephrosis (nephrotic syndrome), **3**-1071
Reproduction
  See Sex
Respiration, **2**-574, **3**-904
Respiratory arrest, **2**-508
Respiratory distress syndrome, **2**-404

Respiratory system, **1**-63, **3**-899
Rest
  State of, **1**-53
Retina, disorders of
  Macular degeneration, **3**-1139
  Retinal detachment, **3**-1138
  Retinal hemorrhages, **3**-1139
  Retinal vascular disorders, **3**-1139
Retinal vascular disorders
  Diabetic retinopathy, **3**-1139
  Retinal artery occlusion, **3**-1139
  Retinal vein occlusion, **3**-1139
Reye's syndrome, **2**-467, **2**-732
Rh disease
  See Anemia
Rh factor
  See Blood types
Rheumatic fever, **2**-474
Rheumatic heart disease, **3**-795
  Endocarditis, **3**-795
  In children, **2**-457
  In teenagers, **2**-489
  Myocarditis, **3**-795
  Pericarditis, **3**-795
Rhythms, biological, **3**-1001
Rickets, **2**-426, **3**-944
  In children, **2**-475
Rickettsialpox, **2**-735
Ringworm (dermatophytosis), **3**-977
  Athlete's foot, **3**-978
  In children, **2**-464
  Of the beard, **3**-978
  Of the body, **3**-978
  Of the groin, **3**-978
  Of the nails, **3**-978
  Of the scalp, **3**-978
River blindness (onchocerciasis), **2**-763
Rocky Mountain spotted fever, **2**-734
Rosacea (acne rosacea), **3**-984
Roseola infantum, **2**-473
Roundworms (ascariasis), **2**-754
Rubella
  See German measles
Rubeola
  See Measles
Ruddy complexion, as symptom of illness, **2**-618

S

Saint Vitus' dance
  See Sydenham's chorea
Salivary duct stone, **3**-850
Salivary glands, **3**-881
Salivary glands, disorders
  Inflammation of, **2**-729, **3**-849

Swayback (lordosis), **3**-942
Spiritual health, **1**-112
Spirochetal diseases, **2**-720
Spleen, **3**-829
Splinter, removal of, **2**-547
Sporotrichosis, **2**-741
Sprains, **2**-554
Sprains (ankles, knees, wrists), **3**-949
Squint (cross-eye), **3**-1140
Starvation, **1**-226, **1**-227
    Kwashiorkor (protein-calorie malnutrition), **1**-227
    Marasmus (protein-energy malnutrition), **1**-227
    Treatment of, **1**-228
STD
    See Sexually transmitted diseases
Stimulants
    Amphetamines, **1**-301
    Cocaine, **1**-301
Stings
    Bee, wasp, hornet, yellowjacket, **2**-535
    Marine animals, **2**-536
    Scorpion, **2**-536
Stomach, **3**-839
    Cancer of, **3**-857
    Foreign body in, **2**-547
    Obstruction of, **3**-856
    Obstruction of, in infants, **2**-425
    Perforation of, **3**-856
Strangling
    See Choking
Strep throat, **3**-913
Stress
    As risk factor in heart disease, **3**-778
    See Emotional stress
Striae, **2**-393
Stroke, **3**-1031
    See Arteries, diseases of: Stroke
    In the elderly, **2**-502
    Ministroke (transient ischemic attack), **3**-801
    Vasospasm, **3**-801
    What to do in event of, **2**-541
Strongyloidiasis
    See Threadworms
Stupor, **2**-635
Stuttering, **2**-451
Sty, **3**-1130
SIDS (Sudden Infant Death Syndrome), **2**-423
Sugar, refined, **1**-90
Sugars
    Hexoses, **1**-89
    Pentoses, **1**-89
Suicide, **3**-1057
Sulfonamides, **1**-5
Sun bath, **2**-600
Sunburn, **3**-988
Sunglasses, **1**-73

Cosmetic, **1**-74
General purpose, **1**-74
Special purpose, **1**-74
Sunlamps, **2**-600
Sunlight
    Action of on pituitary gland, **1**-71
    And bilirubin levels in premature infants, **1**-72
    And biologic rhythms, **1**-71
    And levels of melatonin, **1**-71
    As purifier of environment, **1**-71
    Exposure to, **1**-69
    Hazards of, **1**-73
    Lifegiving properties of, **1**-71
Sunscreen
    Use of, **1**-70
Sunscreens
    SPF ratings of (''sun protection factor''), **1**-73
Surfactant, **1**-271, **2**-422
Swallowing, difficulty in
    Bulbar palsy, **2**-635
    Cancer of the esophagus, **2**-635
    Cardiospasm (achalasia), **2**-635
    Corrosive injury and stricture of esophagus, **2**-635
    Emotional conditions, **2**-636
    Esophagitis, **2**-636
    Foreign body within the esophagus, **2**-635
    Lesions, **2**-636
    Pressure against esophagus, **2**-636
Sweat glands, **3**-968
Sweating disorders
    Bromhidrosis, **3**-987
    Emotional hyperhidrosis, **3**-987
    Excessive sweating (hyperhidrosis), **3**-987
    Lack of sweat (anhidrosis), **3**-987
    Thermogenic hyperhidrosis, **3**-987
Sydenham's chorea, **2**-467
Sympathetic nervous system, **3**-1026
Syphilis, **3**-1044, **3**-1117
    Endemic (bejel), **2**-721
    General paresis, **3**-1045
    Tabes dorsalis (locomotor ataxia), **3**-1045
Systemic fungal diseases
    Characteristics of, **2**-739

T

T cells
    See Lymphocytes
Tapeworms, **2**-755
    Beef and fish tapeworms, **2**-756
    Dwarf tapeworm, **2**-756
    Hydatid disease (echinococcosis), **2**-758
    Pork tapeworm, **2**-756
Target heart rate, **1**-39
Taste buds, **3**-1155

U

Ulcerative colitis, 3-865
Ulcers, 2-637, 3-975, 3-986
Ulcers (stomach or duodenal), 3-855
    Complications of, 3-856
    In children, 2-461
Ultrasound, 1-14
Ultraviolet lamps
    See Sunlamps
Umbilical cord, 2-381
Unconsciousness (coma), 2-557, 2-637
    Caused by diseased blood vessels, 2-638
    Caused by reduced blood supply to brain, 2-639
    Due to head injury, 2-637
    From taking alcohol, drugs, or poisons, 2-637
    In "diabetic coma," 2-638
    In association with brain tumor or abscess, 2-638
    In epilepsy, 2-638
    In hepatic coma, 2-638
    In hypoglycemic coma, 2-638
    In hysteria, 2-639
    In meningitis and encephalitis, 2-638
    In uremic coma, 2-638
Undulant fever (brucellosis), 2-706
Uremia, 3-1070
Ureter disorders
    See Bladder and ureter disorders
Ureters, 3-1066
Urethra, diseases of
    Gonorrheal urethritis, 3-1080
    Nongonococcal or nonspecific urethritis (NSU), 3-1081
    Urethritis, 3-1080
Urinal, 2-574
Urinary system
    Bladder, 3-1066
    Kidneys, 3-1065
    Ureters, 3-1066
    Urethra, 3-1067
    Urine, 3-1067
Urine, 3-1067
    Analyses of, 1-19
Urticaria
    See Hives
Uterine tubes
    See Fallopian tubes
Uterus (womb), 3-1087
    "Uterine milk," 2-381, 3-1089, 3-1090
    Cervix, 3-1087
    Endometrium, 3-1089
Uterus, disorders of
    Absence of periods (amenorrhea), 3-1100
    Cancer, 3-1105
    Displacements of the uterus, 3-1102
    Endometriosis, 3-1103

    Fibroid tumors, 3-1104
    Heavy periods (menorrhagia), 3-1101
    Infrequent periods (oligomenorrhea), 3-1101
    Painful periods (dysmenorrhea, cramps), 3-1101
    Premenstrual syndrome (PMS), 3-1102
    Trophoblastic disease, 3-1103

V

Vaccinations, 2-407, 2-728
    DTP (diphtheria, tetanus, pertussis), 2-407
    MMR (measles, mumps, rubella), 2-407
    Risks and side effects of, 2-407
    TOPV (trivalent oral polio vaccine), 2-407
Vaccines, 1-335
Vagina, 3-1087
    Hymen, 3-1088
Vagina, disorders of
    Vaginal cysts, 3-1109
    Vaginal discharge, 3-1107
    Vaginal fistulas, 3-1109
    Vaginitis, 3-1108
Vaginal discharge, 3-1107
Vaginitis
    Chlamydial infections, 3-1108
    Leukorrhea, 3-1108
    Nonspecific, 3-1108
    Postmenopausal, 3-1108
    Trichomoniasis, 3-1108
    Yeast infections (candidiasis, moniliasis), 3-1108
Valley fever
    See Coccidiomycosis
Varicella
    See Chickenpox
Varicose veins
    See Veins, diseases of
Vas deferens, 2-480, 3-1084
Vascular nevus
    See Birthmarks
Veins, 3-769, 3-770
Veins, diseases of, 3-806
    Hemorrhoids, 3-807
    Phlebitis, 3-808
    Thrombophlebitis, 3-808
    Varicose veins, 3-806
Venipuncture (for blood analysis)
    Blood count, 1-19
    Blood culture, 1-19
    Chemical analyses, 1-19
    Clotting time, 1-19
Vertigo, 3-1052
Vincent's infection
    Trench mouth, 3-849
Viruses
    Viral diseases, 2-723

Incubation period, **2**-723
Latent, **2**-723
Visceral leishmaniasis
See Leishmaniasis: Kala-azar
Vitamin A
Storage of in liver, **3**-843
Vitamin B$_{12}$, **3**-815
Deficiency anemia, **3**-815
Deficiency of, **1**-228
Pernicious anemia and, **1**-228
Sources of, **1**-95
Storage of in liver, **3**-843
Total vegetarians and, **1**-95
Vitamin C
Deficiency of, and osteoporosis, **3**-944
Vitamin D
Deficiency of, and osteomalacia, **3**-944
Deficiency of, and rickets, **3**-944
Lack of, and osteomalacia, **1**-71
Lack of, and osteoporosis, **1**-71
Storage of in liver, **3**-843
Sunlight as source of, **1**-69
Vitamin K, **3**-821
Deficiency, **3**-821
Role in blood clotting, **3**-821
Vitamins, **1**-94
Deficiencies of, **1**-241
Vitiligo, **3**-986
Voice box
See Larynx
Vomiting
First aid for, **2**-561, **2**-639
In children, **2**-455
In infants, **2**-419
Initiating, as emergency procedure, **2**-512
Toxicity, **2**-639
Vomiting, causes of
Disturbances of abdominal organs, **2**-639
Drugs, **2**-639
Excessive stimulation of semicircular canals, **2**-639
Increased intracranial pressure, **2**-639
Poisons, **2**-639
Pregnancy, **2**-639
Psychic reactions, **2**-638
Vulva, **3**-1088
Bartholin's glands, **3**-1088
Clitoris, **3**-1088
Major labia, **3**-1088
Minor labia, **3**-1088
Mons veneris, **3**-1088
Vulva, disorders of
Bartholin's cyst, **3**-1110
Bartholin's gland infection, **3**-1110
Cancer, **3**-1110
Itching (pruritis), **3**-1109

Vulvitis, **3**-1109
Vulvovaginitis
In female children, **2**-466

W

Walleye, **3**-1140
In children, **2**-469
Warts (verrucae), **3**-980
Common, **3**-981
In children, **2**-463
Plantar, **3**-981
Venereal or genital (condyloma), **3**-981
Washing
Hair, **2**-577
Hands, **2**-580
Waste disposal, **2**-581
Water
Benefits of abundant, **1**-81
Compartments of, in human body, **1**-77
Dehydration, **1**-80
Extracellular fluid, **1**-78
Functions performed by, in human body, **1**-76
How to determine if you are drinking enough, **1**-81
Intracellular fluid, **1**-78
Loss of body water, **1**-79
Maintaining balance of, in human body, **1**-79
Necessity of for life, **1**-75
Problems of dehydration, **1**-80
Waterways of the body, **1**-75
When to drink, **1**-81
Weakness, **2**-639
Weaning, **2**-414
Weight
Sudden change in, **2**-640
Weight reduction
Advantages of, **1**-238
Booby traps to avoid in, **1**-235
See also Diets, Obesity
Formulating a program for, **1**-237
Time of meals in relation to, **1**-236
Wells, Horace, **3**-889
Wen
See Skin, tumors of: Epidermal inclusion cyst
Wernicke-Korsakoff syndrome, **3**-1040
Whiplash, **3**-1036
Whipworms, **2**-758
White blood cells, **3**-773
Granulocyte, **3**-773
Lymphocyte, **3**-773
Macrophage, **3**-773
Whooping cough (pertussis), **2**-420, **2**-474
Wilms' tumor
See Kidney tumors: Nephroblastoma
Windpipe